Canine Internal Medicine

Canine Internal Medicine

Canine Internal Medicine

What's Your Diagnosis?

Jon Wray BVSc DSAM Cert VC MRCVS,
RCVS-recognised Specialist in Small Animal Medicine (Internal Medicine)
Consultant Specialist in Small Animal Internal Medicine and Head of Cardiology
Dick White Referrals, Station Farm, Six Mile Bottom, Cambridgeshire

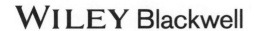

Registered Offices
John Wiley & Sons, Inc., 111 River Street, Hoboken, NJ 07030, USA
John Wiley & Sons Ltd, The Atrium, Southern Gate, Chichester, West Sussex, PO19 8SQ, UK

Editorial Office
9600 Garsington Road, Oxford, OX4 2DQ, UK

For details of our global editorial offices, customer services, and more information about Wiley products visit us at www.wiley.com.

Wiley also publishes its books in a variety of electronic formats and by print-on-demand. Some content that appears in standard print versions of this book may not be available in other formats.

Library of Congress Cataloging-in-Publication Data
Names: Wray, Jon (Jonathan David), 1973- author.
Title: Canine internal medicine : what's your diagnosis? / by Jon Wray.
Description: Hoboken, NJ : Wiley, 2018. | Includes bibliographical references
  and index. |
Identifiers: LCCN 2017030339 (print) | LCCN 2017034096 (ebook) |
  ISBN 9781118917787 (pdf) | ISBN 9781118918166 (epub) | ISBN 9781118918173 (pbk.)
Subjects: | MESH: Dog Diseases | Internal Medicine–methods | Case Reports
Classification: LCC SF991 (ebook) | LCC SF991 (print) | NLM SF 991 | DDC
  636.7/0896–dc23
LC record available at https://lccn.loc.gov/2017030339

Cover image: Courtesy of Jon Wray
Cover design by Wiley

Set in 10/12.5pt MinionPro by Thomson Digital, Noida, India

Printed and bound in Singapore by Markono Print Media Pte Ltd

10 9 8 7 6 5 4 3 2 1

Contents

Acknowledgements

I have the tremendous privilege to work with a truly fantastic group of Specialists, now numbering some 33 in total, in one of the largest referral hospitals in Europe. The Specialists are ably supported by a large number of talented, knowledgeable and caring Residents, Interns, Nurses, Laboratory technicians, Receptionists and others, without whom our practice would quickly grind to a halt. The patients we see (and the patients in this book) all benefit from a group approach and Internal Medicine is a collaborative subject. I could not give my patients the care they deserve without the input of my Specialist colleagues in other disciplines such as Surgery, Diagnostic Imaging, Clinical Pathology, Anaesthesiology, Ophthalmology, Neurology and Dermatology, the daily input from fellow Specialists and Residents in internal medicine and the dedication and care of our brilliant nursing team.

To quote (the often misquoted) Kurt Koffka, the whole really *is other* than the sum of its parts, and our hospital founder, Professor Dick White, has both recognised and encouraged this, both in his vision and in his assembly of a team of like-minded individuals who share a common belief in a multi-disciplinary Specialist approach to veterinary medicine and in our practice ethos of 'Excellence, Trust, Care'.

It is a genuine privilege to work in an environment where everyone's expertise in working towards a common goal yields tangible combined results that can be seen on a daily basis. I should also like to acknowledge the veterinary practices that refer patients to us, in the knowledge that it is not simply having facilities, but more importantly the Specialist expertise to apply them, that counts, and who recognise the distinction between Residency-trained ('apprenticeship') Specialists and other qualifications which, whilst of a good standard, are essentially self-taught. We believe that clinical standards of excellence are worth striving for, even if that means travelling a longer and more arduous personal route to get there, and in this 'post-truth' world (where anyone with an opinion can make it appear as though it is an incontrovertible fact on the world-wide web) critical appraisal and evidence-based approaches are more important than ever to defend.

Specific acknowledgements are due to colleagues Jackie Demetriou for Figure 10.4, Anna Adrian for Figure 11.3, Andrew Holloway for Figure 11.4 and Simon Tappin for case material for Case 34.

Jon Wray
Dick White Referrals
Cambridgeshire
United Kingdom, 2017

Dedication

For those who have left us: big brother SAJ, Dad and Mum who gave me so much and Ross who was taken too young.

For my darling Vicky and our children Ella, Daniel and Sophie, who are my Universe and make me laugh until it hurts, and my brother Matthew.

For my mentors, colleagues, residents, interns, nurses and students who have taught (and continue to teach) me so very many things.

For our patients, who make it all worthwhile.

How to Use this Book

What's your diagnosis? How did you reach it? Through logical deductive reasoning or through 'clinical shortcuts'? Which methods work best? Internal Medicine (IM) is a subject that relies on problem solving so test your problem-solving skills by perusing these cases and see...

This book is neither intended to be an Internal Medicine textbook, nor to include examples of every disease situation encountered in an Internal Medical caseload. What I have intended to do, by use of examples from my clinical practice, is to provide a wide 'spread' of clinical problems in which the case itself becomes 'the teacher'. This book is intended for anyone with an interest in Internal Medicine, whether at undergraduate or post-graduate level, General Practice or Speciality Practice. Inevitably there will be some, relatively common, case presentations that there has not been room to include or where the clinical skills challenged by them are replicated in another case example.

It is a frequent, and in many ways valid, criticism of undergraduate teaching, that by situating it mostly in referral hospitals (where the caseload is by nature highly selected and clients generally motivated and financially secure to expedite diagnosis and therapy) the cases may not offer a 'realistic substrate' for learning the *art* as well as the *science* of small animal medicine. However, I would counter this by stating that, in my experience, these hospitals are usually staffed by very talented clinicians who are both well-adept at drawing attention to specific case details that are important 'learning points' but also at focusing on those basic skills of history taking and physical examination that are the cornerstones of medical diagnosis. This is a point that is often missed – critics may remember that such cases are unusual and may not be representative of the vast majority of their own caseload, but usually forget the basic (and transferable) steps that led to diagnosis of the unusual problem in the first place. Furthermore, none of these cases miraculously 'appear out of the ether' in the reception area of a referral hospital – all have walked (or been carried) through the door of a general veterinary practice and the presenting complaint will be one encountered every day in a practice *somewhere*. You might be the vet who encounters it; are you ready?

Similarly, post-graduate education has become much more widely available and there are a plethora of excellent CPD courses, post-graduate qualifications, modular programs, etc., for the interested and committed individual. However, what none of these can do is replicate a busy Internal Medicine caseload and it is all too easy to fall into the trap of being well-informed, but never having the chance to experience the practical caseload that a busy IM department sees and thus not generating the 'right sort' of case *experience*. These cases are all taken from our Internal Medicine caseload at Dick White Referrals. We are a very busy department with 10 full-time Internal Medicine Clinicians and a tremendous and varied caseload. Our Residents have the luxury of being totally immersed in large numbers of these cases every day and I hope to share some of these with you. Where there are 'take-home' messages (which have become popular to refer to as 'pearls', and who am I to argue?), which I believe are pertinent to each case, I have tried to highlight these. I've also tried to include some useful additional information in the form of common differential diagnoses and case approaches, which, whilst not intended to be as complete as a textbook, will hopefully be easier to remember when attached to an interesting case. I always learn better with the immediacy and constant cue of a patient with which I am dealing and I hope the reader also finds refreshing their memory in the context of a clinical case that much more engaging than an abstract text.

I am a busy Specialist clinician having spent the last nineteen years exclusively in small animal Internal Medicine (canine and feline – I am not a particular advocate of a 'species-ist' restriction of one's caseload) referral practice at four major UK referral centres and being continuously 'on clinics' during that time. During this time I have also examined many veterinary surgeons in their pursuit of post-graduate qualifications at both Certificate and Diploma level. Partly the choice of which case subjects to include in this book is informed by this experience of those clinical problems that often seem to cause the most diagnostic difficulty and conversely in the exclusion of some common scenarios that really do not present much of a diagnostic 'challenge'.

In the same vein, whilst the cases here vary in their complexity, the features they all have in common are that they provide useful 'take-home messages' and challenge areas of clinical skill that are worth emphasising and learning from. In this way I hope that this book acts as a 'self-assessment' guide, but one that provides a little more detail than most. The cases are divided into subject area/body systems chapters. I have summarised the areas where there is further explanation of key clinical skills and approaches in the table in Appendix 1, which can then be cross-referenced with the cases. The table in Appendix 2 lists the diagnosis for each case for easy reference. Finally, the table in Appendix 3 lists conversion from SI units to common units for the reference of those readers from outside Europe.

After each case presentation there are a series of questions to prompt the reader in thinking about/problem solving a particular aspect of the case. I would recommend performing these before reading on. After answers to these questions, the actual findings and outcome of the case described are presented along with a brief discussion. As with all cases, there may be several routes to the appropriate diagnosis and it is often the case that no two clinicians might manage or investigate a case in exactly the same way.

Also, as with any case-based text, one of the inherent drawbacks is that the cases are derived from a population that may have different prevalence of some diseases from other parts of the world. The reader is urged to apply their own experience and clinical commonsense in modifying their approach accordingly.

Before the cases is a brief introductory section on medical problem solving.

Jon Wray
Dick White Referrals
Cambridgeshire
United Kingdom, 2017

Introduction

Approach to medical problem-solving and laboratory interpretation

All medical problem solving succeeds or fails on the history and the physical examination. Without performing these properly, all diagnostic attempts are doomed to being based more on luck than judgment. These skills tend to, in my humble opinion, be ignored/marginalised/undervalued by many veterinary surgeons who are keen to explore more technologically 'glamorous' avenues of diagnosis. This is a mistake. Honing the skills of asking the *right questions*, in the *right way* and interpreting the findings of this and a thorough, skillful and objective physical examination are the *sine qua non* of Internal Medicine diagnosis.

The problem list

The initial approach to medical diagnosis starts with the problem list. In this context a medical 'problem' may be a clinical sign exhibited by the animal or concern expressed by their owner, a physical examination abnormality or the result of a diagnostic test that differs from the expected normal. Great care must be taken to define the *nature* of the problem, especially where different problems may appear, or at least be described, similarly. An example of this would be the need to distinguish regurgitation (which is often due to oesophageal disease) versus vomiting (which is usually associated with pathology distal to the oesophagus). Careful 'open' (that is not leading) questioning and unbiased interpretation of responses during the initial history taking is an important skill to cultivate. A good thorough clinical history should often allow a judicious clinician to both define *what* the problem is and often *where* the problem is. This latter is especially important in refining the diagnostic approach to the likely area of interest, especially where diagnostic imaging is to be performed. For example, performing thoracic radiographs alone to look for a cause of dyspnoea in an older Labrador with laryngeal paralysis is not only going to lead to misdiagnosis but belies a lack of recognition of the site of disease because of poor observational/physical examination skills.

By defining a problem list that is complete, the clinician can avoid potential errors of omission and 'anchoring bias' (see below) that may prevent accurate diagnosis. By using this problem list to develop a set of relevant differential diagnoses for each problem, areas of potential commonality may be reviewed and can help marshal the differential diagnosis more rapidly into an order of likelihood than might otherwise be the case. The law of parsimony (Occam's razor) is usefully employed (see Case 3 for a further explanation) to focus on the simplest hypothesis/that which involves the fewest assumptions first.

Although a problem list should be complete, there is sense in considering both those problems that are the most serious/impactful on the patient and also those that have a limited or well-defined differential diagnosis and affording these greater emphasis when it comes to construction of a differential diagnosis list. For instance, in an animal whose clinical signs (problems) include vomiting, lethargy, jaundice and inappetence, the problems of vomiting and jaundice have more easily defined and limited differential diagnoses than those of lethargy and inappetence, which are common to so many clinical illnesses that the differential diagnosis of them would be huge (and meticulous consideration and exclusion of all of them would result in an unnecessarily lengthy, broad-based and potentially medically overintrusive diagnostic course). Thus whilst it is encouraged to maintain an open mind in producing a problem list that is genuinely reflective of all problems identified, equally clinicians are encouraged to perform some initial 'sorting' of these into problems that may rationally be afforded greater emphasis ('pivotal' problems) or be a more effective 'substrate' for medical problem-solving, versus those that, whilst not dismissed, are of a more general/broad nature.

The differential diagnosis

Differential diagnoses can be problematic in many ways, not least because there is variation in how these can be considered. One can consider a 'mechanistic' differential diagnostic approach such as may be appropriate for considering icterus/jaundice (to divide it into pre-hepatic, hepatic and post-hepatic causes) or polyuria/polydipsia, but this may not be suitable for many other types of clinical problem. There are various useful mnemonics, such as VITAMIN-D or DAMNIT-V to help the clinician consider broad aetiologies of differential diagnosis and thus to avoid errors of omission. Whilst these have their place, it is important to recognise that these, and commonly lists of differential diagnoses reproduced in reference textbooks, fail to take into account the prevalence of diseases and geographical and practice-type variability. These have a profound effect on pre-test probability (see below) and, by-and-large, it is sensible to start with a relatively broad differential diagnostic list and then to 'marshal' these into some sort of order of likelihood based on factors such as known prevalence and geography, as well as considering those problems whose differential diagnoses are limited as offering the greatest possibility of successful medical problem solving. This book is written in the United Kingdom and in particular there are many infectious diseases that are not endemic to our shores, so readers in other countries are encouraged to elevate diseases native to their own countries to their appropriate position based on prevalence. Where I have used mnemonics I have used the DAMNIT-V system, not because it is particularly better than any other, but because that is what I was taught and am most familiar with. The DAMNIT-V mnemonic describes broad aetiological subdivisions as:

D	Degenerative
A	Anomalous, Anatomical
M	Metabolic
N	Neoplastic, Nutritional
I	Infectious (including parasitic), Inflammatory, Immune-mediated
T	Traumatic, Toxic
V	Vascular

One notable absence from both DAMNIT-V and VITAMIN-D classifications is genetic disorders, though these may variably fall under one of the categories such as 'Metabolic' or be considered an 'Anomaly'.

The usefulness of such mnemonics is that they help reduce the fallacies of omission and 'anchoring' bias that may beset clinical problem solving. The primary disadvantage of them is that they may appear to afford equal emphasis to all possibilities whereas the thoughtful clinician will construct a list that takes into account not only *possibility* but also *likelihood*.

Sources of diagnostic error, recognition of diagnostic styles, bias and cognitive error and heuristics

It should go without saying that the success of any treatment relies on applying it to patients in which an accurate diagnosis has been made first of all. It behoves clinicians to recognise those potential causes of diagnostic error, which may then limit the effectiveness of any future treatment strategy if it is thus consequently misapplied to the wrong diagnosis. Sources of diagnostic error may include:

- So-called 'no fault error', for example where willful misleading of a veterinary surgeon by an owner occurs or where a new variation of disease occurs.
- 'System error', where organisational, technical problems or production of spurious results hampers diagnosis.
- 'Cognitive error', which is due to flawed clinical reasoning.

The clinical approach to diagnostic reasoning has been previously described in terms of 'Intuitive' reasoning (sometimes called 'System 1 thinking') and 'Analytical' reasoning (sometimes called 'System 2 thinking'). Clinicians who employ purely Intuitive reasoning rely heavily on experience, prior case exposure, intuition, pattern recognition, heuristics (mental shortcuts that make intuitive diagnostic sense) and long-term memory. Those who employ Analytical thinking rely on systematic problem solving, analysis, reasoning and hypothesis or data-driven consciously controlled decision making. The former approach risks errors of omission and fallaciously limited consideration based on potentially very limited prior case exposure; the latter may risk clinicians overthinking problems, missing the obvious/commonsensical approach and may lead to overly laborious, expensive, medically intrusive and 'throwing the kitchen sink at it' approaches to medical diagnosis. Of course, in reality these two different styles of diagnostic reasoning are seldom practiced one to the exclusion of the other and most clinicians will employ a range of approaches that often use a combination of these styles. By considering those aspects of medical problem solving that are best served by one or other of these approaches and by critically appraising those features that may lead to errors of diagnostic judgment (cognitive errors), thoughtful clinicians can guard against making mistakes that may hamper accurate diagnosis.

Cognitive error (flawed clinical reasoning) has many forms and causes and whilst it is often stated that cognitive error is more common in System 1-based thinking it is erroneous to consider System 2-based thinking as free of the shackles of cognitive errors. As clinicians, our level of tiredness, stress, anxiety and distractions of everyday life can enhance our risk of falling into traps of cognitive error but, nonetheless, recognition of the types of error we may be prone to allows clinicians to be mindful of these and reduce our chances of falling prey to them.

Although not an exhaustive list, common sources of cognitive error in diagnostic reasoning include:

- *Confirmation bias*. This is the tendency to look for and interpret information in a way that supports prior-held preconceptions about a case. This is often most risked by individuals who have a limited case-exposure or experience (note that it is difficult for an individual to be aware that this is the case since by definition that is the the working environment they are accustomed to) and who may prematurely cease a search for a correct diagnosis based on initial findings. Often this may result in a clinician being satisfied by finding '*an* answer' rather than '*the* answer'. In diagnostic imaging this phenomenon is well-recognised as premature 'satisfaction of search', that is an individual may inadvertently eschew thorough evaluation of an entire radiograph, for example, when they spot an obvious lesion initially. Confirmation bias may not be 'all bad' and the counterpoint to it is that sometimes the immediately obvious (Gestalt recognition) is correct and there may be danger of 'talking oneself away' from the correct diagnosis in pursuit of an open-minded broad investigation. 'Sutton's Law' describes the sometimes unarguable veracity of the obvious (Sutton was an American bank-robber whose name is enshrined in the annals of history for supposedly stating in court when asked why he robbed banks, 'Er, because that's where the money is!').

- *Availability bias* is the tendency to overestimate likelihood of a diagnosis based on how memorable previous examples of that diagnosis were.
- *Anchoring bias* is the fallacy of weighting too much of the clinical argument for a diagnosis on one particular piece of information or diagnostic trait, rather than considering other possibilities.
- *Attribution error* is the tendency to leap to conclusions rapidly that serve to reinforce a negative stereotype or afford less diagnostic emphasis in a patient that is unpleasant, aggressive or uncooperative (or whose owners show similar traits).
- *Affective error ('rose-tinted spectacles' thinking)* is the error caused by clinicians (unintentionally) blinding themselves to the possibilities of negative outcomes, less appealing alternative diagnoses or the prospect of needing to perform procedures that are perceived unpleasant. Clinicians are particularly prone to this error in patients with which they have formed emotional attachments/owners in whom good rapport has been established, especially if this is over a long period of time.
- *Commission bias* is the tendency to err towards action 'for the sake of it', often in the absence of a firm idea of what is being treated. It is often more profitable to the patient and safer not to do anything but to take further time considering a patient's needs.
- *Vertical line failure* (thinking inside the box) is a tendency to be contrained by a sequential/narrow field of search, often anchored (see above) on a previous diagnostic test or heavily constrained by overreliance on one particular form of diagnostic testing. A particular danger here is clinicians who may overrely on tehcniques such as MRI or CT, which, whilst undoubtedly powerful diagnostic techniques, have limitations that if not appreciated may lead to cognitive effort. Failure to keep an open mind and to continually review the initial problem list based on accurate history and physical examination are the principle initiators of this error.

Biases in clinical thinking are more likely to occur with System 1 (pattern-recognition) thinking but also somewhat in System 2 thinking if it is untrained. However, not all bias necessarily has a negative impact on the diagnostic process, and when recognised and harnessed, bias may provide clinically useful and appropriate shortcuts in thinking logically that we term 'heuristics' (see below). One of the first steps in avoiding harmful bias is in recognising sources of cognitive error and taking steps to avoid them once aware. However, some 'tools' of clinical thinking (sometimes referred to as 'metacognitive strategies') can also help in avoiding such diagnostic pitfalls. Examples of metacognitive strategies include (in addition to education and awareness of cognitive error and types of clinical thinking) recognising a need to observe the broad clinical picture, carving out time and head-space to both reflect upon and to rationalise clinical thinking but also in recognising the impact of affective states (such as tiredness, anxiety, mood) on one's critical thinking. Creation of time and also forcing oneself to 'slow down' on occasion is inherent to this and we will often exhort our Residents to find a quiet area, clear their desk and their mind and spend some time in quiet reflection about a case; using pen-and-paper to organise one's thoughts, write checklists and review/rewrite/reorder problem lists and differential diagnosis lists can be helpful in this. Above all, in situations where immediate action is not critical to the wellbeing of the patient, having the self-determination to do nothing medically but to expend effort on critical thinking, is often the correct strategy. This has sometimes been described by reversing a common phrase into 'don't just do something, stand there'.

Medical professionals generally do not think or process thought in a linear fashion in the same way that, for example, economists do, by first receiving data then analysing it in its entirety. In Donald Shön's 'The Reflective Practitioner' clinicians are described as displaying (though not uniquely among professionals) 'reflection-in-action', synthesising information, inquiry and intervention, interlaced with each other. In order to make cognitive sense of such a simultaneous confluence of processes, clinicians often develop cognitive shortcuts, known as heuristics, which may help rapidly navigate through seemingly highly complex situations in a way that marshals probability without closing off less common cognitive routes and so committing fallacies of omission. Heuristics are clinically useful provided they are balanced by knowledge, recognition of cognitive error and frequent reflection, and tend to thrive in environments of 'commonsense' thinking and where cost and technological constraints force logical deductive reasoning rather than a defensive, 'throw the (diagnostic) kitchen sink' at a problem, approach.

Reference intervals, appropriate diagnostic testing and dangers of the Ulyssees syndrome

Interpretation of diagnostic test results depends on having a reference interval for that analyte; that is the range of results we might expect to find in a healthy animal. In this book the reference intervals are selected from our own clinical pathology laboratory at Dick White Referrals staffed by a team of Specialist Clinical Pathologists. Reference intervals should be established by any individual laboratory by assessment of a number (usually at least 60, preferably 120) of normal animals. The criteria used to assess 'normality' should be selected prior to data collection (including age, sex, breed, etc). A reference interval is based on the values obtained in 95% of this sample population and clinicians should always remember that *even if the reference population is exactly representative of the population 'at large'* 2.5% of clinically normal animals will have values of an analyte that fall below this reference interval and 2.5% have values of the analyte that fall above it.

This should lead to cautious interpretation of values that fall just outside reference intervals and prompt the realisation amongst clinicians that whilst 'panels' of diagnostic tests are convenient and economic for laboratories to provide, they also magnify the chances of detecting apparently abnormal results in individuals where the value recorded is not due to a pathological process. For instance, if a panel of 20 biochemical tests is performed on a healthy individual, there is a 64% chance of at least one value falling outside the reference interval. With a panel of just 5 biochemical tests, the chance is still 23%. Thoughtful clinicians can minimise the chance of overinterpretation of such meaningless results, by selecting those tests:

a. that help answer a clinical question that they have in mind; i.e. a 'test' should always be performed in order to answer a clinical question, not performed to 'trawl' for abnormalities upon which to act.
b. that have the most chance of being abnormal in the population in which they are applied (see the pretest probability below). For example, performing an ACTH stimulation test for detection of canine Cushing's syndrome (a test that may be rendered abnormal by any non-adrenal illness) in animals with weight loss and anorexia (two clinical signs that are not expected in the majority of patients with canine Cushing's syndrome) is going to increase the chances of detecting

spuriously abnormal results, compared with applying this test to animals with polyuria/poly-dipsia, polyphagia and weight gain (which are expected signs).

There is an inherent problem (other than it completely goes against the principles of thought-ful problem solving based on presenting problem, history and physical examination findings) of employing a strategy of 'obtaining a minimum database'. This phrase has become popular in vet-erinary medicine and the problem with this sort of 'database recognition' approach is that it both bypasses considered testing based on clinical likelihood and leads to the sorts of errors of judgment caused by misinterpretation of values that fall outside the 95% reference interval in unaffected ani-mals. Often the phrase 'minimum database' or 'I'll do *full* bloods' is used to imply thoroughness or indeed that this is 'the expected standard of care' rather than (let's be clinically honest here) in lieu of thoughtful problem solving. Whilst there are circumstances in which such an approach may be justified (the unconscious emergency patient for example) really the 'minimum database' should be a thoughtful history and physical examination from which a problem list and differential diagnosis is derived!

Clinicians should develop an awareness of just 'how' abnormal a level of significance is reached at. In any population to which a clinical pathology test is applied there is an overlap in values be-tween those individuals who are ill and those who are healthy. In the case of some analytes (electro-lytes would be an example), relatively small deviations from reference intervals can have a profound clinical impact and relevance and consequently a low degree of latitude is clinically afforded to them in interpretation. Other analytes (such as serum transaminases, e.g. ALT) may need to be more significantly elevated before laboratory findings are considered to merit further investigation due to a poor degree of correlation of lesser values with identifiable pathology. For example, in the case of ALT a cut-off of >3–4 × the upper reference limit is often interpreted as a significant level, with values below this being of more debatable clinical importance. Compare this with serum po-tassium where such a value would be fatal to the patient. A complete discussion of the interpretive thresholds of significance of diagnostic tests is beyond the scope of this book, but clinicians should avail themselves of a good clinical pathology textbook for a description of these.

Failure to take into account these thresholds of significance for different analytes may lead clinicians into errors of diagnostic judgment and in particular inadvisable unquestioning pursuit of a laboratory abnormality that may in fact be irrelevant to the patient. This is referred to as the 'Ulysses syndrome' (Ulysses' adventures were undertaken at great cost to his men with little tangi-ble to demonstrate for it) and may at the very least result in patients being exposed to unnecessary (and expensive) diagnostic testing and may result (in the case of the clinician proposing liver biopsy for a very mild elevation in ALT) in risk of morbidity or even mortality of the patient for no sound clinical reason.

Similarly, any repetition of diagnostic tests (for instance to chart the course of a disease state improvement, persistence, response to medical management, etc.) should be undertaken with knowledge of the expected time-course for changes in these analytes (which is a function primarily of their half-lives). Overexuberant unnecessarily frequent diagnostic testing serves no clinical pur-pose and again exposes patients and owners to inappropriate testing and should not be condoned.

Pretest probability, sources of analytic error, diagnostic properties and predictive value

When any diagnostic test is applied to a patient, four possible outcomes are possible, which are shown in the table below:

		Patient's disease status is	
		Positive	Negative
Diagnostic test result	Positive	True positive (TP)	False positive (FP)
	Negative	False negative (FN)	True negative (TN)

The probability of a test result being an accurate reflection of an animal's disease status ('post-test probability') is dependent on a number of variables, one of the most important of which is the 'pre-test probability' of disease. Essentially, the greater the disease prevalence in a population to which the test is being applied, the less likely false-positive test results are likely and the greater the proportion of positive findings are true positives. Another method of evaluating the impact of pre-test probability on the impact on test performance is to consider the likelihood of disease.

Sources of analytic error of diagnostic tests are not limited to the performance of the test itself ('laboratory error') but include pre-analytical sources of error (for example, failure to apply the right test in the right situation, failure to collect a sample or prepare the patient properly) and post-analytical (for example, errors of transcription or quality control on reports generated by a laboratory or poor interpretive skills by the clinician reading the report).

The diagnostic value of a particular test may be described by its:

Sensitivity
- Defined as the frequency with which a test is positive in patients with positive disease status.
- It is the same as the number of true positive results divided by the number of true positives plus false negatives.
- A highly sensitive test makes a good screening test – there will be few false negative results and if the animal has the disease there is a high chance that the test result will be positive. This will be at the expense of an increased number of false positive results.

Specificity
- Defined as the frequency with which a test is negative in patients with negative disease status.
- It is the same as the number of true negative results divided by the number of true negatives plus false positives.
- A highly specific test is not a good screening test but is a good confirmatory diagnostic test. Positive results have a low chance of being a false positive and thus correlate with a high chance of the animal having the disease. This will be at the expense of an increased number of false negative results.

Predictive value
A positive predictive value is the probability that a positive test result indicates the animal has the disease. A high positive predictive value indicates that a positive test result strongly implicates presence of the disease.

A negative predictive value is the probability that a negative test result indicates the animal does not have the disease. A high negative predictive value indicates that a negative test result strongly implicated absence of the disease.

By considering factors such as disease prevalence and likelihood, pre-test and post-test probability, test performance and predictive value, clinicians can become educated consumers of the tests used as tools to chart a course through the differential diagnosis of the problems identified whilst avoiding errors of interpretation (including overinterpretation).

		Patient's disease status is		
		Positive	Negative	
Diagnostic test result	Positive	True positive (TP)	False positive (FP)	**Positive predictive value (PPV) =** $\dfrac{\text{True positive (TP)}}{\text{TP + FP}}$
	Negative	False negative (FN)	True negative (TN)	**Negative predictive value (NPV) =** $\dfrac{\text{True negative (TN)}}{\text{TN + FN}}$
		Sensitivity = $\dfrac{\text{True positive (TP)}}{\text{TP + FN}}$	**Specificity =** $\dfrac{\text{True negative (TN)}}{\text{TN + FP}}$	

Summary

The history and physical examination underpin the diagnostic process by allowing the thoughtful clinician to define 'what is (are) the problem(s)?' and 'what is (are) the location(s)?' Differential diagnoses must be considered before planning a diagnostic route. Any diagnostic test must be performed in order to answer a clinical question. Performing broad-based testing as a means of 'trawling' for diagnoses or as part of a 'minimum database' does not involve deductive reasoning or System 2 thinking and risks errors of overinterpretation and false positive diagnoses as well as being economically wasteful. Cognitive error may hamper diagnosis but some cognitive bias may be harnessed and incorporated into System 2 thinking to provide useful heuristic navigation aids, *provided* these are anchored firmly in a broad knowledge base and appreciation of pre-test probability and informed judgment regarding test performance and interpretation.

Recommended reading

The interested reader is directed to the following excellent texts, popular science books and articles about the diagnostic process:

Canfield, P. et al. (2016) Case-based clinical reasoning in feline medicine. 1: Intuitive and analytical systems. *Journal of Feline Medicine and Surgery* (2016) **18**, 35–45

Canfield, P. et al. (2016) Case-based clinical reasoning in feline medicine. 2: Managing cognitive error. *Journal of Feline Medicine and Surgery* (2016) **18**, 240–247

Gawande, A. (2008) *Complications*, Profile Books

Groopman, J. (2007) *How Doctors Think*, Houghton Mifflin Harcourt Publishing, New York

Maddison, J.E., Volk, H.A. & Church, D.B. (2015) *Clinical Reasoning in Small Animal Practice*, Wiley-Blackwell, Chichester

Philips, C. (1988) *Logic in Medicine*, British Medical Journal Publications, London

Polya, G. (2014) How to Solve It, Princeton University Press, Princeton, New Princeton Library Edition

Popper, K.R. (1959) The Logic of Scientific Discovery, Basic Books, New York

Shön, D.A. (1991) The Reflective Practitioner. How Professionals Think in Action, Ashgate Books, Farnham

Whitehead, M. et al. (2016) Case-based clinical reasoning in feline medicine. 3: Use of heuristics and illness scripts. *Journal of Feline Medicine and Surgery* (2016) **18**, 418–426

Endocrinology

Clinical presentation

An 11 year-old male-neutered Border terrier (**Figure 1.1**) weighing 10.4 kg is presented with a history of lethargy, anorexia, vomiting and progressive dullness resulting in a reluctance to walk. His owners report that he has had previous episodes of self-limiting vomiting lasting 2–3 days of which he has had four episodes over the previous 6 months. They have noticed both his water consumption and urination increased dramatically over the previous 2 weeks. No haircoat or skin abnormalities have been noted but he has lost some weight over this time. His appetite up until 48 hours ago has been excellent. He has vomited, accompanied by abdominal effort, 8 times in the last 24 hours and the vomitus has been bile-stained fluid.

Physical examination demonstrates a very depressed dog in overweight body condition (body condition score 4/5) who is reluctant to walk. The eyes are sunken and normal skin turgor is lost. Mucous membranes are very tacky to the touch but are of a normal colour with a capillary refill time of 2.5 s. Heart rate is 144/min, respiratory rate is 32/min and rectal temperature is 38.3 °C. Peripheral pulse quality is slightly poor. Auscultation of the heart and respiratory tract is normal and abdominal palpation generates reproducible cranial abdominal discomfort but no palpable structural abnormalities. The urinary bladder is moderately full and after palpation the dog spontaneously voids urine without apparent difficulty, and some is collected for analysis.

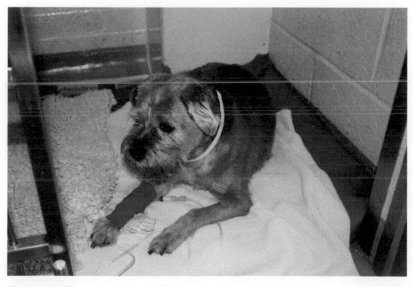

Figure 1.1 The patient at presentation.

Canine Internal Medicine: What's Your Diagnosis? First Edition. Jon Wray.
© 2018 John Wiley & Sons Ltd. Published 2018 by John Wiley & Sons Ltd.

A blood sample is also taken and the following results were obtained:

Haematology

Parameter	Value	Units	Range
RBC	6.89	$\times 10^{12}$/l	(5.5–8.5)
Haemoglobin	14.4	g/dl	(12.0–18.0)
Haematocrit	0.49	l/l	(0.37–0.55)
Mean cell volume	71.3	fl	(60–77)
Mean cell haemoglobin cconcentration	30	g/dl	(30.0–38.0)
Mean cell haemoglobin	20.9	pg	(19.5–25.5)
Total white cell count	**19.26**	$\times 10^{9}$/l	(6.0–15.0)
Neutrophils	**16.37**	$\times 10^{9}$/l	(3.0–11.5)
Lymphocytes	**0.96**	$\times 10^{9}$/l	(1.0–4.8)
Monocytes	**1.96**	$\times 10^{9}$/l	(0.2–1.4)
Eosinophils	**0**	$\times 10^{9}$/l	(0.1–1.2)
Basophils	0	$\times 10^{9}$/l	(0.0–0.1)
Platelets	223	$\times 10^{9}$/l	(200–500)

Biochemistry

Parameter	Value	Units	Range
Total protein	**78**	g/l	(54–77)
Albumin	39	g/l	(25–40)
Globulin	39	g/l	(23–45)
Urea	**13.5**	mmol/l	(2.5–7.4)
Creatinine	132	µmol/l	(40–145)
Potassium	3.6	mmol/l	(3.4–5.6)
Sodium	143	mmol/l	(139–154)
Chloride	118	mmol/l	(105–122)
Calcium	2.2	mmol/l	(2.1–2.8)
Inorganic phosphate	0.9	mmol/l	(0.60–1.40)
Glucose	**34**	mmol/l	(3.3–5.8)
ALT	**385**	IU/l	(13–88)
AST	**96**	IU/l	(13–60)
ALKP	**2130**	IU/l	(14–105)
GGT	**32**	IU/l	(0–10)
Bilirubin	3	µmol/l	(0–16)
Cholesterol	**10.2**	mmol/l	(3.8–7.0)
Triglyceride	**2.4**	mmol/l	(0.56–1.14)
Creatine kinase	168	IU/l	(0–190)

Urinalysis

Parameter	Value	Units	Range
Appearance	Clear, straw		
Chemistry			
Specific gravity	1.032		
pH	8.1		
Protein	Trace		
Nitrite	–		
Blood / Hb	–		
Glucose	++++		
Ketones	++++		
Bilirubin	–		
Urobilinogen	–		
Cytology			
Red cells	2	/hpf	(0–2)
White cells	1	/hpf	(0–2)
Epithelial cells	0	/hpf	(0–5)
Casts	–		
Crystals	–		
Bacteria	–		
Other			

Questions

1. How would you interpret these laboratory results in the context of the history and clinical examination findings, and what is this dog's clinical diagnosis?
2. How might this have arisen and what further information might be gained to plan appropriate treatment?
3. What are this dog's immediate fluid and other medical therapy needs and what problems may be anticipated/pre-empted during the initial stages of treatment?

Answers

1. How would you interpret these laboratory results in the context of the history and clinical examination findings, and what is this dog's clinical diagnosis?
   - The haematology shows a mild neutrophilia, a monocytosis and concurrent lymphopenia and eosinopenia, all components of a stress leukogram. Inflammation may also account for neutrophilia and monocytosis but would not be expected to cause the concurrent lymphopenia and eosinopenia.
   - The biochemistry demonstrates:
     ○ A marked hyperglycaemia which, with concurrent glucosuria, is consistent with diabetes mellitus.
     ○ A rise in urea without a concomitant rise in creatinine, which suggests that a pre-renal azotaemia may be present and indeed the urine SG of 1.032 (i.e. > 1.030) is supportive of this.

- ◦ Total protein is marginally elevated, though albumin and globulin are just within the upper end of their respective reference intervals. With the pre-renal azotaemia, haematocrit that is in the upper end of the reference interval and clinical examination findings, this is most likely due to dehydration.
- ◦ A moderate rise in ALT and AST together with a more marked raise in ALKP and GGT is seen. This is likely to represent hepatopathy with a cholestatic component or response to endogenous or exogenous glucocorticoids.

The similarity in biochemistry between diabetic and Cushingoid patients

It is important to remember that such changes in hepatocellular and cholestatic markers are common in untreated diabetic patients due to the effects of hepatic lipidosis induced by insulin deficiency. Such biochemical findings are very similar to those seen in patients with hyperadrenocorticism (in which hepatic glycogen is stored in excess, not lipid) and it is common in the author's experience that veterinary surgeons commonly have suspicion aroused of concurrent hyperadrenocorticism by such findings, rather than considering them an expected effect of untreated diabetes mellitus. Improvement in these with serial biochemical monitoring after institution of insulin therapy is the key differentiator.

- ◦ A hyperlipidaemia comprising rises in both cholesterol and triglyceride is present. This may be present in diabetes mellitus, pancreatitis, hypothyroidism, hyperadrenocorticism, protein-losing nephropathy and cholestasis (though more usually cholesterol only is elevated in these last two).
- Urinalysis demonstrates glucosuria and ketonuria.
  - ◦ Remember that urine test strips detect acetoacetate and acetone but not β-hydroxybutyrate.

The patient has been demonstrating polyuria, polydipsia, weight loss and until very recently a healthy appetite. In conjunction with the hyperglycaemia and glucosuria a diagnosis of **diabetes mellitus** can be confidently made. It is unnecessary to perform a fructosamine level to confirm this diagnosis although many clinicians advocate assessment of a fructosamine level at diagnosis for future comparison with subsequent fructosamine levels.

The patient is ketonuric and may be described as diabetic and ketotic. Diabetic ketoacidosis (DKA) has not been established at this time by measurement of blood acid-base status, but the clinical findings of depression, vomiting and recumbency strongly implicate DKA and diagnosis of DKA on clinical grounds may be confidently made.

2. **How might this have arisen and what further information might be gained to plan appropriate treatment?**

Diabetic ketoacidosis represents part of a continuum of severity of diabetes mellitus from uncomplicated diabetes mellitus to diabetic ketosis (animal is well but ketonuria +/− serum ketones are detectable) to diabetic ketoacidosis (animal is sick and has identifiable ketonuria and serum ketones).

The initial ketone produced is acetoacetate, which is then either converted to β-hydroxybutyrate (BHB, which accumulates and is the principle ketone body in dogs and cats with DKA) or is spontaneously decarboxylated to acetone. Most urine reagent strips only detect acetoacetate and acetone and beyond initial detection of ketonuria, serial use is limited by the fact that BHB

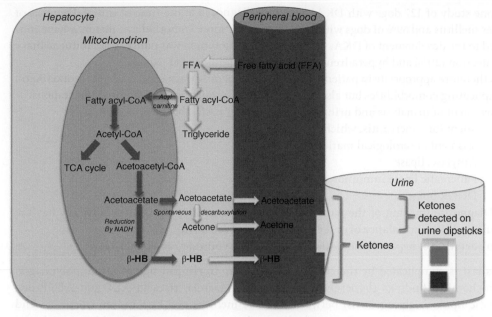

Figure 1.2 Generation of ketone bodies in diabetic ketoacidosis (DKA).

will accumulate due to conversion of acetoacetate over time. β-hydroxybutyrate may be directly measured on a serum blood sample.

Diabetic ketoacidosis develops when the extent of acetyl CoA production after beta-oxidation of free fatty acids liberated by peripheral lipolysis (in response to insulin deficiency and when storage as triglyceride is maximal) exceeds the capacity of the tricarboxylic acid (Krebs') cycle to metabolize to carbon dioxide and water (**Figure 1.2**). Frequently development of DKA is precipitated by a physiologically stressful comorbidity and it is though that development of DKA is usually seen in the setting of both hypoinsulinism and increased counter-regulatory hormone (glucagon, catecholamines, cortisol, growth hormone) production. Examples of comorbidities commonly implicated in DKA are shown in **Table 1.1**.

Table 1.1 Comorbidities commonly associated with development of DKA in dogs

- Pancreatitis
- Urinary tract infection
- Cholangiohepatitis
- Inflammatory bowel disease
- Respiratory tract infection
- Congestive heart failure
- Bacterial pyoderma
- Renal insufficiency
- Administration of insulin-antagonistic medications such as corticosteroids or progestogens
- Hyperadrenocorticism
- Hypothyroidism

In one study of 127 dogs with DKA, 65% were diagnosed at the time of initial diagnosis of diabetes mellitus and 69% of dogs with DKA had one or more comorbidities that may have contributed to the development of DKA. Of these the most common was pancreatitis (41%), urinary tract infection (20%) and hyperadrenocorticism (15%) (Hume et al. 2006).

It is therefore appropriate in patients with DKA to not only warn owners about the likelihood of complicating comorbidities but also to assess for these. Such assessment might include:

- Assessment of urinalysis and urine culture, the latter preferably by cystocentesis
- Assessment for pancreatitis, which may be by
  - Assessment of serological markers
    - Amylase, lipase
    - Pancreatic lipase immunoreactivity (PLI)
    - DGGR lipase
  - Diagnostic imaging of the pancreas, of which pancreatic ultrasound currently has the most utility and balance of cost effectiveness and sensitivity
- Consideration of hyperadrenocorticism (Cushing's syndrome) as a comorbidity

This last is complicated by the considerable overlap in clinical signs (pu/pd, polyphagia) and biochemical findings (hyperglycaemia, hyperlipidaemia, rises in ALT and ALKP due to hepatic lipidosis/glycogenosis) between diabetes mellitus and hyperadrenocorticism and the knowledge that all diagnostic tests for hyperadrenocorticism are affected by non-adrenal illness.

Diabetes mellitus is a 'non-adrenal' illness, which affects tests for Cushing's syndrome

It is important to remember that a positive ACTH stimulation test or low-dose dexamethasone suppression test (LDDST) is compatible with a diagnosis of hyperadrenocorticism *but also* with non-adrenal illness, and diabetic ketoacidosis is a *potent* inducer of false positive results in these tests. Extreme caution must therefore be undertaken with interpretation of these tests in a newly diagnosed sick diabetic dog and the author would recommend against performing tests for hyperadrenocorticism initially.

Certain features, which might lend supportive evidence to the possibility of concurrent hyperadrenocorticism (since they are not usually expected in diabetes mellitus alone), would be development of non-pruritic flank alopecia or development of calcinosis cutis. If abdominal ultrasound examination is undertaken to evaluate the pancreas the opportunity to evaluate both adrenal glands should not be missed (but bearing in mind that normal adrenal gland size does not exclude the possibility of hyperadrenocorticism and that adrenal gland 'incidentalomas' (non-functional benign tumours of the adrenal glands) are not infrequently seen in dogs. If raises in ALKP are provoking consideration of hyperadrenocorticism it is sensible to re-evaluate this after institution of insulin therapy since an improving biochemical picture suggests the waning effects of hepatic lipidosis rather than continued untreated hyperadrenocorticism.

In recognizing that development of DKA usually involves concurrent production of counter-regulatory and insulin-antagonistic hormones, one should also anticipate that with direct therapy (such as in the case of urinary tract infection) or spontaneous resolution with supportive care (such as in pancreatitis), as the source of insulin-antagonism subsides, so the relative insulin sensitivity of the patient is likely to change dramatically. This should be predicted and monitored for lest insulin overdose result due to failure to account for this.

3. **What are this dog's immediate fluid and other medical therapy needs and what problems may be anticipated/pre-empted during the initial stages of treatment?**
   The dog's initial medical needs can be summarised as:

A. Correction of fluid deficit

B. Provision of insulin

C. Correction of acid–base and electrolyte disturbances

D. Management of concurrent disease

A. Fluid needs
- Fluid loss in diabetic ketoacidosis may be prodigious because
  ○ Presence of glucosuria prior to onset of DKA causes osmotic diuresis and associated loss of large volumes of total body water.
  ○ Presence of hyperglycaemia draws fluid from the interstitial compartment to the intravascular compartment.
  ○ Ketoacids, primarily β-hydroxybutyrate and acetoacetate, not only act to cause further osmotic diuresis, but their strong negative charge causes substantial excretion of cations such as sodium, which in turn 'draws' further water loss with it.
  ○ Nausea and vomiting cause increased gastrointestinal fluid loss and diminished intake of water and moisture in food.
- An initial fluid plan should assess
  ○ The degree of dehydration of the patient (often referred to as *replacement requirement*).
  ○ The ongoing losses, which are
    - Predictable normal losses (often referred to as *maintenance requirement*).
      -- Sensible losses (urine, faeces)
      -- Insensible losses (respiration, metabolism)
    - Pathological losses (often referred to as *contemporary losses*)
      -- Vomit
      -- Diarrhoea
  ○ From what fluid compartments this loss is likely to have occurred/be occurring and to plan to restore this.

Fluid therapy is an 'iterative' process and an accurate prescription, not a guess!

Fluid therapy is not a 'set-up and leave-it' endeavour but an 'iterative' (constantly re-evaluated) prescription. That is, the clinician should base an initial prescription on knowledge of the above and a hands-on physical examination, plan 'way-points' at which to assess the effectiveness of the initial prescription (i.e. is it doing what was intended, at the time expected?) and to then adjust therapy accordingly. Failure to do this, or worse to fall into the unconscionably sloppy habit of considering 'multiples of maintenance' as an adequate prescription of fluids, often results in under-treatment. One of the biggest problems we see in our clinic is patients that have received inadequate fluid therapy because the initial clinician has sought to avoid making what are often perceived as 'tricky' assessments of fluid need, and have instead sought to take simplified 'short-cuts'. In reality these assessments are not tricky at all.

Table 1.2 Physical examination parameters of hydration and perfusion

Parameters that are altered in dehydration	Parameters that are altered in perfusion
Mucous membrane dryness / membrane 'slip'	Mucous membrane colour
Skin turgor	Capillary refill time
Sunken eyes	Extremity temperature
Total body weight	Peripheral pulse pressure and quality / distance
	Heart rate
	Arterial blood pressure*
	Urine output*

*Note. These fall late in the progression of intravascular volume depletion and normal blood pressure or urine output does not preclude severe intravascular volume depletion.

- An estimate of dehydration is based on the physical examination findings. Remember that dehydration is an assessment of loss of total body water. About two-thirds of total body water is intracellular and one-third is extracellular, of which about one-third is intravascular and two-thirds is interstitial. The interstitial compartment is depleted of fluid to maintain vascular fluid volume and thus perfusion and because of this and the relative amount of total body water stored here, signs of interstitial dehydration tend to occur more noticeably before alterations in perfusion. With severe interstitial dehydration, shift of fluid into the intravascular compartment cannot occur and alterations in perfusion are noted. Different physical examination parameters (**Table 1.2**) may tell the clinician about different aspects of these, which is why the hands-on physical examination, its objective and accurate interpretation, recording of this, and serial evaluation (the 'iterative' process of fluid therapy) is essential.

The degree of dehydration may be estimated by evaluating physical examination and historical findings and are listed in **Table 1.3**. Alteration in parameters of perfusion tends to occur with loss of ≥10% of total body water.

Table 1.3 Estimated level of dehydration

Estimated dehydration	History and physical examination findings
≤5%	History of increased gastrointestinal fluid loss but normal physical examination findings
5–7%	Dry mucous membranes, mild loss of skin turgor, normal heart rate and pulse quality, normal mucous membrane colour and capillary refill
7–10%	Dry mucous membranes, loss of skin turgor, sunken eyes, mild increase in heart rate, normal mucous membrane colour and capillary refill, normal pulse quality, normal extremity temperature, normal arterial blood pressure
10–12%	Dry mucous membranes, loss of skin turgor, sunken eyes, tachycardia, pale mucous membranes and extended capillary refill, poor peripheral pulse quality peripherally, clammy extremities, normal arterial blood pressure, depressed habitus
12–15%	Dry mucous membranes, loss of skin turgor, sunken eyes, tachy-or bradycardia, very pale mucous membranes and difficult to discern capillary refill, weak pulses, cool extremities, subnormal arterial blood pressure, altered level of consciousness
>15%	Death

Replacement requirement. In this patient the history and physical examination findings would suggest both interstitial dehydration (dry mucous membranes, sunken eyes, loss of skin turgor) and reduced perfusion (extended capillary refill, raised heart rate, poor peripheral pulse quality, depressed mental habitus) and a 10–12% total body water deficit can be comfortably estimated

- In this patient: $(0.12 \times 10.4 \times 1000) = $ **1248** ml

Ongoing *maintenance requirement* may be estimated as a function of resting energy expenditure (REE) with 1 ml of body water being metabolized for each kcal of REE, calculated by $30 \times$ body weight (kg) + 70

- In this patient being: $(30 \times 10.4) + 70 = $ **382** ml/24 hours

This patient is vomiting currently 8 times/24 hours and if we estimate 50–100 ml of fluid/vomit we may predict a further *contemporary loss* of

- In this patient: **800** ml/24 hours

Thus, unless the vomiting ceases immediately the overall replacement deficit is 1248 ml and the predicted ongoing losses in the next 24 hours (maintenance + contemporary losses) is a further 1182 ml. This does not, of course, take account of the fact that the underlying pathology leading to such prodigious loss of fluid is unlikely to be corrected immediately, so this total fluid requirement of 2430 ml is likely to represent, if anything, an underestimation of fluid need. This is why it is essential to re-evaluate *by hands-on physical examination*, at frequent way-points whether the physical exam parameters are changing in a way that denotes a positive impact of fluid therapy. Laboratory tools such as blood gas analysis and serum lactate may have their place in offering objective measurements of the success of fluid resuscitation but it behoves clinicians not to be seduced by the frequent performance of these in neglect of more important, cost-effective and physiologically appropriate parameters of goal-led fluid resuscitation such as physical examination parameters. As an instructive exercise, try calculating what the likely deficiency between fluid need and amount of fluid actually given if this animal was simply placed on 'three times maintenance fluid rate' in the first 24 hours of therapy.

- Crystalloid fluid therapy is principally indicated and 0.9% NaCl is usually the fluid of choice since whole-body sodium depletion is frequently present. Potassium supplementation is usually required (see below). Occasionally patients with hypernatraemia may be encountered in which use of a lower sodium fluid such as Hartmann's may be preferred.
- One common strategy is to replace 25% of the total deficit over the first 1–2 hours of therapy, 25% over the next 4–5 hours and then the remaining 50% over the rest of the first 24 hour period.
- The intravenous route is preferred and because of the fluid volume required a securely placed short length, wide bore peripheral intravenous cannula or a central venous line may be considered. Because of the frequently debilitated state of these patients, strict attention to an aseptic technique should be adhered to. Advocates of central venous line placement cite the ability to frequently measure central venous pressure and a limitation of the need for repeat venepunctures for blood glucose assessments, especially with

multi-port central venous lines. This must be weighed up against the risk of complications including thrombosis and sepsis, the need for increased nursing vigilance and the expense associated with these. Ultimately choice depends on appropriateness in the clinical circumstances.

B. Provision of insulin
- Insulin is necessary to
    - ○ Correct hyperglycaemia and provide cellular metabolism with carbohydrate substrate.
    - ○ Reverse the effects of massive lipolysis.
    - ○ Reverse the metabolic effects of ketonemia, ketonuria and glucosuria causing dehydration and metabolic acidosis.
- Short-acting soluble/neutral insulin is preferred initially because
    - ○ Its dosage can be rapidly adjusted dependent on need, allowing the clinician a great deal of control in correction of hyperglycaemia.
    - ○ It may be delivered by the intravenous or intramuscular route and absorption of longer-acting insulins from subcutaneous depot injections may be unpredictable in severely dehydrated patients.
    - ○ It is sensible to initially provide fluid therapy to re-expand the extracellular fluid compartment for 1 to 2 hours prior to instituting insulin therapy to prevent glucose and water shifting from the vascular space intracellularly. Provision of fluid therapy will immediately start to decrease blood glucose levels and start to reverse acidosis.
    - ○ There are two tried-and-tested strategies in neutral insulin administration, the continuous intravenous method and the intermittent intramuscular method.
    - ○ For intravenous method (**Table 1.4**)
        - - 2.2 units/kg of neutral insulin is diluted in 250 ml of normal saline and 50 ml of this is run through the giving set.
        - - Using an accurate infusion pump, this insulin solution is infused at a rate dependent on the previous blood glucose level. The timing of blood glucose assessment is initially every 1–2 hours with gradual lengthening of this as the rate of insulin administration is decreased.
        - - In the original report of this method, once blood glucose decreased below 14 mmol/l, the principle fluid replacement was changed to 0.45% NaCl with dextrose added at 2.5% (blood glucose 8–14 mmol/l) or 5% (blood glucose <8 mmol/l) to prevent hypoglycaemia.

Table 1.4 Intravenous insulin infusion method

Previous blood glucose measurement	Infusion rate of neutral insulin 2.2 units/kg in 250 ml 0.9% NaCl	Reassess blood glucose
>14 mmol/l	10 ml/h	Every 2 h
11–14 mmol/l	7 ml/h	Every 4 h
8–11 mmol/l	5 ml/h	Every 4 h
5.5–8 mmol/l	2 ml/h	Every 2 h
<5.5 mmol/l	Discontinue	Every 2 h

  ◦ For the intramuscular method

    - 0.2 units/kg neutral insulin is administered intramuscularly once then 0.1 units/kg neutral insulin is repeated i.m. every 1–2 hours after measurement of blood glucose.

    - Once blood glucose is <14 mmol/l but >5 mmol/l, a dose of 0.1 units/kg is administered i.m. every 4–6 hours

  ◦ With either method, during this interval fluid deficit correction should be well underway and patients will usually be feeling very much better. Once this occurs, consideration should be given to administration of a longer-acting insulin, such as lente, given subcutaneously twice daily.

C. Correction of acid–base and electrolyte disturbances

- On presentation severe metabolic acidosis (due to both cellular dehydration and the accumulation of ketoacids), severe dehydration and whole-body depletion of potassium and sodium can be anticipated.

- Regular assessment of venous pH, base excess and serum electrolytes is useful to gauge correction and need for supplementation but should be performed at a frequency that is commensurate with the patient's needs and with sensitivity to the likely time-frame of changes in these analytes, not based on overzealous/defensive or protocol-driven recommendations.

- The serum potassium levels may initially appear normal but this may be due to translocation of intracellular potassium into the extracellular compartment as buffering for hydrogen ions, accumulating during metabolic acidosis, in exchange for intracellular potassium.

- With the introduction of both fluid therapy (correction of acidosis) and of insulin (which will drive both glucose and potassium intracellularly), a profound drop in circulating potassium can be anticipated within the first 24 hours of therapy, and should be pre-empted by supplemental potassium administration.

- Potassium in the form of potassium chloride may be added to fluids, but it should be borne in mind that initial fluid resuscitation rates may be necessarily very high and the clinician should take time to calculate the likely rate of potassium administration at any concentration – a dose exceeding 0.5 mmol/kg/h of potassium chloride may be fatal and recommendations include both the amount to be added to fluid and the maximal rate of administration. It is often preferable that this is either given via a separate fluid delivery line/pump or that initiation of potassium supplementation is deferred for the first 1–2 hours of fluid therapy when fluid rates are likely to be at their highest. One recommendation for rate of fluid administration is given in **Table 1.5**.

- Phosphate may also fall rapidly in DKA patients during the initial phases of treatment due to a combination of prior depletion, correction of metabolic acidosis and transcellular shifts. Decreases in serum phosphate <0.5 mmol/l may be associated with haemolytic anaemia,

Table 1.5 Potassium supplementation rate

Serum potassium	Amount added to fluids (mmol/l)	Maximum fluid administration rate (ml/kg/h)
3.6–5.0 mmol/l	20	25
2.6–3.5 mmol/l	40	12
2.1–2.5 mmol/l	60	10
≤2.0 mmol/l	80	7

especially in smaller patients. Decreases in phosphate are less predictable and less common than those in potassium and are frequently delayed 24–72 hours after the onset of treatment. Daily monitoring for phosphate decreases <0.5 mmol/l is recommended during this period and supplementation instituted with potassium phosphate given at 0.02–0.05 mmol/kg/h in normal saline considered if levels fall below this threshold. Great care needs to be taken with phosphate supplementation since hypocalcaemia and tetany may develop from overzealous application.

- The use of bicarbonate in an attempt to hasten correction of metabolic acidosis is controversial and in most circumstances judicious use of fluid therapy and institution of insulin treatment will correct this. Potential detrimental effects of bicarbonate administration include hypotension, decreased oxygen tissue delivery due to the Bohr effect, paradoxical CNS acidosis and so-called 'overshoot' metabolic alkalosis due to coinciding iatrogenic delivery of bicarbonate and metabolism of lactic acid and ketones, which result in endogenous bicarbonate elaboration. Nonetheless, in severely acidotic states (venous pH <7.1, HCO_3 <12 mmol/l), then bicarbonate administration may be considered. Recommendations vary but a dose of 0.1–0.2 × body weight × base excess over 20–30 minutes has been proposed.

D. Management of concurrent disease

- If urinary tract infection is identified, appropriate antimicrobial treatment of this should be initiated, but it should be borne in mind that the insulin-antagonism so resulting from the infection will be reversed. In animals that are already receiving treatment for diabetes mellitus this may result in a lower insulin requirement subsequently than before recognition of the infection.
- This dog has been vomiting frequently and antiemetics such as maropitant, metoclopramide or ondansetron would be helpful in modifying this.
- Management of pancreatitis is essentially supportive and is discussed further in **Case 14.**

Discussion

Diabetic ketoacidosis is a common emergency presentation and such patients challenge many aspects of medical emergency decision making. However, this challenge equally makes such cases extremely rewarding to treat and with appropriate therapy ≥70% of such patients survive to discharge from the hospital. The single factor most closely correlated with outcome is the severity of metabolic acidosis at presentation. Initial fluid therapy and close attention to pre-empting the metabolic consequences of correction of DKA are the keys to a successful outcome and fluid therapy planning and re-evaluation needs to be undertaken carefully.

Reference

Hume, D.Z., Drobatz, K.J. & Hess, R.S. (2006) Outcome of dogs with diabetic ketoacidosis: 127 dogs (1993–2003). *J Vet Intern Med* **20**, 547–555

Further reading

Boysen, S.R. (2008) Fluid and electrolyte therapy in endocrine disorders: diabetes mellitus and hypoadrenocorticism. *Vet Clin North Am Small Anim Pract* **38**, 699–717, xiii–xiv

Durocher, L.L., Hinchcliff, K.W., DiBartola, S.P. & Johnson, S.E. (2008) Acid–base and hormonal abnormalities in dogs with naturally occurring diabetes mellitus. *J Am Vet Med Assoc* **232**, 1310–1320

Hess, R.S., Saunders, H.M., Van Winkle, T.J. & Ward, C.R. (2000) Concurrent disorders in dogs with diabetes mellitus: 221 cases (1993–1998). *J Am Vet Med Assoc* **217**, 1166–1173

Macintire, D.K. (1993) Treatment of diabetic ketoacidosis in dogs by continuous low-dose intravenous infusion of insulin. *J Am Vet Med Assoc* **202**, 1266–1272

Macintire, D.K. (1995) Emergency therapy of diabetic crises: insulin overdose, diabetic ketoacidosis, and hyperosmolar coma. *Vet Clin North Am Small Anim Pract* **25**, 639–650

O'Brien, M.A. (2010) Diabetic emergencies in small animals. *Vet Clin North Am Small Anim Pract* **40**, 317–333

Clinical presentation

A 7 year-old female-neutered Airedale terrier (**Figure 2.1**) is presented with a history of seizures. 48 hours before presentation the dog was investigated by a colleague due to the owner's concern that the dog had developed a rather stilted/stiff hindlimb gait on walks and general lethargy. Radiographs of the spine, pelvis and proximal hindlimbs had been performed and were unremarkable. A blood sample had been taken to try and aid diagnosis of the lethargy but results were not yet available.

The night before presentation three generalised tonic–clonic seizures had been witnessed by the owner, each lasting approximately 60 seconds.

Questions

1. What are the major causes of seizures in the dog and what initial approach should be taken to try and establish the cause of seizures in this patient?
2. The results of the haematology and biochemistry from this patient are hurriedly obtained from the laboratory to which they were sent. Look at the results below. What are the most important abnormalities and do they proffer a cause for the observed clinical signs?
3. What differential diagnoses would you consider for the most pivotal of these abnormalities and what diagnostic approach would you recommend to the owners?

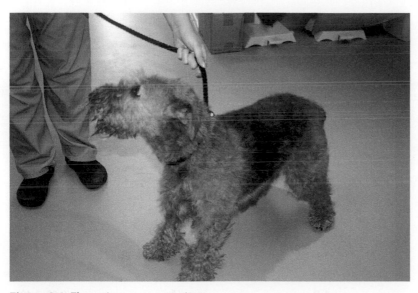

Figure 2.1 The patient at presentation.

Canine Internal Medicine: What's Your Diagnosis? First Edition. Jon Wray.
© 2018 John Wiley & Sons Ltd. Published 2018 by John Wiley & Sons Ltd.

Haematology

Parameter	Value	Units	Range
RBC	7.23	$\times 10^{12}$/l	(5.5–8.5)
Haemoglobin	17.9	g/dl	(12.0–18.0)
Haematocrit	0.55	l/l	(0.37–0.55)
Mean cell volume	76.1	fl	(60–77)
Mean cell haemoglobin concentration	32.5	g/dl	(30.0–38.0)
Mean cell haemoglobin	24.8	pg	(19.5–25.5)
Total white cell count	10.26	$\times 10^9$/l	(6.0–15.0)
Neutrophils	7.68	$\times 10^9$/l	(3.0–11.5)
Lymphocytes	1.88	$\times 10^9$/l	(1.0–4.8)
Monocytes	0.51	$\times 10^9$/l	(0.2–1.4)
Eosinophils	0.16	$\times 10^9$/l	(0.1–1.2)
Basophils	0.02	$\times 10^9$/l	(0.0–0.1)
Platelets	368	$\times 10^9$/l	(200–500)
Film comment:	Unremarkable smear examination		

Biochemistry

Parameter	Value	Units	Range
Total protein	73	g/l	(54–77)
Albumin	40	g/l	(25–40)
Globulin	33	g/l	(23–45)
Urea	2.8	mmol/l	(2.5–7.4)
Creatinine	95	μmol/l	(40–145)
Potassium	3.8	mmol/l	(3.4–5.6)
Sodium	142	mmol/l	(139–154)
Chloride	**100**	mmol/l	(105–122)
Calcium	**1.0**	mmol/l	(2.1–2.8)
Magnesium	0.79	mmol/l	(0.62–0.90)
Inorganic phosphate	**1.8**	mmol/l	(0.60–1.40)
Glucose	**6.1**	mmol/l	(3.3–5.8)
ALT	**194**	IU/l	(13–88)
AST	**97**	IU/l	(13–60)
ALKP	46	IU/l	(14–105)
GGT	**21**	IU/l	(0–10)
Bilirubin	5	μmol/l	(0–16)

Parameter	Value	Units	Range
Cholesterol	4.4	mmol/l	(3.8–7.0)
Triglyceride	0.6	mmol/l	(0.56–1.14)
Creatine kinase	**590**	IU/l	(0–190)

Answers

1. **What are the major causes of seizures in the dog and what initial approach should be taken to try and establish the cause of seizures in this patient?**

   Seizures (and epilepsy – recurrent seizures) may be classified by various methods and several approaches are valid. This may be:

   - According to the type or symptomology
     - For example generalised, partial, partial-complex.
   - According to the broad likely aetiology
     - Many classification systems exist but commonly are referred to as
       - 'Primary'/'idiopathic'/'genetic'.
       - 'Structural'/'symptomatic'/'secondary', which is due to structural brain disease.
       - 'Reactive', which is due to systemic, metabolic or toxic causes.
       - Unknown or cryptogenic seizures (seizures in the absence of or prior to, investigative efforts).
     - According to intra- or extracranial location of the cause.
   - Examples of common causes of seizures, classified by the terms 'primary', 'secondary' and 'reactive', are tabulated in **Table 2.1**.

   An initial approach to establishing a cause of the seizure in this dog should include:

   - Questioning the owner about the seizure event and the period before, during and after it. This is vitally important since other episodic events such as syncope, arrhythmia, vestibular episodes, regional hypoxaemia or narcolepsy may all be confused with seizures. It is also important to establish whether any asymmetrical signs (i.e. discernible neurological deficits / signs affecting only one side / region of the head or body) were identified that might be more suggestive of a secondary seizure event.
   - Ascertaining a good medical and environmental history, which should include
     - Previous vaccination, dietary, travel, anti-parasitic and medication history.
     - Any history of trauma, especially head trauma.
     - Any history of exposure to potential toxins including recreational drugs.
     - Whether the animal has been in otherwise good general health.
     - Whether, if seizures are recurrent and separated by a reasonable length of time, complete recovery between episodes has been seen or whether some signs persist as might be expected with secondary or reactive seizures.

Table 2.1 Example of causes of seizures

Primary seizures	Secondary seizures	Reactive seizures
Idiopathic epilepsy	Tumours	Toxins
	Congenital/anatomical abnormalities	Hypoglycaemia
	Inflammatory and infectious diseases	Hypocalcaemia
	Vascular disorders (haemorrhage, infarct)	Hepatic encephalopathy
		Polycythaemia

Performing a thorough neurological examination. In general, persistence of abnormal findings on the neurological examination might suggest secondary seizure (though caution should be exercised because post-ictal neurological impairment may persist for many hours after a seizure).

Basics of a neurological examination

A neurological examination does not require any equipment that is not found in every veterinary practice merely time, patience, an open mind and application.

The neurological examination should include

- Observation of mentation (both the level of consciousness and content of consciousness).
- Posture, including head, body and limb posture.
- Presence/absence of spontaneous involuntary movement such as tremor.
- Gait.
- An ophthalmic examination.
- Systematic assessment of
  - Cranial nerves
  - Postural reactions
  - Spinal/myotatic reflexes
  - Spinal hyperaesthesia.
- Performing a thorough general physical examination.

- Laboratory tests that are helpful to perform to assess for the most common causes of reactive seizures would include
  - A packed cell volume to assess for polycythaemia.
  - Serum glucose to assess for hypoglycaemia.
  - Serum calcium to assess for hypocalcaemia.
- Performance of a bile-acid stimulation test to assess for hepatic functional impairment or portosystemic shunting (but also remember that bile acids will increase in the presence of obstructive biliary disease).

2. **The results of the haematology and biochemistry from this patient are hurriedly obtained from the laboratory to which they were sent. Look at the results below. What are the most important abnormalities and do they proffer a cause for the observed clinical signs?**

The haematology is essentially unremarkable. Numerous abnormalities are seen on evaluation of the biochemistry and this is very common when a broad 'panel' of tests is performed. What is more important than just identifying abnormalities is knowing how *relevant* any changes are. For instance, whilst the glucose, ALT, AST, GGT and creatine kinase are all elevated, none are so much to the extent that they are likely to be clinically relevant (commonly primary hepatic disease causes elevations in hepatic enzymes exceeding 3–4 times the upper reference limit). The marginally raised glucose makes hypoglycaemia as a cause of the seizures very unlikely. The chloride is only marginally low but may be consistent with increased loss or altered distribution with metabolic alkalosis, respiratory acidosis or hypoventilation.

By far the most significant finding is the profound hypocalcaemia of 1.0 mmol/l (2.1–2.8). This is certainly low enough that, if genuine, clinical signs such as seizure, stiffness, vocalization, facial pruritus and muscle fasciculations may occur. Most commonly these are seen when serum calcium levels are below 1.6 mmol/l or so.

Spurious calcium measurements are common

It is important to recognize that calcium measurement may be prone to error and levels are often spuriously abnormal, mandating that abnormally low or high calcium levels should always be double-checked with a reference laboratory. If treatment is instituted prior to confirmation of this, it is essential that clinicians collect sufficient samples (and of correct type) to allow further diagnostic testing, especially frozen EDTA plasma for PTH assessment. It is helpful to interpret calcium levels in conjunction with phosphate levels, which here are marginally increased, and albumin, which is normal.

3. What differential diagnoses would you consider for the most pivotal of these abnormalities and what diagnostic approach would you recommend to the owners?

Differential diagnoses for hypocalcaemia are shown in **Table 2.2**.

Approximately 45% of calcium circulates in a 'bound' form (protein-bound about 35% and complexed to citrate, lactate, bicarbonate and phosphate about 10%). The remaining 55% circulates as 'free' (ionised) calcium and is the biologically 'available' portion. Measurement of ionised calcium may be useful in confirming the presence of significant hypocalcaemia, though in this case with such a low total calcium it would be expected to be very low (and in fact it was only 0.45 mmol/l where it should be approximately 50–55% of the total calcium, i.e. approximately 1–1.6 mmol/l).

Symptomatic hypocalcaemia is a rare finding with a limited differential diagnosis

When symptomatic hypocalcaemia is identified in a non-whelping bitch and where exposure to ethylene glycol is not suspected, primary hypoparathyroidism is the most likely diagnosis.

Table 2.2 Differential diagnosis of hypocalcaemia in dogs

Commonly associated with clinical signs of hypocalcaemia	Not usually associated with clinical signs of hypocalcaemia
• Puerperal tetany	• Spurious
• Primary hypoparathyroidism	• Pancreatitis
• Iatrogenic hypoparathyroidism	• Chronic kidney disease
• Ethylene glycol toxicity	• Citrated blood or EDTA contamination
• Intestinal hypovitaminosis D	• Hypoalbuminaemia
	• Hypomagnesaemia

Diagnosis of primary hypoparathyroidism requires demonstration of an inappropriately subnormal parathyroid hormone (PTH) level or inappropriately normal PTH when the calcium is low. It is essential to remember the following:

Measurement of PTH: essentials to remember

- That in order to interpret PTH results, a sample must be taken at the same time that it is known that calcium is abnormal, since the calcium–PTH axis can change rapidly.
- The relationship between PTH and serum calcium is sigmoidal and follows a pattern as in the simplified curve below, whereby at low serum calcium levels, PTH production should be elevated, and at high levels of calcium, PTH production should be suppressed (Figure 2.2).

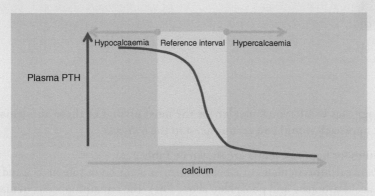

Figure 2.2 Calcium / PTH axis.

- That samples are collected and assayed appropriately. PTH is labile and most laboratories will advise that EDTA plasma is collected and immediately separated and the plasma frozen thoroughly prior to transportation to the lab. It should be ensured that the sample arrives frozen by transport in a chilled pack and is not sent just prior to weekends or public holidays.

PTH assays are not generally performed every day and emergency management of symptomatic hypocalcaemia (see below) is required in most circumstances prior to the receipt of results.

There is little benefit in performing diagnostic imaging and primary hypoparathyroidism cannot be diagnosed by performing ultrasound or other high-definition soft tissue imaging of the parathyroid region.

Diagnosis

Repeat assessment of total calcium in this dog was 0.9 mmol/l and ionised calcium was 0.45 mmol/l. A sample for PTH assessment was taken at the same time that was below the limit of detection (the sample arrived at the laboratory properly frozen) at <10.0 pg/ml (20–65). Since PTH should be elevated in response to hypocalcaemia this is an inappropriate level and confirms the diagnosis of **primary hypoparathyrodism**.

As a curiosity, this patient also demonstrated a finding of punctate lenticular cataracts on ophthalmic examination (see **Figure 2.3**), a finding that has been reported in dogs with primary hypoparathyroidism but which does not, in the author's experience, appear to be particularly common.

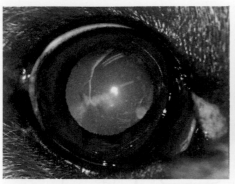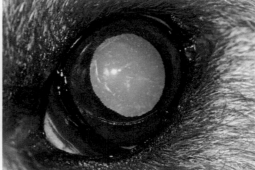

Figure 2.3 Bilateral punctate lenticular cataracts.

Treatment

This dog was not symptomatic at the time of presentation but nonetheless total and ionised calcium were very low and several seizures had been witnessed in the preceding 24 hours. Management of hypoparathyroidism requires emergency replacement of calcium but establishment of longer-term oral therapy.

> ### The need for activated vitamin D
>
> Hypoparathyroidism results in failure of activation of vitamin D_3 to active 1,25 dihydroxyvitamin D_3 (calcitriol), which is required for calcium absorption in the gut. Supplementation of calcium alone is therefore ineffective at controlling clinical signs and a form of activated vitamin D_3 is required for long-term maintenance. Note that giving forms of vitamin D that are not activated is ineffective as PTH will not be present to produce the activated form (see **Figure 2.4**).

This dog was treated with 10% calcium borogluconate delivered at a total 24 hour dose of 60–90 mg/kg of elemental calcium in normal saline as a constant rate infusion whilst oral medications were started and for the first 4 days of treatment. If acute hypocalcaemic tetany or seizures are occurring then 10% calcium borogluconate can be administered slowly intravenously at a dose of 1 ml/kg body weight. This agent is a vesicant/causes phlebitis and is best diluted approximately 1:3 with normal saline and the heart rate should be monitored for development of calcium-induced bradycardia during infusion. Calcium chloride products should be avoided as they can cause marked tissue damage if extravasated. Oral calcium (as calcium carbonate) was administered at a dose of 1 g/day in divided doses and activated vitamin D3 was administered in the form of 0.25 mg calcitriol (Rocaltrol, Roche) p/o BID. Ionised calcium was 1.0 mmol/l at the time of discharge and no further seizures had been seen. After 7 days the ionised calcium had risen to 1.6 mmol/l and the serum phosphate was 2.0 mmol/l. Calcitriol dosage was reduced to 0.25 mg p/o SID and after a further 7 days ionised calcium was measured at 1.27 mmol/l and phosphate at 1.8 mmol/l.

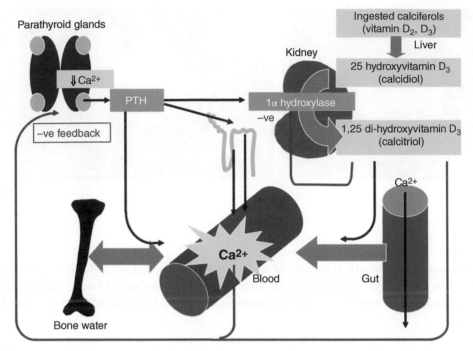

Figure 2.4 Absorption and mobilisation of calcium. Activation of vitamin D_3 to calcitriol by the actions of the renal enxyme 1-alpha hydroxylase is required for absorption of calcium from dietary sources via the gut. Note that both actions of parathyroid hormone (PTH) and calcitriol are needed to mobilise and reabsorb calcium and that whilst low ionised calcium stimulates PTH release, both the presence of ionised calcium and calcitriol inhibit PTH production. Negative feedback is shown by red arrows, positive by black arrows.

Discussion

Primary hypoparathyroidism is a rare condition caused by immune-mediated destruction of parathyroid tissue, but nonetheless it is an important differential diagnosis for dogs presenting with tetanic muscular activity and fasciculation and seizures. Clinically affected patients will also sometimes show facial pruritus, sneezing and behavioural changes, sometimes becoming short-tempered. There are few clinically relevant differential diagnoses for hypocalcaemia but documentation of a subnormal or inappropriately normal PTH level (when the sample has been properly collected and stored and is contemporaneous with the hypocalcaemia) is essential for diagnosis.

Long-term management requires an activated vitamin D replacement. Dosing can be problematic in smaller dogs due to inflexible capsule strengths but use of alfacalcidol (One Alpha, Leo) drops 2 µg/ml (1 drop contains approximately 100 nanograms) can be useful in smaller patients. It is dosed at 40–80 ng/kg/day. Alfacalcidol is hydroxylated to activated vitamin D_3 in the liver and does not require renal activation in the presence of PTH.

Therapy is required lifelong, though most animals, provided that activated vitamin D is supplied, will derive adequate calcium from dietary sources and will not necessarily need extra oral calcium supplements. Regular monitoring of calcium and phosphate, ensuring that the calcium × phosphate product is kept below 6, is advised in the longer term.

Further reading

Bruyette, D.S. & Feldman, E.C. (1988) Primary hypoparathyroidism in the dog. Report of 15 cases and review of 13 previously reported cases. *J Vet Intern Med* **2**, 7–14

Feldman, E.C. & Nelson, R.W. (2004) Chapter 17: Hypocalcaemia and primary hypoparathyroidism. In *Canine and Feline Endocrinology and Reproduction*, 3rd edn. Saunders, St Louis, pp. 717–742

Russell, N.J., Bond, K.A., Robertson, I.D., Parry, B.W. & Irwin, P.J. (2006) Primary hypoparathyroidism in dogs: a retrospective study of 17 cases. *Aust Vet J* **84**, 285–290

A 3 year-old male-neutered Staffordshire bull terrier cross (**Figure 3.1**) is presented with a one-month history of appearing anxious, lethargic, and having lost 1.5 kg in weight. Appetite has become reduced to the point where the dog is no longer eating for the last 48 hours and the dog is drinking a normal amount. Occasional intermittent bouts of vomiting digested food at variable intervals after eating has been reported by the owners, but no change in faecal consistency has been reported. The dog had been seen one week previously and a colleague had identified evidence of dehydration (tacky oral mucous membranes with extended capillary refill time). Balanced crystalloid intravenous fluid therapy had been administered over 24 hours and the owner reported very marked improvement. This was, however, short lived and the dog has become progressively more depressed over the previous week.

On physical examination the dog is noticeably subdued for the breed type, is 23.3 kg in body weight and has a heart rate of 144/min, respiratory rate of 24/min and rectal temperature of 38.2 °C. Peripheral pulse quality is normal. Mucous membranes are pink but are noticeably tacky to the touch and capillary refill time is 2 s; the eyes are a little sunken. Thoracic auscultation is unremarkable and abdominal palpation demonstrates no abnormalities. The dog vomits a small amount of bile-stained fluid during abdominal palpation.

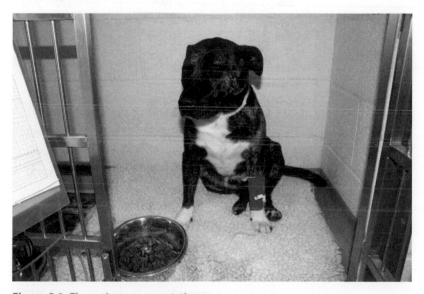

Figure 3.1 The patient at presentation.

Canine Internal Medicine: What's Your Diagnosis? First Edition. Jon Wray.
© 2018 John Wiley & Sons Ltd. Published 2018 by John Wiley & Sons Ltd.

A sample is taken for haematology and a serum biochemistry and the following results are obtained:

Haematology

Parameter	Value	Units	Range
RBC	8.38	$\times 10^{12}/l$	(5.5–8.5)
Haemoglobin	**21.1**	g/dl	(12.0–18.0)
Haematocrit	**0.59**	l/l	(0.37–0.55)
Mean cell volume	70.4	fl	(60–77)
Mean cell haemoglobin concentration	35.8	g/dl	(30.0–38.0)
Mean cell haemoglobin	25.2	pg	(19.5–25.5)
Total white cell count	**16.3**	$\times 10^9/l$	(6.0–15.0)
Neutrophils	7.1	$\times 10^9/l$	(3.0–11.5)
Lymphocytes	**7.1**	$\times 10^9/l$	(1.0–4.8)
Monocytes	0.7	$\times 10^9/l$	(0.2–1.4)
Eosinophils	**1.4**	$\times 10^9/l$	(0.1–1.2)
Basophils	0	$\times 10^9/l$	(0.0–0.1)
Platelets	255	$\times 10^9/l$	(200–500)
Film comment:	No abnormal cells seen		

Biochemistry

Parameter	Value	Units	Range
Total protein	64.2	g/l	(54–77)
Albumin	34.8	g/l	(25–40)
Globulin	29.4	g/l	(23–45)
Urea	**19.8**	mmol/l	(2.5–7.4)
Creatinine	**189**	µmol/l	(40–145)
Potassium	**5.8**	mmol/l	(3.4–5.6)
Sodium	**126.7**	mmol/l	(139–154)
Chloride	**95**	mmol/l	(105–122)
Calcium	**3.02**	mmol/l	(2.1–2.8)
Magnesium	–	mmol/l	(0.62–0.90)
Inorganic phosphate	**2.0**	mmol/l	(0.60–1.40)
Glucose	5.5	mmol/l	(3.3–5.8)
ALT	**241**	IU/l	(13–88)
AST	59	IU/l	(13–60)
ALKP	14	IU/l	(14–105)
GGT	4	IU/l	(0–10)
Bilirubin	11	µmol/l	(0–16)

Parameter	Value	Units	Range
Cholesterol	3.8	mmol/l	(3.8–7.0)
Triglyceride	0.8	mmol/l	(0.56–1.14)
Creatine kinase	121	IU/l	(0–190)

Questions

1. How would you interpret this dog's physical examination findings with regards to fluid status?
2. Interpret the laboratory findings.
3. What further investigation should be performed in this dog?

Answers

1. **How would you interpret this dog's physical examination findings with regards to fluid status?**

The relevant clinical examination findings are that the heart rate is 144/min with normal peripheral pulse quality and normal capillary refill time but with tacky mucous membranes and slightly sunken eyes. In **Case 1, Table 1.2** we established that tacky mucous membranes and sunken eyes are features of dehydration but not of decreased circulating intravascular volume. The findings are consistent with dehydration of 5–7%. The patient's heart rate, considering how subdued he is, is a little high, though some care must be taken to assess heart rate in the context of the patient and its presentation, rather than absolute values.

Often it has been described that heart rates in excess of 120/min in dogs is excessively high; most cardiology textbooks will, however, list normal heart rates as varying between 60 and 160/min in dogs and one very large study, which included 5000 apparently healthy dogs presenting in first-opinion practice for vaccination, the mean heart rate (± standard deviation) was 127.2/min (±19.8) with relatively small differences in mean heart rate between the smallest and largest patients.

Shock

Although the primary findings are of dehydration, the relative increase in heart rate is likely to be a compensatory mechanism to reduced tissue perfusion severe enough to fail to meet cellular metabolic demands. This is defined as 'shock'. Three 'stages' of shock are recognized and may be defined as shown in **Table 3.1**.

Table 3.1 Stages of shock

Stage of shock	Physical parameter	Alterations
Compensatory	Heart rate	Increased
	Mucous membrane colour	Normal to hyperaemic
	Capillary refill	Normal to rapid
	Blood pressure	Normotensive
	Core body temperature	Normothermic

Stage of shock	Physical parameter	Alterations
Early decompensatory		Increased
		Normal to pale
		Rapid
		Normo- to slightly hypotensive
		Normo- to slightly hypothermic
Late decompensatory		Normal to reduced
		Pale
		Prolonged
		Hypotensive
		Hypothermic

2. **Interpret the laboratory findings.**

Haematology findings:

- The haematology shows a mild raise in haematocrit. This may be relative of absolute. Although the serum proteins are not elevated, in the setting of the animal's tacky mucous membranes and previous positive response to fluid therapy, a relative erythrocytosis due to dehydration is most likely. Repetition of this after provision of intravenous fluid therapy could help determine this with more confidence
- The differential white blood cell counts show concurrent lymphocytosis and eosinophilia.

Clues from a 'reverse' of a stress leukogram

Both lymphocytosis and eosinophilia are unusual to find in a sick animal since it is more usual to detect a 'stress leukogram' comprising a combination of one or more of neutrophilia, lymphopenia and eosinopenia.

Lymphocytosis may be seen in chronic antigenic stimulation, shifting of lymphocytes from the marginating lymphocyte pool to the circulating lymphocyte pool, lymphoproliferative disorders and lymphocytosis of hypoadrenocorticism. Eosinophilia may be seen in hypersensitivity disorders, parasitism, mast cell disease, hypoadrenocorticism, eosinophilic leukaemias and in systemic disorders with peripheral eosinophilia (e.g. eosinophilic bronchopneumonopathy). In this case the magnitude of the eosinophilia is very mild.

Biochemistry findings:

- Azotaemia is seen and the magnitude of the elevation in the urea is proportionately greater (approximately double the reference interval upper limit) than the elevation in creatinine (approximately 1.3 times the reference interval upper limit). Azotaemia (elevation in urea, or creatinine or both) may be pre-renal, renal or post-renal (**Table 3.2**).
- Because urea is re-absorbed in the proximal renal tubules in the setting of diminished renal blood flow, in dehydrated animals (where renal plasma flow decreased) urea may become proportionately more elevated than creatinine. This may also happen with incomplete starvation

Table 3.2 Distinguishing causes of azotaemia

	Pre-renal	Renal	Post-renal
Mechanism	• Reduced renal blood flow	• Reduction in glomerular filtration rate due to intrinsic renal diseases	• Diminished urea or creatinine excretion due to obstruction or rupture of urinary tract distal to the nephron
Typical causes	• Hypovolaemia (including hypoadrenocorticism) • Shock	• Inflammatory and infectious renal diseases • Chronic kidney disease • Toxic nephropathies • Congenital and metabolic renal diseases • Renal neoplasia • Ischaemia • Hydronephrosis	• Urinary tract obstruction distal to kidneys due to urolithiasis, matrix plux, tumour, stricture, foreign body, prostatic disease • Urinary tract rupture distal to kidneys due to trauma or erosive disease
Supportive findings	• Concurrent clinical examination findings of dehydration or hypovolaemia • Typically proportional magnitude of urea elevation, greater than that in creatinine • Urine SG >1.030 in the dog (except where impairment of medullary interstitial concentration is present) • Improvement or resolution with fluid therapy	• Typically urine SG in isosthenuric range of 1.008–1.012 but urine SG <1.030 in the setting of clinical dehydration is supportive • Usually history of polyuria/polydipsia • May be accompanied by evidence of structural renal disease • May be accompanied by anaemia or chronic kidney disease	• History of dysuria, stranguria, pollakiuria • History of abdominal/pelvic trauma or recent surgery in area of urinary tract • Enlarged urinary bladder if obstruction distal to it • Uroabdomen

and in the setting of gastrointestinal haemorrhage. Azotaemia should be interpreted in light of the patient's hydration status and in conjunction with measuring urine specific gravity at the same time (and before any fluid or diuretic therapy).

- Concurrent hyperkalaemia, hyponatraemia and hypochloridaemia may be detected in the presence of mineralocorticoid deficiency (hypoadrenocorticism), renal insufficiency, severe gastrointestinal disease, especially haemorrhage, intestinal *Trichuris vulpis* infection, repeated drainage of chylous effusions, severe metabolic acidosis (especially in diabetic ketoacidosis) and pregnancy. Common causes of hyperkalaemia, hyponatraemia or both are listed in **Table 3.3**.
- Mild hypercalcaemia (see also Table 30.5) may be seen as a spurious result (analytical error, lipaemia, physiological growth), in the setting of disease that is pathogenic but does not usually cause clinical signs directly related to hypercalcaemia (hypoadrenocorticism, chronic kidney disease, granulomatous disease, angiostrongyliasis), those disorders that generally cause clinical signs due to hypercalcaemia (primary hyperparathyroidism, hypercalcaemia

Table 3.3 Differential diagnosis of hyperkalaemia, hyponatraemia and both hyperkalaemia and hyponatraemia

Causes of hyperkalaemia	Causes of hyponatraemia	Causes of both hyperkalaemia and hyponatraemia
Increased K^+ fluid administration Shift of K^+ from intracellular to extracellular fluid compartment: • Metabolic acidosis • Rhabdomyolysis/muscle trauma, reperfusion • Massive tissue necrosis or haemolysis Decreased excretion of K^+ • Acute renal failure • Urinary tract obstruction • Hypoaldosteronism (including hypoadrenocorticism and hyporeninaemia hypoaldosteronism) Miscellaneous causes • Trichuriasis, salmonellosis, perforated duodenal ulcer • Chylothorax with repeated drainage • Some drugs, e.g. ACE inhibitors, potassium sparing diuretics	Spurious/analytic error in presence of • Hyperlipidaemia • Hyperproteinaemia With volume depletion in • Hypoadrenocorticism • Gastrointestinal loss due to vomiting and diarrhoea • Loss into body cavities ('third space') in pleural effusion, peritonealeffusions, uroabdomen, pancreatitis) • Burns • Excessive diuresis, especially loop diuretics such as furosemide With volume excess in • Congestive heart failure • Hepatic failure • Nephrotic syndrome • Fluid overload in oliguric renal failure With normovolaemia • Primary polydipsia • Syndrome of inappropriate ADH secretion • Administration of ADH analogues such as DDAVP • Myxoedema	• Hypoadrenocoticism • Acute renal failure • Urinary tract obstruction • *Trichuris vulpus* (whipworm) infestation • Gastrointestinal fluid loss • Uroabdomen • Chylous effusion with repeated drainage

of malignancy) and hypercalcaemia-inducing toxins (grapes, raisins, vitamin D containing medical products and rodenticides). Mild hypercalcaemia may also be seen with reduced glomerular filtration rate.

- Hyperphosphataemia may be due to metabolic acidosis, cell lysis, trauma, intoxication or decreased renal excretion.
- A raise in ALT usually signifies release from hepatocyte cytosol due to hepatocellular damage, small amounts being released also from damaged skeletal muscle. Raises in ALT of > 3–4 x the upper limit of the normal reference range are more specific for primary hepatic disease in the dog, levels below this, as in this patient, being commonly seen with 'reactive hepatopathies', endocrinopathies, hypoxia and congestion of the liver, or local gastrointestinal pathology.

3. **What further investigation should be performed in this dog?**

   This dog's current problem list is:
   - Lethargy
   - Weight loss
   - Intermittent vomiting
   - Hyporexia
   - Episodes of dehydration, which are responsive to fluid therapy (along with clinical signs) but which quickly relapse
   - A likely relative polycythaemia
   - A 'reverse' of a stress leukogram, with lymphocytosis and eosinophilia
   - Azotaemia with disproportionate raise in urea compared with creatinine
   - Hyperkalaemia
   - Hyponatraemia
   - Hypochloridaemia
   - Mild hypercalcaemia
   - Mild hyperphosphataemia
   - Mild raise in ALT

   This list is lengthy and may appear daunting, but in considering medical problem solving two basic tennets will often help.

Marshalling the problem list: pivotal problems and Occam's Razor

a. Consider those 'problems' from the original problem list which are 'pivotal'. By pivotal, we mean not necessarily the ones that are most life-threatening or medically important, but those that are most *useful* to act as a springboard for problem solving because they have a very limited differential diagnosis, or a differential diagnosis made of components that can very quickly be ruled out. For instance, in this animal, concurrent hyperkalaemia and hyponatraemia has a more restricted differential diagnosis list than many of the other 'problems' such as relative polycythaemia or intermittent vomiting.

b. Always employ the principle of 'Occam's Razor' (also known as the 'Law of Parsimony'). William of Ockam was a thirteenth to fourteenth century English Franciscan friar and theologian who posited that amongst competing hypotheses, the one that should be initially pursued was that which resulted from the fewest assumptions, that is the simplest (a 'razor' is a philosophical 'rule of thumb'). In other words, always look for the simplest explanation first, and if all the problems can be explained by one disease process (and this will usually come up again and again if you write out the differential diagnosis for each problem, which is why it is such a useful exercise) then it is most likely that this is the diagnosis.

In this case,
- Performance of a urinalysis to assess urine specific gravity in the light of the azotaemia is sensible though it should be borne in mind that in patients with hyponatraemia, the ability to mount a concentrated medullary interstitium within the kidney and so concentrate urine is impaired.

Effect of hyponatraemia on urine SG

This is an important exception to the usual rule that dogs with pre-renal azotaemia should have a urine SG >1.030. In dogs with decreased renal plasma flow *and* hyponatraemia, urine SG will often be <1.030.

- Hypoadrenocorticism is present on the differential diagnosis list for all the abnormalities detected. Whilst further investigation for other causes of hypercalcaemia, for instance, might be appropriate in the longer term, in this patient hypoadrenocorticism should be excluded before any further diagnostic testing. Not to do so, not only defies clinical 'common sense' but would result in unnecessary expense and delay in treatment were the patient to have hypoadrenocorticism. This is an important difference between 'database-recognition' approaches to medical problem-solving and 'deductive reasoning'. Various tests for hypoadrenocorticism have been considered.
  - Most tests involve assessment of cortisol. Although the principle clinical signs of hypoadrenocorticism are due to a mineralocorticoid deficiency (principally aldosterone), since cortisol is the glucocorticoid whose secretion is most impaired in hypoadrenocorticism and this is relatively cheap to assay, it is used as a 'surrogate' for global decrease in adrenal cortical 'reserve'. Disadvantages include that this does not differentiate between those animals with isolated glucocorticoid deficiency and combined glucocorticoid/mineralocorticoid deficiency and that the effects of exogenous glucocorticoids, including topical skin/eye/otic products, can render false positive test results in animals without hypoadrenocorticism for many weeks, even after only brief administration. It is therefore imperative that clinical history taking includes such details prior to interpretation of cortisol assays.
  - Traditionally ACTH stimulation testing, with assessment of serum cortisol before and 60–90 minutes after intravenous administration of an ACTH analogue, usually tetracosactrin or cosytropin has been used, with affected dogs showing levels of cortisol before and after stimulation of <55 nmol/l, and usually below the limit of detection of this analyte (usually <27 nmol/l). Expense of these analogues in the United States has led to evaluation of alternate testing using a low dose (5 mcg/kg body weight compared with the traditional method of 250 mcg/dog or 125 mcg/dog if under 5 kg) of analogues and assessment of basal cortisol alone. Intramuscular injection and the use of ACTH analogue gels is also popular in some countries and despite concerns that the intramuscular route in hypovolaemic patients may result in variable absorption, this seems to yield similar results.
  - A basal serum cortisol as a sole test is helpful in excluding hypoadrenocorticism if it is >55 nmol/l. However, many normal dogs will have a basal cortisol below this level and the specificity for a serum cortisol of <55 nmol/l in diagnosing hypoadrenocorticism is only 78%; therefore at this level an ACTH stimulation test becomes mandatory.
  - Measurement of endogenous ACTH may be useful in differentiating primary hypoadrenocorticism from secondary hypoadrenocorticism in those patients without electrolyte abnormalities.

Diagnosis

In this patient urine SG was measured at 1.028, which is inappropriately low in the setting of azotaemia and might suggest either renal azotaemia or pre-renal azotaemia with concurrent poor renal concentrating ability due to hyponatraemia.

An ACTH stimulation test was performed and pre- and post-stimulation cortisol levels were <27 nmol/l, <27 nmol/l respectively. It was definitively established that no history of administration of glucocorticoids had occurred.

A diagnosis of **hypoadrenocorticism** (Addison's disease) was made.

Treatment

As the dog was inappetent and vomiting, and dehydration (primarily of the interstitial compartment) was present, intravenous fluid therapy was given with 0.9% sodium chloride to correct a volume deficit of approximately 12%. Ongoing insensible losses and occasional vomiting was also accounted for and the dog was administered the fluid at a rate of 300 ml/h for the first 6 hours and then 100 ml/h thereafter. Hydrocortisone was administered as a constant rate infusion at an initial rate of 0.3 mg/kg/h for 12 hours (adjusting for the decrease in fluid administration rate after 6 hours). No further vomiting was seen and by 12 hours post-admission, it was felt possible to start the dog on oral medication. Fludrocortisone tablets were administered orally at a dose of 0.02 mg/kg p/o SID and prednisolone at a dose of 0.2 mg/kg p/o SID (desoxycorticosterone pivalate, DOCP, was not licenced or available in the United Kingdom at the time of diagnosis but has since become so).

The dog was eating well and evidence of interstitial dehydration had dissipated by 48 hours after initial assessment and the dog was discharged home to continue to receive oral medication.

Reassessment by history, physical examination and by assessing serum electrolytes occurred after a further week, then monthly for 3 months and then every 3–6 months thereafter. Based on recurrence of hyponatraemia, the fludrocorticosone dose was gradually increased and by 12 months post-initiation the fludrocortisone dose was 0.03 mg/kg/day.

Discussion

Hypoadrenocorticism may present with somewhat vague and non-specific signs. Episodes of collapse are relatively uncommon and probably occur in <10% of patients. Similarly, it should not be expected that patients with hypoadrenocorticism necessarily will be bradycardic on presentation. Whilst bradycardia is a potential effect of hyperkalaemia, in more instances dogs have normal heart rates at presentation (though this may be 'inappropriate' in the face of volume depletion). The biggest impediments to diagnosis of hypoadrenocorticism are failure to appreciate the wide variety of presentations of it and any prior glucocorticosteroid use (and this is one of many reasons why glucocorticosteroids should never be given out of desperation to be seen to be doing something in lieu of a diagnosis). Iatrogenic adrenal cortical suppression may last for many weeks, even after a short-term administration of glucocorticoids of any sort, and whilst a normal ACTH stimulation test or a cortisol >55 nmol/l effectively excludes hypoadrenocorticism, it is not possible to distinguish prolonged iatrogenic suppression from naturally occurring disease. Approximately 10% of dogs with hypoadrenocorticism can have normal electrolyte values on presentation due to a variety of reasons, not least the effects of ion shifts occurring during acidosis and effects of prior fluid administration. Thus hypoadrenocorticism should never be excluded on the grounds of normal serum sodium and potassium. A subset of dogs may present with primarily evidence of glucocorticoid deficiency and these dogs have been termed 'atypical' Addisonians, with the implication made that isolated glucocorticoid deficiency exists in these patients. However, many are found to be mineralocorticoid deficient also and although many of these dogs will retain potassium and sodium haemostasis for some time, they will usually eventually develop electrolyte abnormalities.

Profound volume depletion accompanies mineralocorticoid deficiency and patients with hypoadrenocorticism require rapid replacement of this if they are not to succumb to shock. Note that fluid prescriptions in this, and indeed all situations requiring fluid therapy, should be considered a careful and 'iterative' form of treatment in which treatment goals are planned, assessed for and the plan re-assessed if the expected outcome is not seen. Use of 'multiples of maintenance', which has become a depressingly common feature of veterinary fluid prescriptions and which bypasses all critical planning of fluid therapy, is inadequate in these settings.

A solution of 0.9% sodium chloride is an appropriate fluid in most settings since the combined goals of fluid replacement, sodium and chloride replacement and potassium reduction through dilution with potassium-free fluid are all met. However, it is a fallacy to assiduously avoid potassium-containing fluids if they are all that is available since even those balanced electrolyte solutions that contain potassium will usually contain no more than 4 mmol/l and rapid dilutional reduction in serum potassium levels of hyperkalaemic patients will result from their use. Care should be taken in animals with profoundly low serum sodium levels (<120 mmol/l). These patients have central nervous system adaptation to low serum osmolality, which, if the sodium level is rapidly elevated, can result in neuronal dehydration and demyelinosis. It is recommended that in animals with sodium levels in this range, rises of no more than 10–12 mmol/l over the first 24 hours, and no more than 18 mmol/l over the first 48 hours, are achieved. These figures are somewhat arbitrary and techniques to try and achieve this may include more prolonged fluid replacement or use of a fluid such as Hartmann's solution, which contains 130 mmol/l sodium rather than 154 mmol/l as is found in 0.9% saline. Marked hyperkalaemia, usually >7 mmol/l, may cause severe cardiac depression by the increase in extracellular potassium, resulting in decreased resting membrane potential of the cardiac myocyte decreasing phase 0 of the action potential upstroke and delayed conduction. Emergency therapy may include administration of calcium gluconate slowly intravenously (at a dose of 0.5ml / kg of 10% calcium borogluconate solution) or combining insulin and dextrose (at a dose of 1-2g of dextrose per unit of insulin, and insulin given at 0.2 units/kg of neutral insulin), but these measures are very seldom needed if fluid therapy is judiciously given; the authors' observation would be that many inexperienced clinicians become distracted by the desire to provide these therapies when it would behove them more to concentrate on the basics of life-saving fluid therapy!

Short-term glucocorticoid and mineralocorticoid administration may be helpful until the animal can tolerate oral medications, though it is generally fluid therapy rather than pharmaceuticals that is initially life-saving. The glucocorticoids most commonly given are dexamethasone sodium phosphate (0.1–2.0 mg/kg), prednisolone sodium succinate (1–10 mg/kg) or hydrocortisone given at a dose of 0.5 mg/kg and then as a constant-rate infusion of 0.3–0.5 mg/kg/h. These doses may be repeated every 6 hours, but their wide range is reflective of the largely anecdotal derivation of these doses.

In the long term, both mineralocorticoid and glucocorticoid replacement is effective. The former is achieved by desoxycorticosterone pivalate (DOCP) (also known as deoxycorticosterone or desoxycortone pivalate) at 2.2 mg/kg s.c. or i.m. q25 days in countries where this is available or fludrocortisone 0.01–0.02 mg/kg p/o daily in other countries. DOCP dosage may require to be given more frequently in some dogs. Concurrent glucocorticoid replacement at an equivalent dose of 0.2 mg/kg of prednisolone daily is required in most dogs, though since fludrocortisone also has some glucocorticoid activity, this one product may be sufficient to meet both needs in some animals. Mineralocorticoid requirement is based on serial evaluation of serum potassium and sodium and it is common to see this need increase over the first year or so of treatment (so-called 'fludrocortisone drift'), likely due to continued destruction of adrenal cortices.

Further reading

Baumstark, M.E., Sieber-Ruckstuhl, N.S., Muller, C., Wenger, M., Boretti, F.S. & Reusch, C.E. (2014) Evaluation of aldosterone concentrations in dogs with hypoadrenocorticism. *J Vet Intern Med* **28**, 154–159

Boysen, S.R. (2008) Fluid and electrolyte therapy in endocrine disorders: diabetes mellitus and hypoadrenocorticism. *Vet Clin North Am Small Anim Pract* **38**, 699–717, xiii–xiv

Greco, D.S. (2007) Hypoadrenocorticism in small animals. *Clin Tech Small Anim Pract* **22**, 32–35

Kintzer, P.P. & Peterson, M.E. (1997) Primary and secondary canine hypoadrenocorticism. *Vet Clin North Am Small Anim Pract* **27**, 349–357

Kintzer, P.P, & Peterson, M.E. (2014) Canine hypoadrenocorticism In: *Kirk's Current Veterinary Therapy*, Vol. XV, eds J.D. Bonagura and D.C. Twedt. Elsevier, St Louis, pp. 233–238

Kintzer, P P. & Peterson, M.E. (1997) Treatment and long-term follow-up of 205 dogs with hypoadrenocorticism. *J Vet Intern Med* **11**, 43–49

Meeking, S. (2007) Treatment of acute adrenal insufficiency. *Clin Tech Small Anim Pract* **22**, 36–39

Van Lanen, K. & Sande, A. (2014) Canine hypoadrenocorticism: pathogenesis, diagnosis, and treatment. *Top Companion Anim Med* **29**, 88–95

A 9 year-old entire male Giant Schnauzer, weighing 46 kg, presents with a 5 month history of progressive alopecia and a four week history of progressive polyuria/polydipsia and increased appetite (**Figure 4.1**). He is described as being otherwise very bright and well by his owner. His owner quantifies his water intake as in excess of 6 litres/24 hours.

Physical examination demonstrates a bright dog in good body condition. Bilateral non-pruritic alopecia affecting the whole trunk and proximal limbs is noted, as are cystic lesions along the dorsum. Both testicles are present and no mass lesions are palpated within them though both feel rather flaccid in texture. The prostate cannot be palpated per-rectum.

Questions

1. How is polyuria/polydipsia defined in the dog?
2. What are the differential diagnoses for polyuria/polydipsia and which of these are most common?
3. How would you investigate this dog further?

Answers

1. How is polyuria/polydipsia defined in the dog?

Defining polyuria/polydipsia (pu/pd)

Most normal dogs will intake 40–80 ml/kg/24 hours of water and polyuria/polydipsia is usually defined as intake >100 ml/kg/24 hours. It is hugely important before embarking on investigation for pu/pd that it is confirmed that the dog is indeed polydipsic, not just assumed to be so. Without doing this, extensive, expensive and sometimes intrusive investigations might be undertaken without good basis to expect that a medical abnormality is present or answer likely to be forthcoming.

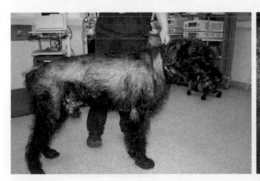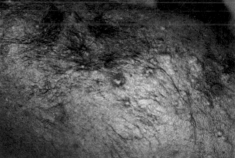

Figure 4.1 The patient at presentation with close-up of alopecia along dorsum (right image).

Canine Internal Medicine: What's Your Diagnosis? First Edition. Jon Wray.
© 2018 John Wiley & Sons Ltd. Published 2018 by John Wiley & Sons Ltd.

It is important for owners to measure water intake, or at least quantify 'number of bowls/day' and to then measure the normal amount to which they fill one bowl. This disparity between 'normal' and pu/pd is usually not a subtle one, and the author finds it useful to ask owners who are unable to quantify water intake but are reporting increased thirst 'would you say that water intake has more than doubled or thereabouts?'; usually owners of animals merely showing slight variation in water intake will refute such an increase. It is also important to rule out influences of medications that may cause diuresis at an early stage, both prescribed and 'home remedies'. The author has been presented with several dogs for investigation of pu/pd that have been given remedies to protect owners' lawns against 'urine scald' and on further investigation many of these act as diuretics and their purported 'lawn-sparing' properties are principally by this mechanism.

2. **What are the differential diagnoses for polyuria/polydipsia and which of these are most common?**
   There are several ways of classifying causes of pu/pd in the dog but it is useful to consider these 'mechanistically' as
   a. Those disorders that cause polyuria primarily and polydipsia is a 'compensatory response' to prevent clinical dehydration (these account for the majority of causes) and
   b. Those disorders in which polydipsia occurs primarily (these are uncommon).

In addition there are some clinical situations in which an apparent polydipsia is seen without polyuria. These are largely situations in which either the 'dipsogenic drive' to drink is provoked by hypovolaemic shock (the classical example in which this is commonly seen is dogs with acute whole blood loss due to ruptured splenic mass lesions who regularly are reported to become polydipsic after an episode of collapse) or where baroreceptor-driven increase in thirst occurs due to cardiac tamponade in pericardial effusion. Mechanisms by which thirst and water balance are regulated are summarised in **Figure 4.2**.

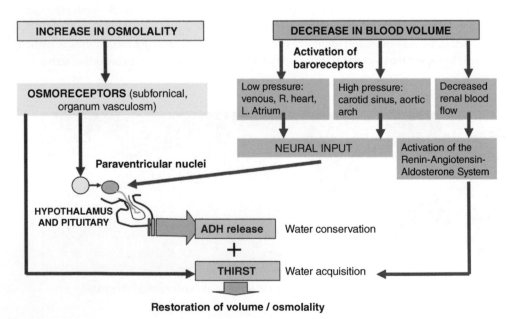

Figure 4.2 Control of thirst and water conservation. The two principle mechanisms of this are detection of decreased circulating blood volume and the detection of rising plasma osmolality. The principle effector hormone of water conservation is antidiuretic hormone (ADH, vasopressin) through its actions in the collecting ducts of the kidneys.

Confusing terms

It bears mentioning three areas of frequent confusion when it comes to the differential diagnosis of pu/pd.

a. The term 'diabetes insipidus' often causes confusion. The term stems from differences in urine taste (insipidus = insipid or tasteless urine, mellitus = sweet-tasting urine) from a time when (a now thankfully obsolete!) diagnostic method was popular. Diabetes insipidus therefore essentially refers to the production of large amounts of dilute urine and is probably best thought of as a descriptive term rather than 'a disease'. *Primary* diabetes insipidus refers to situations of either complete lack of production of antidiuretic hormone (ADH, vasopressin), which is known as primary central diabetes insipidus, or a congenital lack of either renal ADH receptors or the aquaporin channels through which water is conserved (primary nephrogenic diabetes insipidus). Many causes of pu/pd involve some degree of impairment of these mechanisms.

b. The term 'psychogenic polydipsia' may often be misapplied in canine medicine. Whilst there may be some animals that truly do have a behavioural cause of primary polydipsia, the psychological causes of primary polydipsia in man are few and relatively well defined by criteria that are not applicable in veterinary medicine. Furthermore, some dogs with primary polydipsia have been demonstrated to have an altered sensitivity of vasopressin response to plasma tonicity. The author would therefore recommend that the term 'primary polydipsia' be used in preference.

c. Urine specific gravity (SG) is often overinterpreted. There is really no such thing as a 'normal' urine specific gravity in dogs, the SG is reflective of the state of extracellular water balance and should always be interpreted in the context of the patient's hydration status. Urine SG in healthy dogs has been shown to vary between 1.006 to >1.040 within a 24 hour period and one would be ill-advised to make assumptions about health status from single urine SG results (other than that a urine SG <1.030 in a clearly dehydrated animal is abnormal, that an SG <1.030 in the presence of azotaemia is abnormal and that an SG >1.030 is unlikely to be seen in a genuinely polyuric/polydipsic dog). Furthermore, when urine SG ranges for dogs with a variety of causes of pu/pd have been evaluated there is considerable overlap between causes.

The most common causes of pu/pd in dogs encountered in first opinion veterinary practice are

- Diabetes mellitus
- Chronic kidney disease
- Pyometra
- Hyperadrenocorticism
- Hypercalcaemia

Note that, of these, hyperadrenocorticism is both very common and extremely challenging to diagnose, a combination that commonly leads to its erroneous premature exclusion (in favour of rarer diagnoses) during diagnostic evaluation of pu/pd. A full differential diagnosis of pu/pd by mechanism is shown in **Table 4.1**.

Table 4.1 Table of major causes of pu/pd by mechanism. Those that are most common are highlighted in **bold**.

	Mechanism	Disorder or disease
Disorders causing primarily polyuria, with compensatory polydipsia	Osmotic diuresis	**Diabetes mellitus** (in which is included that secondary to acromegaly)
		Chronic kidney disease
		Post-obstructive diuresis
		Primary renal glucosuria
	Inadequate:	
	• Production of ADH	Primary central diabetes insipidus
	• Renal response to ADH	Primary nephrogenic diabetes insipidus
	• Maintenance of a concentrated medullary interstitium	Acquired secondary nephrogenic diabetes insipidus
		• **Hyperadrenocorticism***
	Leading to failure of water conservation	• **Hypercalcaemia**
		• Bacterial endotoxin
		◦ **Pyometra**
		◦ Pyelonephritis
		• Hypokalaemia
		• Hepatic insufficiency and portosystemic shunts*
		• Pyelonephritis
		• Primary hyperaldosteronism
		• Hypoadrenocorticism
		• Hyperthyroidism (may also be psychogenic and osmotic diuresis)
		• Polycythaemia*
		*Probably also caused by acquired partial central diabetes insipidus.
Disorders that cause primary polydipsia with secondary polyuria	Primary dysfunction of thirst centre	Primary polydipsia caused by defective 'osmostat' function of abnormal ADH (vasopressin) response to hypertonicity
	Psychological compulsion to dipsogenesis	Primary polydipsia caused by psychogenic polydipsia
Miscellaneous causes or obscure mechanism		Exocrine pancreatic insufficiency
		Drugs
		• Glucocorticoids
		• Anticonvulsants
		• Diuretics
		• Thyroid hormone supplementations
		• Progestins
		• Lithium
		• Amphotericin B
		• Sodium bicarbonate
		Natural vegetable/mineral diuretics ('lawn-sparing' products)
		Dietary salt

3. **How would you investigate this dog further?**

The problem list for this dog includes polyuria / polydipsia, increased appetite and non-pruritic alopecia. Alopecia is discussed in the following case (Case 5). Here polyuria / polydipsia may be considered a 'pivotal' problem. Investigation should always be preceded by determining that pu/pd is genuinely present by measurement of water intake and excluding obvious iatro-genic/environmental causes. Interpretation of diagnostic tests in the context of other clinical signs and constitutional health is essential, especially

- Whether appetite is normal, increased or decreased.
- Whether weight loss or gain has been seen.
- Whether the animal seems clinically well other than the pu/pd.
- Whether dermatological abnormalities are present.

Note that diagnostic testing for hyperadrenocorticism may be frustrating, may need to be repeated and may change over the protracted time-course of development of this endocrinopathy and it is sensible to warn owners of this at the commencement of investigation to pre-empt frustration with repetitive/non-diagnostic attempts to rule-in/out this common disorder. Remember that 'diabetes insipidus' is neither a single disorder (see above) nor water deprivation testing is not a 'diagnostic test' for it (see below). Water deprivation testing should be rarely undertaken in investigation of pu/pd and is both potentially hazardous and fraught with interpretive difficulty, largely through inappropriate application. Investigation into confirmed pu/pd may rationally be performed in three 'steps':

First step: basic physical examination and laboratory testing
A rational first step might be as given in **Figure 4.3**.

Second step: testing for hyperadrenocorticism
Tests for hyperadrenocorticism may be divided into those tests that are used to support a diagnosis, which are
  - ACTH stimulation test
  - Low-dose dexamethasone suppression test (LDDST)
  - Urine cortisol:creatinine ratio (UC:Cr)

and those that are 'discriminatory' tests that help distinguish between pituitary and adrenal-dependent forms of hyperadrenocorticism. Note that these tests should not be performed until a diagnosis of hyperadrenocorticism has been made. These include
  - High-dose dexamethasone suppression test
  - Combined measurement of endogenous ACTH with ultrasound examination of *both* adrenal glands (in pituitary-dependent disease eACTH should be high and in adrenal-dependent disease it should be low; special sample handling is required and should be checked with the laboratory)

Third step: further specific diagnostic testing as indicated (for example diagnostic imaging for evidence of pyelonephritis) and possibly modified water deprivation test (see below)
The high-dose dexamethasone suppression test is now only rarely performed since it only contributes diagnostic information in about 12% of cases. This tests should *never* be used as an initial diagnostic test. The low-dose dexamethasone suppression test is unique in being both a diagnostic test and, in certain situations, a discriminatory test also.

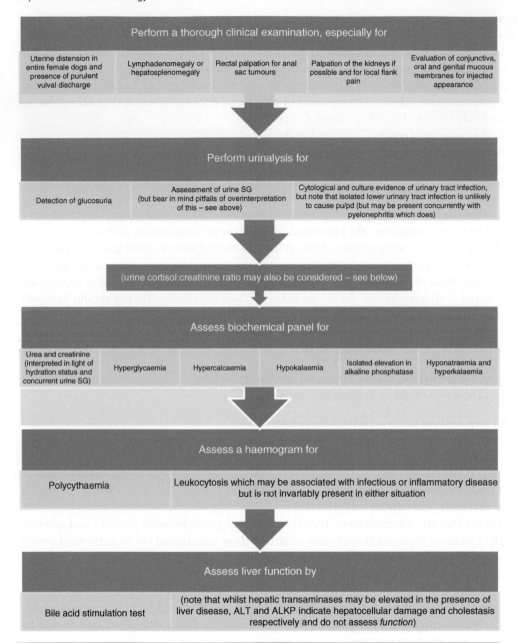

Perform a thorough clinical examination, especially for

| Uterine distension in entire female dogs and presence of purulent vulval discharge | Lymphadenomegaly or hepatosplenomegaly | Rectal palpation for anal sac tumours | Palpation of the kidneys if possible and for local flank pain | Evaluation of conjunctiva, oral and genital mucous membranes for injected appearance |

Perform urinalysis for

| Detection of glucosuria | Assessment of urine SG (but bear in mind pitfalls of overinterpretation of this – see above) | Cytological and culture evidence of urinary tract infection, but note that isolated lower urinary tract infection is unlikely to cause pu/pd (but may be present concurrently with pyelonephritis which does) |

(urine cortisol:creatinine ratio may also be considered – see below)

Assess biochemical panel for

| Urea and creatinine (interpreted in light of hydration status and concurrent urine SG) | Hyperglycaemia | Hypercalcaemia | Hypokalaemia | Isolated elevation in alkaline phosphatase | Hyponatraemia and hyperkalaemia |

Assess a haemogram for

| Polycythaemia | Leukocytosis which may be associated with infectious or inflammatory disease but is not invariably present in either situation |

Assess liver function by

| Bile acid stimulation test | (note that whilst hepatic transaminases may be elevated in the presence of liver disease, ALT and ALKP indicate hepatocellular damage and cholestasis respectively and do not assess *function*) |

Usually by this stage, of the common differential diagnoses for pu/pd, chronic kidney disease, hypercalcaemia and diabetes mellitus can be reasonably excluded. Hyperadrenocorticism (usually patient is otherwise well) and pyometra (patient is unwell and is an entire female) may remain common considerations and depending on signalment and the health status of the animal, either genital tract ultrasound or testing for hyperadrenocorticism may be considered.

Figure 4.3 Suggested first step of investigation of pu/pd.

Remember the effects of 'non-adrenal' illness

It is of great importance to bear in mind (and in the author's view many diagnostic laboratories are guilty of not emphasising this enough in reports) that all diagnostic tests may be positive in the face of other illness and a positive result should be interpreted as *'supportive of a diagnosis of hyperadrenocorticism or non-adrenal illness'*.

The relative sensitivities and specificities of the diagnostic tests are tabulated in **Table 4.2**. For a guide to interpretation of these tests, the reader is advised to consult the 'Further reading' citations.

Beware: ACTH stimulation tests are convenient but insensitive

Note that although very popular due to the short time course over which it can be performed, the ACTH stimulation test suffers from lack of sensitivity and false negative results are extremely common with this diagnostic test in the presence of hyperadrenocorticism, often resulting in clinicians forsaking a justifiable suspicion of hyperadrenocorticism in favour of much rarer diagnoses.

In the author's opinion, the low-dose dexamethasone suppression test should be considered the diagnostic test of choice for hyperadrenocorticism (but bearing in mind the caveat of 'non-adrenal illness'). Lastly 17-OH progesterone measurement before and after administration of synthetic ACTH analogues (so-called sex hormone alopecia profile, or SHAP test) has been proposed as a diagnostic test of 'occult' hyperadrenocorticism. Interpretation of this test is fraught with difficulty and the diagnosis is a controversial one; for a discussion of evidence for and against this test see Behrend (2015). Pituitary imaging by MRI or CT may be useful in some circumstances, usually where it informs treatment of pituitary-dependent disease, but is not recommended as a diagnostic test or that it be performed where imaging is not being performed by individuals with specialist expertise in neuro-diagnostic imaging.

ACTH stimulation testing is much less sensitive in the presence of a functional adrenal tumour than it is when pituitary-dependent disease is present. One can see the 'trade-off' between these tests from the table:

- The low-dose dexamethasone suppression test is very sensitive, but suffers from reduction in specificity; confidence (and all of these tests) in it is enhanced by application to patients

Table 4.2 Approximate sensitivities and specificities of commonly used diagnostic tests for canine Cushing's syndrome

Test	Sensitivity	Specificity
Low-dose dexamethasone suppression test	95%	73%
ACTH stimulation test	57–83%	86%
Urine cortisol:creatinine ratio	75–100%	20–77%

with compatible clinical signs of hyperadrenocorticism. When positive, it also helps differentiate between pituitary-dependent hyperadrenocorticism (PDH) and adrenal-dependent hyperadrenocorticism (ADH) in 60% of cases.

- The ACTH stimulation test is a relatively insensitive test for hyperadrenocorticism and many false negatives are seen. However, positive results in animals with compatible signs have only a low chance of being false positives.
- The urine cortisol:creatinine ratio is abnormal in most dogs with hyperadrenocorticism but is also abnormal in most ill dogs.

A comparison between the tests and their interpretation is shown in **Table 4.3**.

Due to the common occurrence of hyperadrenocorticism in the dog and the frequency of false negative results with diagnostic tests, the author would always commend that where it remains a differential diagnosis, repeat testing using another diagnostic test, or repetition of tests after a delay should always precede further diagnostic tests. Note that an ACTH stimulation test does not need to be performed before commencement of medical treatment in order to use it to guide therapy if a secure diagnosis of hyperadrenocorticism has been made by other means; in this latter instance the test can be thought of as assessing 'adrenal reserve', whereas in the former case a test is needed to diagnose cortisol excess.

Water deprivation testing

Much misunderstanding surrounds water deprivation testing, leading to inappropriate usage and rendering interpretation impossible if not correctly employed.

The water deprivation test is not (and has never been) a 'diagnostic' test, and it is certainly not a diagnostic test for diabetes insipidus (see above). A water deprivation test is a *discriminatory* test used to distinguish between three possibilities: primary central diabetes insipidus, primary nephrogenic diabetes insipidus and primary polydipsia. It can *only* ever be diagnostically useful, and correct interpretation applied, if all other differential diagnoses of pu/pd except these three have been confidently excluded and thus should really only ever be the last diagnostic step employed. Therefore the author would boldly state that an absolute contraindication to performing this test is accurate diagnostic exclusion of all other causes of pu/pd, bearing in mind that almost all of these are far more common than the somewhat rarer differentials that this test seeks to distinguish between. Water deprivation testing is potentially very dangerous and in the author's opinion it should never be performed where round-the-clock nursing care and observation is not available or where practices do not perform their own emergency provision out of hours. The author has seen fatalities due to wrong application of this test.

For a complete description of modified water deprivation testing see the texts in Further reading.

An alternative to water deprivation testing that has gained popularity recently is application of trial treatment with DDAVP (Desmopressin). However, in the same way that a water deprivation test can only be used to discriminate between three possibilities once the differential diagnosis has been sufficiently and accurately narrowed to them, similarly trial treatment can also *only* be interpreted also once the same degree of diagnostic rigour has been applied.

Table 4.3 Guide to performance and interpretation of common diagnostic tests for hyperadrenocorticism (HAC, canine Cushing's syndrome)

Test	Performance	Interpretation
ACTH stimulation test	Serum cortisol is measured before and 1 h after administration of an analogue of ACTH (such as tetracosactrin or cosyntropin) at a dose of 5 mcg/kg (to a maximum of 250 mcg/dose) intravenously For monitoring of efficacy of medical treatment for hyperadrenocorticism (HAC) ACTH stimulation testing 2–4 hours post-pill is advised (though performance of this test at other times may also be used to explore duration of action of medications)	*For diagnosis of canine Cushing's syndrome (HAC):* A post-ACTH cortisol level within the laboratory-specific reference range does not support a diagnosis of HAC (but cannot be used to exclude it) A post-ACTH cortisol level greater than the laboratory-specific reference range supports a diagnosis of HAC in a dog with compatible clinical signs (*or non-adrenal illness*) *For assessment of adrenal functional 'reserve' in animals undergoing medical treatment:* A post-ACTH cortisol level >27 nmol/l but <126 nmol/l is expected to document both adequate adrenal functional reserve and adequate suppression of cortisol excess
Low-dose dexamethasone suppression test (LDDST)	Samples are collected for serum cortisol measurement before and at 3 and 8 hours after intravenous administration of 0.01 mg/kg dexamethasone sodium phosphate It is recommended to carefully label collection tubes with time of collection and to be certain of dosage since in smaller patients the volume of dexamethasone required is extremely small	*For diagnosis of canine Cushing's syndrome (HAC):* The 8 hour sample result is examined: • An 8-hour post-dexamethasone sample <40 nmol/l shows suppression and does not support a diagnosis of HAC (but cannot be used to exclude it) • An 8-hour post-dexamethasone sample >40 nmol/l supports a diagnosis of HAC in a dog with compatible clinical signs (*or non-adrenal illness*) *For differentiation between pituitary- and adrenal-dependent HAC (PDH, ADH), only when a diagnosis has been made,* the 0- and 3-hour samples are also examined: • Suppression of the 3-hour sample below 40 nmol/l (but 8-hour >40 nmol/l) *or* • Suppression of the 3-hour sample or the 8-hour sample below 50% of the 0-hour result (but 8-hour >40 nmol/l) Are both compatible with PDH • Any other combination with an 8-hour sample >40 nmol/l may be compatible with either PDH or ADH
Urine cortisol: creatinine (UC:Cr) ratio	A urine sample is collected at home, not within 2 days of a veterinary visit or other predictable stressful event and submitted to a laboratory to measure UC:Cr	Results above the laboratory-specific reference interval are supportive of, but not specific for, HAC. This test is highly influenced by any non-adrenal illness or stressor. Negative results are usually interpreted as making HAC unlikely

Diagnosis

This patient was referred after some initial diagnostic tests were performed. Results from this patient were as shown in the table below.

Haematology

Parameter	Value	Units	Range
RBC	6.35	$\times 10^{12}$/l	(5.5–8.5)
Haemoglobin	16.8	g/dl	(12.0–18.0)
Haematocrit	0.449	l/l	(0.37–0.55)
Mean cell volume	70.7	fl	(60–77)
Mean cell haemoglobin concentration	37.4	g/dl	(30.0–38.0)
Mean cell haemoglobin	**26.5**	pg	(19.5–25.5)
Total white cell count	6.6	$\times 10^9$/l	(6.0–15.0)
Neutrophils	5.2	$\times 10^9$/l	(3.0–11.5)
Lymphocytes	1	$\times 10^9$/l	(1.0–4.8)
Monocytes	0.2	$\times 10^9$/l	(0.2–1.4)
Eosinophils	0.2	$\times 10^9$/l	(0.1–1.2)
Basophils	0	$\times 10^9$/l	(0.0–0.1)
Platelets	397	$\times 10^9$/l	(200–500)

Biochemistry

Parameter	Value	Units	Range
Total protein	74	g/l	(54–77)
Albumin	36	g/l	(25–40)
Globulin	38	g/l	(23–45)
Urea	6	mmol/l	(2.5–7.4)
Creatinine	101	μmol/l	(40–145)
Potassium	4.4	mmol/l	(3.4–5.6)
Sodium	145	mmol/l	(139–154)
Chloride	110	mmol/l	(105–122)
Calcium	2.7	mmol/l	(2.1–2.8)
Magnesium	0.8	mmol/l	(0.62–0.90)
Inorganic phosphate	1.4	mmol/l	(0.60–1.40)
Glucose	5.8	mmol/l	(3.3–5.8)
ALT	**162**	IU/l	(13–88)
AST	55	IU/l	(13–60)
ALKP	**182**	IU/l	(14–105)

Parameter	Value	Units	Range
GGT	10	IU/l	(0–10)
Bilirubin	5	μmol/l	(0–16)
Cholesterol	**7.8**	mmol/l	(3.8–7.0)
Triglyceride	1.1	mmol/l	(0.56–1.14)
Creatine kinase	180	IU/l	(0–190)

Urinalysis

Parameter	Value	Units	Range
Appearance	Clear, straw coloured		
Chemistry			
Specific gravity	1.015		
pH	7.5		
Protein	Trace		
Nitrite	Negative		
Blood/Hb	Negative		
Glucose	Negative		
Ketones	Negative		
Bilirubin	Negative		
Urobilinogen	Negative		
Cytology			
Red cells	0	/hpf	(0–2)
White cells	0	/hpf	(0–2)
Epithelial cells	0	/hpf	(0–5)
Casts	Negative		
Crystals	Negative		
Bacteria	Negative		
Other			
Quantitative protein			
Urine protein:creatinine	**0.6**	Ratio	<0.5
Total T4	21	nmol/l	15–50

ACTH stimulation test

Sample	Result	Reference interval
Cortisol pre-injection	82 nmol/l	110–250 nmol/l
Cortisol 1 hour post-injection	257 nmol/l	150–550 nmol/l

Low-dose dexamethasone suppression test

Sample	Result	Reference interval
Cortisol before dexamethasone	124 mol/l	
Cortisol 3 hours post-injection	**142** nmol/l	<40
Cortisol 8 hours post-injection	**110** nmol/l	<40

4. How would you interpret these results?

The haematology result is essentially unremarkable – there is a marginal increase in mean cell haemoglobin concentration but in the absence of other changes such a marginal change is of debateable significance. Biochemistry demonstrates very modest elevations in ALT and ALKP and in cholesterol. ALT is considered a marker of hepatocellular damage and results from leakage of hepatocyte cytosolic content, but elevations below 3–4 x the upper limit of the reference interval are frequently seen in 'reactive' hepatopathy and are not specific for primary liver disease. Similarly, whilst elevations in ALKP are usually indicative of cholestasis, elevations below the same level are poorly specific for primary liver disease. Note that approximately 10% of dogs subsequently diagnosed with hyperadrenocorticism have normal ALKP levels at presentation and a normal or only modestly increased value should never be used to exclude this common diagnosis. Hypercholesterolaemia is frequently seen in incompletely starved samples, hypothyroidism, hyperadrenocorticism, pancreatitis, protein-losing nephropathies and in familial hyperlipidaemias. In this case the urine protein:creatinine ratio was only very marginally increased and serum T4 was subsequently found to be normal.

Of the common causes of pu/pd that are applicable in a patient with this signalment, hyperadrenocorticism remains the most likely diagnosis in the absence of glucosuria, azotaemia and hypercalcaemia.

The ACTH stimulation test results are within the normal reference range, which neither supports nor excludes any clinical suspicion of hyperadrenocorticism

The low-dose dexamethasone suppression test subsequently performed does not show suppression <40 nmol/l at the 8-hour time-point. This result is supportive of a diagnosis of hyperadrenocorticism or severe non-adrenal illness. If the 8-hour sample is <40 nmol/l adequate and expected suppression has occurred. If the value is >40 nmol/l then the 3-hour sample may be evaluated. A decrease in this 3-hour value to <50% of the starting cortisol or suppression below 40 nmol/l (with subsequent elevation at 8 hours) is consistent with pituitary-dependent hyperadrenocortism (this occurs in about 40% of hyperadrenocorticoid dogs). Failure to suppress to this degree at both 3- and 8-hour samples is consistent with either pituitary- or adrenal-dependent hyperadrenocorticism.

Do not overinterpret lack of 3 hours suppression on the LDDST

Approximately 25% of dogs with PDH do not show suppression on an LDDST and almost 100% of dogs with functional adrenal tumours. Since approximately 85% of dogs with HAC have PDH and 15% have ADH, the percentage of dogs with HAC that have no suppression on an LDDST having adrenal tumours is about 37%. Many laboratories unfortunately seem to equate failure of suppression with a greater likelihood of adrenal-dependent disease than pituitary, which is clearly not the case.

This dog had an abdominal ultrasound examination performed and concurrent assessment of the endogenous ACTH, ensuring that the sample was collected in an EDTA tube, spun and separated and the EDTA plasma rapidly frozen and transported in a manner that ensured arrival in a frozen state.

Ultrasound examination demonstrated a 1.85 cm mass within the cranial pole of the left adrenal gland (**Figure 4.4, left panel**) with no evidence of vascular invasion. The contralateral adrenal gland was small and no evidence of other nodular change was found within the abdomen. Subsequently, thoracic radiographs were normal. An endogenous ACTH was 7 pg/ml, <10 pg/ml being supportive of an adrenal-dependent hyperadrenocorticism.

A diagnosis of **adrenal-dependent hyperadrenocorticism** was made, without evidence of vascular invasion or metastasis. The dog was treated surgically by adrenalectomy (**Figure 4.4, right panel**) without event. Post-operative monitoring of the function of the remaining adrenal was monitored by ACTH stimulation testing and evaluation of electrolytes. Histopathology of the mass confirmed it to be an adrenal cortical adenoma. The dog's clinical signs resolved and the haircoat returned to normal within 6 months of adrenalectomy (**Figure 4.5**).

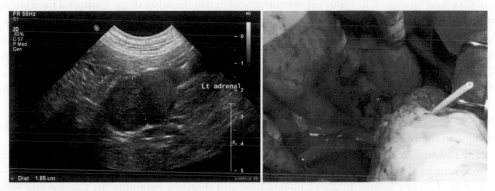

Figure 4.4 (left) Ultrasound examination showing a mass lesion within the left adrenal gland. The contralateral right adrenal gland was decreased in size. (right) The adrenal mass during surgical adrenalectomy.

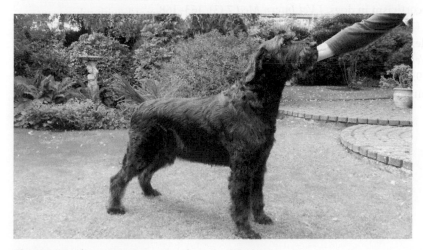

Figure 4.5 The patient 6 months after adrenalectomy.

Discussion

Polyuria/polydipsia can be complex to investigate in dogs but provided that one keeps in mind the most common differential diagnoses and adopts a logical approach, a diagnosis is achieved in most circumstances. The most common error that the author sees is misplaced faith in the sensitivity of an ACTH stimulation test, negative results often leading to premature and inappropriate exclusion of a common disorder (hyperadrenocorticism), which is difficult to diagnose. Adrenalectomy is a highly successful treatment in appropriate cases and in the setting of adrenal adenoma is the only common circumstance in which canine Cushing's syndrome may be permanently cured without the need for long-term expensive medical management.

Reference

Behrend, E.N. (2015) Chapter 10. Canine hyperadrenocorticism. In *Canine and Feline Endocrinology*, 4th edn, eds E.C. Feldman, R.W. Nelson, C.E. Reusch, J.C.R. Scott-Moncrieff and E.N. Behrend, Elsevier, St Louis, pp. 377–451

Further reading

Brown, C.G. and Graves, T.K. (2007) Hyperadrenocorticism: treating dogs. *Compend Contin Educ Vet* **29** (3), 132–134, 136, 138 passim; quiz 144–135

Feldman, E.C. et al. (1996) Use of low- and high-dose dexamethasone tests for distinguishing pituitary-dependent from adrenal tumor hyperadrenocorticism in dogs. *J Am Vet Med Assoc* **209** (4), 772–775

Gilor, C. and Graves, T.K. (2011) Interpretation of laboratory tests for canine Cushing's syndrome. *Top Companion Anim Med* **26** (2), 98–108

Gould, S.M. et al. (2001) Use of endogenous ACTH concentration and adrenal ultrasonography to distinguish the cause of canine hyperadrenocorticism. *J Small Anim Pract* **42** (3), 113–121

Kintzer, P.P. and Peterson, M.E. (1997) Diagnosis and management of canine cortisol-secreting adrenal tumors. *Vet Clin North Am Small Anim Pract* **27** (2), 299–307

Nelson, R.W. (2015) Chapter 1. Water metabolism and diabetes insipidus. In *Canine and Feline Endocrinology*, 4th edn, eds E.C. Feldman, R.W. Nelson, C.E. Reusch, J.C.R. Scott-Moncrieff and E.N. Behrend, Elsevier, St Louis, pp. 1–36

Smiley, L.E. and Peterson, M.E. (1993) Evaluation of a urine cortisol:creatinine ratio as a screening test for hyperadrenocorticism in dogs. *J Vet Intern Med* **7** (3), 163–168

Van Liew, C.H. et al. (1997) Comparison of results of adrenocorticotropic hormone stimulation and low-dose dexamethasone suppression tests with necropsy findings in dogs: 81 cases (1985–1995). *J Am Vet Med Assoc* **211** (3), 322–325

van Sluijs, F.J. et al. (1995) Results of adrenalectomy in 36 dogs with hyperadrenocorticism caused by adreno-cortical tumour. *Vet Q* **17** (3), 113–116

Clinical presentation

A 3 year-old female-neutered Labrador (**Figure 5.1**) is presented with a history of weight gain, lethargy and poor coat quality. The owners have noted weight gain in the previous 3 months, before which weight recorded in her clinical record was 33 kg. Her appetite is normal and there has been no alteration in her drinking or urinating. The owners have noted development of patches of bilaterally sparse hair on the dog's flanks, through which the underlying skin can be easily seen. They feel that she is non-pruritic.

Physical examination demonstrates a very overweight dog of 42 kg. Mucous membranes are pale but the pulse rate is 88/min with normal pulse quality. Bilateral partial flank alopecia and skin scale and scurf over the caudal dorsum is noted. The skin is unbroken in these areas and no pustules, nodules, papules or macules are seen. Remaining physical examination is normal.

Questions

1. **What are the most common causes of weight gain in the dog?**
2. **What are the principle differential diagnoses for non-pruritic, bilaterally symmetrical flank alopecia in the dog?**
3. **How would you investigate this dog further?**

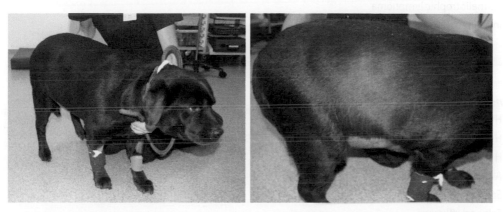

Figure 5.1 The patient at presentation demonstrating overweight body condition and partial flank alopecia with dorsal scale and scurf.

Answers

1. **What are the most common causes of weight gain in the dog?**

The most common cause is overfeeding, causing obesity or at least failure to match calorie intake to expenditure. Medications such as glucocorticoids, progestagens, beta-blockers and phenobarbitone may also cause weight gain.

Pathological causes of apparent weight gain, which are reported to account for less than 1% of cases, are shown in **Table 5.1**.

Canine Internal Medicine: What's Your Diagnosis? First Edition. Jon Wray.
© 2018 John Wiley & Sons Ltd. Published 2018 by John Wiley & Sons Ltd.

Table 5.1 Pathological causes of real and apparent weight gain

Pathological causes of generalised weight gain	Pathological causes of change in body shape that may mimic generalised weight gain
• Hypothyroidism	• Ascites
• Hyperadrenocorticism	• Generalised oedema
• Insulinoma	• Abdominal organomegaly
• Hypogonadism	
• Acromegaly	

Table 5.2 Differential diagnosis of non-pruritic flank alopecia

The principle causes may be described as *non-inflammatory* or *inflammatory*

Inflammatory causes of alopecia

Inflammatory causes are usually not obviously symmetrical in distribution and usually are associated with presence of lesions of the skin (such as nodules, pustules and macules) and may include

- Demodicosis
- Dermatophytosis
- Bacterial folliculitis
- Sebaceous adenitis
- Epitheliotrophic lymphoma
- Immune-mediated dermatopathies
  - Superficial pemphigus
  - Systemic lupus erythematosus
  - Erythema multiforme

Non-inflammatory causes of alopecia

- Hyperadrenocorticism
- Hypothyroidism
- Hypogonadism
- Alopecia X
- Seasonal flank alopecia
- Telogen effluvium
- Acquired pattern alopecia
- Sertoli-cell tumour and other hyperoestrogenism-associated alopecia

2. **What are the principle differential diagnoses for acquired non-pruritic, bilaterally symmetrical flank alopecia in the dog?**

   The differential diagnosis of non-pruritic flank alopecia is shown in **Table 5.2**.

3. **How would you investigate this dog further?**

   The problem list for this dog is
   - Weight gain
   - Lethargy
   - Non-pruritic bilaterally symmetrical flank alopecia

- Mucous membrane pallor
- Skin scale and scurf

Mucous membrane pallor may be due to anaemia or reduced vascular perfusion of the oral mucous membranes, either due to a local reduction in blood flow or a generalised hypoperfusive state.

The bilateral flank alopecia should prompt consideration of endocrinopathy though the owners should be questioned as to whether similar changes have been seen previously and then resolved (as may be the case with seasonal flank alopecia). The lack of change in thirst and urinating behaviour and normal appetite would make hyperadrenocorticism unlikely.

Rational investigation might include:

- Microscopic examination of skin scrapings and hair plucks from the areas of alopecia and examination by Wood lamp (+/– fungal culture)
- Assessment of a haemogram in the light of the mucous membrane pallor
- Assessment of serum biochemistry, specifically of serum cholesterol and triglycerides
- Performance of further testing for hypothyroidism
- Should it be considered that the weight gain may not be generalised but due to possible ascites or abdominal organomegaly, then abdominal imaging might be rationally considered

Difficulties in assessment of hypothyroidism

Assessment of hypothyroidism may be hampered by the fact that development of clinical hypothyroidism is a gradual process and most diagnostic tests are blighted by being affected by non-thyroidal illness. Breed, age, reproductive status and concurrent medications may also alter T4 levels. 'Panels' of tests have become popular but often lead to less, not more, certainty in diagnosis, particularly if these are applied injudiciously to patient populations without supportive clinical signs of hypothyroidism.

A total T4 assessment should be considered initially since this test has high sensitivity and a normal value usually excludes hypothyroidism. Approximately 60–70% of dogs with clinical hypothyroidism will have an elevated thyroid stimulating hormone (TSH) concentration and the finding of concurrently low T4 and elevated TSH is compelling evidence for hypothyroidism. Combined T4/TSH assessment or, more cost-effectively, collecting sufficient sample serum for both tests and requesting TSH only if the T4 is low, is a reasonable first step in investigation of suspected hypothyroidism. The unbound (and biologically active) portion of serum T4, free-T4 may be measured, but whilst this is slightly more specific and sensitive than total T4, it is still affected by non-thyroidal illness. **Table 5.3** below shows comparative sensitivities and specificities (sic) of alterations in T4, TSH and free-T4.

Thyroglobulin autoantibodies are thought to result from leakage of thyroglobulin into circulation secondary to lymphocytic thyroiditis but are found in only 50% of hypothyroid dogs. Furthermore, a significant proportion of dogs in whom positive thyroglobulin autoantibody tests are detected will revert to a negative result when monitored over time.

In cases of discordant results, for example a low total T4 but normal TSH, the clinician has three choices (provided they have clinical grounds to continue to suspect hypothyroidism):

- Do nothing but revisit diagnostic evaluation after a period of time (for example 2–3 months) has elapsed.

Table 5.3 Comparative sensitivity and specificity of different tests for hypothyroidism. ED = equilibrium dialysis

Test findings	Sensitivity (%)	Specificity (%)
↓ Total T4	89–100	75–82
↓ Free T4 (ED)	80–98	93–94
↑ TSH	63–87	82–93
↓ Total T4 *and* ↑ TSH	63–67	98–100
↓ Free T4 (ED) *and* ↑ TSH	74	98

- Perform further diagnostic assessment.
- Commence a treatment trial.

Further diagnostic assessments may include performance of a TSH stimulation test or a TRH stimulation test. The TSH stimulation test comprises an assessment of total T4 before and 6 hours after administration of either bovine TSH (0.1 IU/kg to a maximum of 5 IU) or recombinant human TSH (rhTSH 50 mcg/dog). Failure of total T4 to rise to >20 nmol/l is supportive of hypothyroidism. TSH stimulation can still be affected by non-thyroidal illness and utility is limited by lack of availability of reagents at the time of writing. TRH stimulation testing is not recommended due to more subjectivity in assessment and overlap between normal and affected dogs; it gives little advantage over other tests. In experienced hands the morphology of the thyroid glands by ultrasound can be useful to determine the presence of hypothyroidism but both skill and frequent performance of this are required.

A decision to perform a therapeutic trial should only be undertaken (1) where there is sufficient clinical grounds to suspect hypothyroidism, (2) where there is an objective and measurable parameter by which to assess efficacy (such as gained body weight, coat abnormalities, hyperlipidaemia), (3) with a replacement dose of thyroxine that is sufficient to reliably produce a clinical result and (4) in the knowledge (and after communication with owners) that such a strategy precludes, at least temporarily, further assessment for hypothyroidism and may in some cases lead to clinical signs of (reversible) iatrogenic thyrotoxicosis.

Diagnosis and treatment
In this case skin scrapes and hair plucking results were normal. The haematology and biochemistry results are shown below.

Haematology

Parameter	Value	Units	Range
RBC	**4.25**	× 10^{12}/l	(5.5–8.5)
Haemoglobin	**9.0**	g/dl	(12.0–18.0)
Haematocrit	**0.30**	l/l	(0.37–0.55)
Mean cell volume	69.5	fl	(60–77)
Mean cell haemoglobin Conc	30.4	g/dl	(30.0–38.0)
Mean cell haemoglobin	21.2	pg	(19.5–25.5)

Parameter	Value	Units	Range
Total white cell count	13.3	$\times 10^9/l$	(6.0–15.0)
Neutrophils	9.67	$\times 10^9/l$	(3.0–11.5)
Lymphocytes	2.65	$\times 10^9/l$	(1.0–4.8)
Monocytes	0.40	$\times 10^9/l$	(0.2–1.4)
Eosinophils	0.27	$\times 10^9/l$	(0.1–1.2)
Basophils	0.00	$\times 10^9/l$	(0.0–0.1)
Platelets	224	$\times 10^9/l$	(200–500)
Film comment:		Erythrocytes are normocytic and normochromic	

The haematology demonstrates a mild normocytic, normochromic anaemia. A reticulocyte count was $36 \times 10^9/l$, indicating that the anaemia is non-regenerative. Differential diagnoses for a non-regenerative anaemia of mild nature might include reduced erythropoiesis due to chronic renal disease, inflammatory disease, endocrinopathies (especially hypothyroidism), infectious agents, bone marrow myelophthisis, cytotoxic drug therapy and immune-mediated disease.

Biochemistry

Parameter	Value	Units	Range
Total protein	72	g/l	(54–77)
Albumin	33	g/l	(25–40)
Globulin	39	g/l	(23–45)
Urea	7.1	mmol/l	(2.5–7.4)
Creatinine	136	µmol/l	(40–145)
Potassium	4.5	mmol/l	(3.4–5.6)
Sodium	144	mmol/l	(139–154)
Chloride	109	mmol/l	(105–122)
Calcium	2.8	mmol/l	(2.1–2.8)
Magnesium	-	mmol/l	(0.62–0.90)
Inorganic phosphate	1.2	mmol/l	(0.60–1.40)
Glucose	5.2	mmol/l	(3.3–5.8)
ALT	68	IU/l	(13–88)
AST	**64**	IU/l	(13–60)
ALKP	37	IU/l	(14–105)
GGT	6	IU/l	(0–10)
Bilirubin	3	µmol/l	(0–16)
Cholesterol	**25.8**	mmol/l	(3.8–7.0)
Triglyceride	**3.2**	mmol/l	(0.56–1.14)
Creatine kinase	185	IU/l	(0–190)

The most striking biochemical abnormality is the marked hyperlipidaemia comprising a very marked elevation in serum cholesterol and less marked rise in triglycerides. Post-prandial hyperlipidaemia should always be initially accounted for though it would be highly unlikely at this level. Primary hyperlipidaemias may be seen in some breeds, especially the Miniature Schnauzer but common acquired causes of hypercholesterolaemia that should be considered are hypothyroidism, hyperadrenocorticism, pancreatitis, protein-losing nephropathy, diabetes mellitus and cholestasis. Some drug therapy, especially glucocorticoids, may cause hyperlipidaemia. Very marked hypercholesterolaemia, >15 mmol/l, is most commonly associated with hypothyroidism.

In this case the history, clinical signs, mild non-regenerative anaemia and isolated hyperlipidaemia with a very marked hypercholesterolaemia were all felt to be supportive of hypothyroidism. Other endocrinopathies such as hyperadrenocorticism were considered unlikely due to lack of polyuria, polydipsia or changes in appetite.

A total T4 was very low and TSH was elevated confirming the diagnosis. Additional diagnostic tests for hypothyroidism are unnecessary in this patient.

Parameter	Value	Units	Range
Total T4	**<6.44**	nmol/l	(15–50)
TSH	**1.79**	ng/ml	(0.0–0.60)

L-Thyroxine supplementation was introduced at a dose of 0.02 mg/kg p/o q12 hours. After 6 weeks of commencing therapy the dog had lost 3 kg in weight and the haircoat appeared less scurfy, though partial alopecia still remained. Reassessment of HCt, cholesterol and total T4 was performed approximately 4 hours after the morning medication.

Results were as follows:

Parameter	Value	Units	Range
Cholesterol	**11.3**	mmol/l	(3.8–7.0)
HCt	0.37	l/l	(0.37–0.55)
Total T4	49.5	nmol/l	(15–50)

These results suggest adequate supplementation and whilst cholesterol was not yet within the reference range marked improvement is demonstrated.

Discussion

Weight gain accompanied by bilateral flank alopecia is most commonly seen in hypothyroidism and in hyperadrenocorticism. However, the latter is usually associated with additional clinical signs of polyuria/polydipsia and polyphagia (whilst appetite in hypothyroid dogs usually remains normal). The two syndromes are not mutually exclusive and can occur concurrently in the same dog. Both of these may be associated with hyperlipidaemia, but whilst about a third of hypothyroid dogs have an identifiable normocytic, normochromic non-regenerative anaemia at presentation, anaemia is rarely present in hyperadrenocorticoid dogs, a modest erythrocytosis being a more typical finding. Testing for both of these endocrinopathies is limited by poor specificity in the presence of other non-thyroidal/non-adrenal illnesses and in hyperadrenocorticism by poor sensitivity also. Diagnosis of hypothyroidism is beset by difficulties of false positive diagnoses due to the so-called sick-euthyroid syndrome effects on diagnostic test results. All diagnostic tests for hypothyroidism are to some extent affected by these and the most pragmatic ways to guard against overdiagnosis are assiduous application of such tests only to patient populations with compatible clinical signs and to exert a healthy degree of criticism over interpretation of results. Panels of diagnostic tests offered by commercial laboratories may not yield better diagnostic value than more selective test choice and in particular clinicians should be wary of misinterpretation of positive thyroglobulin autoantibody tests as being synonymous with hypothyroidism. Thyroid histological findings in hypothyroid dogs may show lymphocytic thyroiditis and/or the presence of thyroid atrophy. Whether one merely represents an end-stage in the continuum of the other is unclear and certainly the time-course for development of clinical hypothyroidism may be extremely protracted in some animals, with variation in test results during this natural history. Whilst taken to be indicative of thyroiditis, positive thyroglobulin autoantibodies are only detected in approximately 50% of cases and in longitudinal studies of dogs with positive thyroglobulin autoantibody tests, a similar proportion reverted to negative status, as did progress to overt hypothyroidism.

Further reading

Dixon, R.M., Reid, S.W. & Mooney, C.T. (2002) Treatment and therapeutic monitoring of canine hypothyroidism. *J Small Anim Pract* **43**, 334–340

Graham, P.A., Nachreiner, R.F., Refsal, K.R. & Provencher-Bolliger, A.L. (2001) Lymphocytic thyroiditis. *Vet Clin North Am Small Anim Pract* **31**, 915–933, vi–vii

Graham, P.A., Refsal, K.R. & Nachreiner, R.F. (2007) Etiopathologic findings of canine hypothyroidism. *Vet Clin North Am Small Anim Pract* **37**, 617–631, v

Panciera, D.L. (1999) Is it possible to diagnose canine hypothyroidism? *J Small Anim Pract* **40**, 152–157

Haematology and Immunology

Genetics for Aid Medicine: What's Your Diagnosis? First Edition. Jon Webe...
© 2018 John Wiley & Sons Ltd. Published 2018 by John Wiley & Sons Ltd.

Clinical presentation

A 6 year-old female-neutered Cocker Spaniel (**Figure 6.1**) is presented with sudden-onset lethargy. Her owner reports that the dog was well up until 48 hours ago. The owner had noted pinky-red discolouration of the dog's urine but no dysuria or pollakiuria and had made an appointment for the first available routine appointment thinking that the dog had a urine infection. Overnight the dog had become very listless.

Physical examination demonstrates a quiet and listless dog with normal body condition score (2.5/5). Weight is 18 kg. The dog is ambulatory but weak, mucous membranes are pale pink, mucous membrane hydration appears normal and capillary refill time is less than 2 seconds. Rectal temperature is 39.5 °C and heart and pulse rate are 160/min with sinus rhythm and pulses slightly bounding; extremities feel warm; the respiratory rate is 40/min. Thoracic auscultation demonstrates a soft, grade II/VI early systolic left basilar heart murmur (no murmur was mentioned on physical examination findings 4 months previously at routine vaccination). On abdominal palpation there is an impression that the spleen appears smoothly enlarged but is not painful.

No peripheral lymphadenomegaly or evidence of external haemorrhage or petechiation is present. The dog has not travelled outside the United Kingdom, is not receiving any medications and has been vaccinated annually against distemper, infectious hepatitis, parvovirus, parainfluenzavirus and leptospirosis.

A decision is made to send a haematology and biochemistry sample to a reference laboratory as they have a courier service and you will receive the results in about 4 hours. Your haematology analyser has broken down, although you have access to some laboratory facilities in-house (microscope, centrifuge, 'Diff-quik' modified Romanowsky stain, tubes and slides, equipment for urinalysis).

Questions

1. How would you interpret this dog's clinical examination findings?
2. What could you do to find out more about this patient's problem in the interim whilst you are awaiting the lab results?

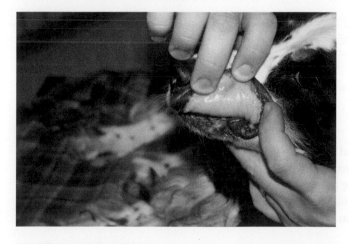

Figure 6.1 Patient at presentation.

Canine Internal Medicine: What's Your Diagnosis? First Edition. Jon Wray.
© 2018 John Wiley & Sons Ltd. Published 2018 by John Wiley & Sons Ltd.

Answers

1. How would you interpret this dog's clinical examination findings?

- Pale mucous membranes may indicate anaemia or hypoperfusion (either regional or generalised).
- However, the dog is normally hydrated, has normal capillary refill and pulse quality is good to slightly bounding with warm extremities. There are therefore no other signs to support hypoperfusion in this dog.
- The patient is tachycardic, tachypnoeic and there is a soft systolic heart murmur, which has not been detected before, over the left basilar region. Murmurs may be acquired due to structural or functional heart disease or due to altered blood viscosity or high output cardiac states. The most common acquired cardiac disease causing a left-sided systolic murmur is myxomatous mitral valve disease, in which the murmur is harsh in quality rather than soft and would be expected to be apical in location. These findings are suggestive of a haemic murmur and response to decreased tissue oxygen delivery due to anaemia.
- Splenomegaly may be due to primary splenic disease (including infiltrative disease processes), due to extramedullary haematopoiesis within the spleen or due to reactive change. Splenomegaly may be further characterised as regional or generalised, nodular or diffuse.
- An elevated rectal temperature is consistent with fever due to inflammation or infection or hyperthermia due to endogenous heat gain or failure of heat dissipation.

2. What could you do to find out more about this patient's problem in the interim whilst you are awaiting the lab results?

Initial basic assessment of anaemias

There are several steps that should be taken in every patient that might be anaemic, which are rapid to perform and will immediately start to narrow the possible differential diagnosis. Such assessment should always be undertaken prior to institution of treatment It should be performed in tandem with assessment of the clinical impact of the anaemia on the patient, keeping in mind the question of whether immediate therapeutic intervention is necessary. In this scenario, where limited resources are available it is still possible to answer:

- Is the patient anaemic and, if so, how severely?
- Is there evidence of haemolysis?
- Is there evidence of in-saline agglutination?
- What is the total protein?
- What does a blood smear evaluation look like? Is the anaemic regenerative or non- (or pre-) regenerative?

These questions can be answered by:

- *Measuring the packed cell volume (PCV).* Taking a well-mixed blood sample (ensuring there are no clots which may produce false positive results) into a microhaematocrit tube centrifuge for 5 minutes at 10 000–15 000 rpm (which will result in adequate cell packing). Severity of anaemia in dogs is classified as:
  - PCV 30–37%   Mild
  - PCV 20–29%   Moderate
  - PCV 13–19%   Severe
  - PCV <13%   Very severe

- *Examining the supernatant.* When the microhaematocrit tube has been spun, examine the supernatant above the packed blood cells and note whether it is
  - Clear/straw coloured
  - Icteric
  - Haemolysed (pink discoloured due to free haemoglobin)
- *Looking for 'in-saline agglutination'.* Taking one drop of whole blood and mixing with one drop of saline on a slide, observe for macroscopic agglutination. The reason for mixing with saline is that it disrupts rouleaux formation (bridging links between red cells by globular proteins or fibrinogen). Agglutination suggests that anti-erythrocyte IgM, or in large quantities IgG, is present and implicates immune-mediated haemolytic anaemia; however, spontaneous agglutinates can also occur in the presence of increased plasma proteins and cold agglutinin disease and this may occasionally lead to false positive results.
- *Measuring total protein/solids.* Whilst laboratory measurement of total protein is preferred, an estimate of total protein may be gained by measuring the total solids (most of which comprises serum proteins) using a refractometer. A drop of spun serum may be placed on a calibrated refractometer and the total solid recorded (normal range in the dog being about 54–75 g/l. Assessment of total solids is useful in differentiating regenerative anaemias due to haemolysis or blood loss since the latter usually result in loss of protein during haemorrhage, if acute. Caution should be applied in interpretation of this in dehydrated animals in which falsely normal total solid may be seen despite haemorrhage.
- *Examining a blood smear.* Examination of a properly performed and stained blood smear which may proffer the following information:
  - Evaluation of erythrocyte size, central pallor and relative 'hue', which may give an indication of whether an anaemia is regenerative or non-regenerative.
    - In general, the presence of polychromasia (variation in erythrocyte staining hue) and anisocytosis (variation in erythrocyte size) on a blood smear is usually an indication of a regenerative response, but
      -- Red cell size also depends on other factors such as iron stores, whether there is spherocyte development and in some breeds microcytosis is seen as a normal finding (Akitas and some other Japanese breeds).
      -- It is at best a semi-quantitative result.
      -- A regenerative response may be delayed for 3–5 days after onset of haemolysis or blood loss so an apparently 'non-regenerative' blood film evaluation may also be 'pre-regenerative' and should be re-evaluated after 2–3 days.
  - Evaluation of red cell morphological changes which might implicate an aetiology of the anaemia.
    - Large numbers of **spherocytes** which are the remnants of red blood cells once a large portion of the membrane has been phagocytosed. It is almost always evidence of immune-mediated haemolytic anaemia (though it will not distinguish primary from secondary).
    - Presence of **schistocytes,** irregular red cell fragments caused by 'shearing' injuries. This happens most commonly in vascular neoplasms, with Disseminated Intravascular Coagulation (DIC) and where high shear stress occurs in arteriovenous fistulae or left-to-right communicating cardiac defects.
    - Presence of **acanthocytes** (spur cells), which are usually found in animals with liver disease and with red cell fragmentation (differentials as for shistocytes above – vascular neoplasms, DIC, high shear stress).

- Intracellular inclusions:
  -- Do not forget that stain precipitate, platelets overlying red blood cells, basophilic stippling of red cells (which is common in regenerative anaemias) and Howell–Jolly bodies (small nuclear remnants) are all very commonly mistaken for infectious intracellular inclusions.
  -- **Heinz bodies** are aggregates of precipitated haemoglobin that stain light blue and are always situated at the cell membrane. Heinz bodies are often due to oxidant injury including onion and garlic toxicity, zinc toxicity, acetaminophen and benzocaine. Many systemic diseases including hyperthyroidism, diabetes mellitus and lymphoma will also cause Heinz bodies to form.
  -- Infectious agents:
    - May see
      ◦ *Anaplasma* spp.
      ◦ *Babesia* spp.
      ◦ *Bartonella* spp.
    - Organisms such as *Ehrlichia* spp. form inclusions in leukocytes.

Differentiating between regenerative and non-regenerative anaemias

The most important initial step in evaluation of anaemia is to determine whether it is regenerative (associated with either blood loss or haemolysis) or non-regenerative. A reticulocyte count above 80×10^9/l demonstrates regeneration but it should be remembered that there is a short delay of 3–5 days before a regenerative response may be seen (so called 'pre-regenerative' phase). Findings should therefore be assessed in context of the clinical presentation and other 'clues'.

An animal that has become acutely unwell is more likely to have a regenerative, rather than a non-regenerative anaemia since the latter are usually slow to develop in onset. Similarly, an animal that is profoundly anaemic yet is clinically compensating well is more likely to have a non-regenerative anaemia since a certain amount of physiological 'adaptation' can occur when anaemia develops gradually. Finally, assessment of total protein, which is expected to drop with acute blood loss, and examination of the supernatant of a spun blood sample to look for red pink staining compatible with haemolysis are essential and simple measures to help distinguish between blood loss and haemolysis.

Further questions and answers

3. Look at the laboratory results that arrived later (see the tables below) and also the blood smear (see Figure 6.2).

Haematology

Parameter	Value	Units	Range
RBC	**1.39**	$\times 10^{12}$/l	(5.5–8.5)
Haemoglobin	**3.7**	g/dl	(12.0–18.0)

Parameter	Value	Units	Range
Haematocrit	**0.11**	l/l	(0.37–0.55)
Mean cell volume	75	fl	(60–77)
Mean cell haemoglobin concentration	35.0	g/dl	(30.0–38.0)
Mean cell haemoglobin	**26.4**	pg	(19.5–25.5)
Total White Cell Count	**20.5**	× 10⁹/l	(6.0–15.0)
Neutrophils	**12.73**	× 10⁹/l	(3.0–11.5)
Band neutrophils	**2.67**	× 10⁹/l	(0.0–0.5)
Lymphocytes	1.64	× 10⁹/l	(1.0–4.8)
Monocytes	**2.67**	× 10⁹/l	(0.2–1.4)
Eosinophils	0.82	× 10⁹/l	(0.1–1.2)
Basophils	0.0	× 10⁹/l	(0.0–0.1)
Platelets	202	× 10⁹/l	(200–500)
Reticulocyte count	**284**	× 10⁹/l	(0–80)

Biochemistry

Parameter	Value	Units	Range
Total protein	60	g/l	(54–77)
Albumin	29	g/l	(25–40)
Globulin	31	g/l	(23–45)
Urea	5.5	mmol/l	(2.5–7.4)
Creatinine	56	µmol/l	(40–145)
Potassium	3.5	mmol/l	(3.4–5.6)
Sodium	140	mmol/l	(139–154)
Chloride	108	mmol/l	(105–122)
Calcium	2.2	mmol/l	(2.1–2.8)
Inorganic phosphate	0.7	mmol/l	(0.60–1.40)
Glucose	5.5	mmol/l	(3.3–5.8)
ALT	47	IU/l	(13–88)
AST	**82**	IU/l	(13–60)
ALKP	**130**	IU/l	(14–105)
GGT	0	IU/l	(0–10)
Bilirubin	**29**	µmol/l	(0–16)
Cholesterol	6.9	mmol/l	(3.8–7.0)
Triglyceride	1.1	mmol/l	(0.56–1.14)
Creatine kinase	167	IU/l	(0–190)

(a)

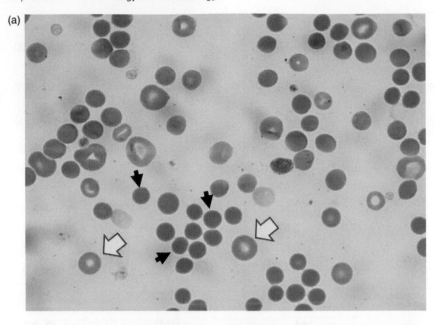

(b)

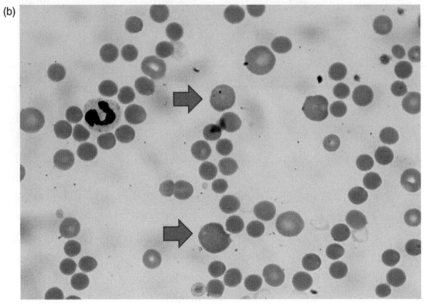

Figure 6.2 Blood smear at presentation, Wright's stain.

a. Interpret the haematology and biochemistry findings.
b. On the blood smear, what are the cells indicated by
    i. The black arrows?
   ii. The yellow arrows?
  iii. The blue arrows?

a. **Interpret the haematology and biochemistry findings**
   ○ A very severe anaemia is present and the anaemia is (based on the erythrocyte indices) normocytic and hyperchromic.
   ○ The reticulocyte count is elevated, indicating that the anaemia is regenerative.
   ○ A mild neutrophilia with a band shift and monocytosis are present. This indicates a regenerative left shift due to increased demand for neutrophils in an inflammatory response. The monocytosis suggests a subacute response to inflammation.
   ○ The biochemistry is most notable in the normal level of proteins, suggesting (in the absence of dehydration) that acute whole blood loss is not responsible for the anaemia and the hyperbilirubinaemia. Hyperbilirubinaemia may be due to pre-hepatic (release of bilirubin from haemolysed or phagocytosed erythrocytes), hepatic or post-hepatic (especially extrahepatic bile duct obstruction) causes. Serum AST and ALKP are only very marginally increased above the reference interval. The combination of anaemia and hyperbilirubinaemia, especially in the presence of only very marginal raises in hepatocellular and cholestatic liver markers, strongly implicates a pre-hepatic cause.

b. **On the blood smear (Figure 6.2), what are the cells indicated by**
   i. **The black arrows?**
      These are spherocytes. They are smaller than normal erythrocytes and lack the central pallor seen in normal erythrocytes.
   ii. **The yellow arrows?**
      These are normal erythrocytes. Note the area of central pallor.
   iii. **The blue arrows?**
      These are polychromatophils. Note the deeper blue/mauve staining. Although this stain does not indicate the internal nucleic acid structure (a new methylene blue stain would be suitable for this), these are likely to represent reticulocytes.

4. **What is the likely diagnosis and how can this be confirmed?**
   • Diagnostic clues in this patient are
      ○ The presence of an acute, regenerative anaemia implicates blood loss or haemolysis.
      ○ There is clinical and laboratory evidence of an inflammatory response (fever, leucocytosis, band shift).
      ○ There is no evidence of external blood loss or decrease in protein level to implicate a haemorrhagic cause.
      ○ The presence of spherocytes indicates that partial erythrocyte phagocytosis has occurred due to surface bound-antibody or complement.

These findings indicate a diagnosis of **immune-mediated haemolytic anaemia (IMHA)**. IMHA may be primary or may occur secondary to pathology such as infectious, inflammatory and neoplastic diseases. Diagnostic imaging such as survey radiography of the thorax and abdomen, and abdominal ultrasound examination, is often helpful in both determining if there is evidence of structural disease or solid or infiltrative neoplasia, and also in evaluating with good sensitivity (in the case of ultrasound) if intracavitary free fluid, which may be compatible with internal blood loss, is present. This is especially useful in situations where there may be less evidence to support that a regenerative anaemia is due to haemolysis or where an underlying disease process is present (e.g. hepatosplenic neoplasia) in which both secondary IMHA and haemorrhage may contribute to anaemia.

Serological and/or PCR testing for infectious organisms implicated in development of IMHA is appropriate and emphasis/specific testing may depend on geographic region. For example, in the United Kingdom, where infectious causes of secondary IMHA in dogs are very rare, rational testing may include assessment for *Anaplasma phagocytophilum* and possibly *Babesia* spp. (*Babesia gibsoni* have been identified in *Ixodes ricinus* ticks in the UK). Leptospirosis may also cause secondary IMHA.

A Coombs' test (direct agglutination test, or DAT) demonstrates the presence of erythrocyte-bound antibody but does not distinguish between primary and secondary IMHA. There is considerable variation in methodology between laboratories and both false negative and also false positive results (in the presence of other inflammatory disorders) are possible.

Diagnosis and outcome

In this patient diagnostic imaging tests demonstrated generalised diffuse splenomegaly with increased echogenicity on ultrasound (**Figure 6.3**), but fine needle aspiration cytology results were merely consistent with extramedullary haematopoiesis. This and the subsequent reduction in splenic size with treatment suggested an appropriate splenic response to severe anaemia rather than, for instance, infiltrative disease such as lymphoma.

Serological and PCR tests for *Leptospira*, *Anaplasma*, *Ehrlichia* and *Babesia* spp. were all negative.

The patient was treated with administration of a packed red blood cell transfusion, after blood-typing DEA 1.1 status, and immunosuppressive therapy was instituted with prednisolone at a dose of 2 mg/kg/day. Post-transfusion haematocrit raised to 0.24 l/l and subsequently declined to 0.18 l/l as continued haemolysis occurred. Thereafter the haematocrit slowly climbed and no further blood transfusion was required. After a further 3 weeks of an immunosuppressive dose of prednisolone the dose was weaned down by approximately 25% every 3–4 weeks, with reassessment of a haematology being performed prior to every dose reduction. After 18 weeks of treatment a dose of approximately 0.3 mg/kg/day prednisolone was reached and this dose was then continued every other day for a further 2 months before trial cessation. No relapse was seen in the dog's condition.

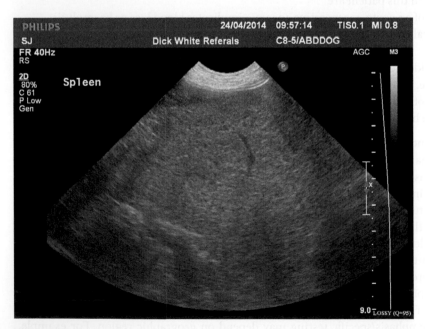

Figure 6.3 Splenic ultrasound in this patient.

Practicalities of transfusion in this dog: what to assess, how much to give and over how long?

A complete discussion of transfusion practice is beyond the scope of this chapter but in this case the patient requires tissue oxygen-delivery in the form of red blood cells (or if available a haemoglobin-based oxygen-carrying solution, HBOC, such as 'Oxyglobin'). Red cells are likely to offer more sustained improvement in oxygen carriage than HBOC solutions but are susceptible to further destruction by the immune-mediated process. Although both packed red blood cell products and whole blood would supply cell-based oxygen delivery, in a eu-volaemic patient packed red blood cells (pRBCs) are preferred.

Blood-typing should be performed prior to transfusion with canine dog erythrocyte antigen (DEA) group 1.1 of positive or negative status being most important. Naturally occurring alloantibodies to DEA 1.1 are not though to occur in animals that have not received prior transfusions but administration of DEA 1.1 positive blood to a negative recipient will sensitise that patient to induce alloantibody formation with any subsequent DEA 1.1 positive transfusion. DEA 1.1 negative dogs should therefore ideally receive transfusion from DEA 1.1 negative dogs for the first transfusion, but certainly for any subsequent transfusions. Whilst DEA 1.1 positive dogs may receive transfusions from either positive or negative dogs, it is ideal to efficiently utilise precious blood-bank stocks if DEA 1.1 positive blood is given to these. Repeat transfusions occurring more than 48 hours after a first transfusion should be cross-matched.

Administration of 2 ml/kg of whole blood or 1 ml/kg of pRBC would be expected to raise the recipient haematocrit by approximately 1% and the amount administered can be calculated more accurately as:

$$\text{For whole blood} = \text{recipient body weight (kg)} \times 85 \times \frac{\text{recipient desired PCV} - \text{current PCV}}{\text{donor PCV}}$$

$$\text{for pRBCs} = \text{recipient body weight (kg)} \times 85 \times \frac{\text{recipient desired PCV} - \text{current PCV}}{80}$$

The transfusion rate is usually slow (usually 0.5 - 1.0 ml/kg/hr) for the first 5–10 minutes whilst observing for transfusion reactions; thereafter, if possible, the transfusion should be completed within 4 hours to reduce chances of bacterial contamination, though in patients sensitive to volume-loading (for instance those with a history of congestive heart failure), more prolonged delivery may be advisable but should be weighed-up against risk of contamination. Rapid administration may be required in haemorrhage.

Discussion

An initial approach to the anaemic patient should always involve distinguishing those anaemias that are regenerative from those that are non-regenerative, whilst bearing in mind the possibility of a 'pre-regenerative' anaemia in those patients with blood loss or haemolysis in which sufficient time for a reticulocyte response has yet to elapse. Common causes of regenerative and non-regenerative anaemias are shown in **Table 6.1**; remember that whilst IMHA is the commonest cause of haemolytic anaemia, not all animals with haemolytic anaemia develop this due to an immune-mediated cause.

Table 6.1 Common regenerative and non-regenerative causes of anaemia in dogs

Regenerative anaemias	Non-regenerative anaemias
• Blood loss	• Anaemia of chronic disease
○ Rapid	• Anaemia of chronic kidney disease
○ Slow	• Myelophthesis
• Haemolysis	○ Lymphoma
○ Immune-mediated	○ Leukaemias
- Primary	○ Multiple myeloma
- Secondary	• Hypoproliferative diseases
○ Non-immune-mediated	○ Myelodysplastic syndrome
- Chemical (copper, zinc, lead, Heinz body, hypophosphataemia)	○ Myelofibrosis
	○ Pure red cell aplasia and non-regenerative IMA
- Erythroenzymopathy	○ Aplastic anaemia
- Red cell destruction due to shear stress	• Infectious diseases affecting the bone marrow

Iron deficiency anaemia (can have characteristics of both depending on when seen)

IMHA is the most commonly reported immune-mediated haematological disease in dogs and the commonest cause of haemolysis. Where IMHA occurs in conjunction with immune-mediated thrombocytopenia (ITP) it is known as Evans' syndrome. The underlying cause of IMHA is loss of self-tolerance by circulating lymphocytes, which become autoreactive, and co-stimulation of these produces autoantibody. IMHA is in effect a type II (antibody-mediated) hypersensitivity in which major targets are erythrocyte membrane glycophorins, the anion exchange molecule (band 3) and the cytoskeletal molecule, spectrin. Evidence for both a seasonal variation in incidence and an association with recent vaccination have been reported in one study (Duval and Giger 1996) but has not been supported by several more studies.

The mainstay of therapy is provision of immunosuppression in the form of prednisolone. Despite the popularity of provision of additional immunosuppressive agents and some weak evidence to support the additional use of azathioprine, as well as weak evidence of a poorer outcome in patients co-administered ciclosporin or cyclophosphamide (Swann and Skelly 2011; Reimer et al. 1999), to date the level of evidence showing improved outcome in multi-drug immunosuppression over prednisolone alone has been poor (Grundy and Barton 2001; Piek et al. 2011; Swann and Skelly 2012). It is very difficult to judge the need to give more than one immunosuppressive agent and very often the decision to do this is prompted more by clinician impatience to see a response than because there is sound evidence behind such treatment. The overall mortality rate in canine primary IMHA has been reported variously between 26% and 70% and up to 15% of patients have been reported to relapse upon or after discontinuation of therapy (Balch and Mackin 2007a, 2007b), although clinical experience would suggest that the actual number may be much lower than this in the author's geographical location.

Supportive care in the form of blood product transfusion may be necessary in order to provide tissue oxygen delivery during the 'time lag', which is usually 5–7 days, before positive effects of immunosuppression are seen. Note that these patients are usually euvolaemic and packed red blood cells are a more appropriate transfusate than whole blood, which may result in volume overload if given too rapidly. There is no particular 'PCV trigger' at which point transfusion should be considered. A decision to transfuse is based upon the clinical examination findings of the patient or other evidence of reduced tissue oxygen delivery and subsequent metabolic decompensation. Certainly not all patients with IMHA require transfusion and blood products are a scarce resource and their use associated with some risk to the recipient of transfusion reaction (especially with second and subsequent transfusions). The amount of packed red blood cells to be transfused depends on the target PCV that one desires, 1 ml/kg or pRBCs being expected to raise the recipient's PCV by 1%. Where and when available, haemoglobin-based oxygen-carrying products such as oxyglobin may also be helpful in raising tissue oxygen delivery but effects are shorter-lived than for blood.

A common feature of many case series describing dogs with IMHA is the contribution to mortality of thromboembolic disease and this has led to a plethora of recent studies advocating the use of anticoagulant or antiplatelet therapies such as unfractionated heparin, low molecular weight heparin, aspirin or clopidogrel. Results of these studies are difficult to interpret in the context of whether a positive benefit of such intervention is apparent and it is likely that individual susceptibility to thromboembolism is variable and dependent on the circumstances of the disease and comorbidities.

References

Balch, A. & Mackin, A. (2007a) Canine immune-mediated hemolytic anemia: pathophysiology, clinical signs, and diagnosis. *Compend Contin Educ Vet* **29**, 217–225

Balch, A. & Mackin, A. (2007b) Canine immune-mediated hemolytic anemia: treatment and prognosis. *Compend Contin Educ Vet* **29**, 230–238; quiz 239

Duval, D. & Giger, U. (1996) Vaccine-associated immune-mediated hemolytic anemia in the dog. *J Vet Intern Med* **10**, 290–295

Grundy, S.A. & Barton, C. (2001) Influence of drug treatment on survival of dogs with immune-mediated hemolytic anemia: 88 cases (1989–1999) *J Am Vet Med Assoc* **218**, 543–546

Piek, C.J., van Spil, W.E., Junius, G. & Dekker, A. (2011) Lack of evidence of a beneficial effect of azathioprine in dogs treated with prednisolone for idiopathic immune-mediated hemolytic anemia: a retrospective cohort study. *BMC Vet Res* **7**, 15

Reimer, M.E., Troy, G.C. & Warnicke, L.D. (1999) Immune-mediated hemolytic anemia: 70 cases (1988–1996) *J Am Anim Hosp Assoc* **35**, 384–391

Swann, J.W. & Skelly, B.J. (2011) Evaluation of immunosuppressive regimens for immune-mediated haemolytic anaemia: a retrospective study of 42 dogs. *J Small Anim Pract* **52**, 353–358

Swann, J.W. & Skelly, B.J. (2012) Systematic review of evidence relating to the treatment of immune-mediated hemolytic anemia in dogs. *J Vet Intern Med* **27**, 1–9

Further reading

Breuhl, E.L., Moore, G., Brooks, M.B. & Scott-Moncrieff, J.C. (2009) A prospective study of unfractionated heparin therapy in dogs with primary immune-mediated hemolytic anemia. *J Am Anim Hosp Assoc* **45**, 125–133

Kidd, L. & Mackman, N. (2013) Prothrombotic mechanisms and anticoagulant therapy in dogs with immune-mediated hemolytic anemia. *J Vet Emerg Crit Care (San Antonio)* **23**, 3–13

Piek, C.J., Junius, G., Dekker, A., Schrauwen, E., Slappendel, R.J. & Teske, E. (2008) Idiopathic immune-mediated hemolytic anemia: treatment outcome and prognostic factors in 149 dogs. *J Vet Intern Med* **22**, 366–373

Scott-Moncrieff, C. (2001) Immune-mediated hemolytic anemia: 70 cases (1988–1996). *J Am Anim Hosp Assoc* **37**, 11

Swann, J.W. & Skelly, B.J. (2015) Systematic review of prognostic factors for mortality in dogs with immune-mediated hemolytic anemia. *J Vet Intern Med* **29**, 7–13

Wardrop, K.J. (2012) Coombs' testing and its diagnostic significance in dogs and cats. *Vet Clin North Am Small Anim Pract* **42**, 43–51

Weinkle, T.K., Center, S.A., Randolph, J.F., Warner, K.L., Barr, S.C. & Erb, H.N. (2005) Evaluation of prognostic factors, survival rates, and treatment protocols for immune-mediated hemolytic anemia in dogs: 151 cases (1993–2002). *J Am Vet Med Assoc* **226**, 1869–1880

Clinical presentation

An aggressive 5 year-old male-neutered Bull Terrier cross (**Figure 7.1**) weighing 16 kg is presented due to lethargy and vomiting. The dog is a known scavenger and has rarely attended veterinary clinics due to his extremely combative behaviour. His owners have noted that he has become extremely lethargic in the previous 48 hours and has vomited bile-stained fluid two to three times daily in the previous five days. The owners report that his stools are black and 'tarry' but are normally formed. No weight loss has been noted and appetite has decreased only slightly.

On physical examination the dog is more docile than previously reported though is still very aggressive. A limited physical examination demonstrates pale and icteric conjunctiva, a heart rate of 136/min with normal peripheral pulse rate and quality, and a soft, grade II/VI systolic left basilar heart murmur. Respiratory rate and effort and respiratory auscultation are not possible to discern due to the dog constantly growling and attempting to bite despite muzzling. Possible cranial abdominal discomfort is elicited on palpation but a satisfactory examination is not possible. A blood sample taken at this time shows the following:

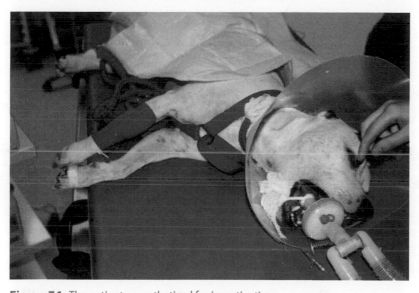

Figure 7.1 The patient anaesthetised for investigation.

Canine Internal Medicine: What's Your Diagnosis? First Edition. Jon Wray.
© 2018 John Wiley & Sons Ltd. Published 2018 by John Wiley & Sons Ltd.

Haematology

Parameter	Value	Units	Range
RBC	1.04	$\times 10^{12}/l$	(5.5–8.5)
Haemoglobin	3.2	g/dl	(12.0–18.0)
Haematocrit	0.09	l/l	(0.37–0.55)
Mean cell volume	82.2	fl	(60–77)
Mean cell haemoglobin concentration	37.2	g/dl	(30.0–38.0)
Mean cell haemoglobin	30.6	pg	(19.5–25.5)
Total white cell count	24.0	$\times 10^9/l$	(6.0–15.0)
Neutrophils	20.43	$\times 10^9/l$	(3.0–11.5)
Lymphocytes	1.68	$\times 10^9/l$	(1.0–4.8)
Monocytes	1.2	$\times 10^9/l$	(0.2–1.4)
Eosinophils	0.00	$\times 10^9/l$	(0.1–1.2)
Basophils	0.00	$\times 10^9/l$	(0.0–0.1)
Nucleated red blood cells	6.5	$\times 10^9/l$	
Platelets	556	$\times 10^9/l$	(200–500)
Reticulocyte count	216	$\times 10^9/l$	(0–60)
Reticulocyte haemoglobin	20	pg	(23.7–29.8)

Film comment:	Very marked polychromasia and anisocytosis. High numbers of hypochromic RBCs. High numbers of nucleated RBCs. Occasional Heinz bodies. Moderate poikilocytosis, including schistocytes and acanthocytes

Biochemistry (note that supernatant of the serum sample is strongly red-brown discoloured)

Parameter	Value	Units	Range
Total protein	54	g/l	(54–77)
Albumin	27	g/l	(25–40)
Globulin	27	g/l	(23–45)
Urea	27.4	mmol/l	(2.5–7.4)
Creatinine	160	mmol/l	(40–145)
Potassium	3.4	mmol/l	(3.4–5.6)
Sodium	150	mmol/l	(139–154)
Chloride	121	mmol/l	(105–122)
Calcium	2.3	mmol/l	(2.1–2.8)
Inorganic phosphate	2.1	mmol/l	(0.60–1.40)
Glucose	3.5	mmol/l	(3.3–5.8)
ALT	85	IU/l	(13–88)

Parameter	Value	Units	Range
AST	55	IU/l	(13–60)
ALKP	100	IU/l	(14–105)
GGT	9	IU/l	(0–10)
Bilirubin	**158**	mmol/l	(0–16)
Cholesterol	3.9	mmol/l	(3.8–7.0)
Triglyceride	1.1	mmol/l	(0.56–1.14)
Creatine kinase	**225**	IU/l	(0–190)

Questions

1. Interpret the haematology and biochemistry findings. What is the likely mechanism of the anaemia in this patient?
2. How would you interpret these findings in light of the patient's history and physical examination findings? How would you investigate this patient further?

Answers

1. Interpret the haematology and biochemistry findings. What is the likely mechanism of the anaemia in this patient?

Haematology

The haematology findings in this patient are fascinating:

- There is an anaemia that is very severe (HCt 0.09 l/l) and the anaemia is regenerative, as indicated by the raised reticulocyte count.
- The anaemia appears to be haemolytic since the supernatant shows haemolysis and the total bilirubin is markedly elevated in the presence of normal hepatic enzymes.
- The mean cell volume is increased, which probably reflects the presence of reticulocytes.
- The mean cell haemoglobin is increased, which is probably artefactual – both the presence of free haemoglobin and Heinz bodies may falsely elevate this.
- There is a stress leukogram present with concurrent neutrophilia and eosinopenia.
- There are large numbers of nucleated red blood cells present, which probably reflects a strongly regenerative response though this can also be seen with lead toxicity and with bone marrow disorders.
- Despite the normal red cell mean haemoglobin concentration there are very many hypochromic red blood cells. This suggests that cell haemoglobin is reduced and is usually indicative of iron deficiency. The low reticulocyte haemoglobin concentration is also suggestive of this.
- Heinz bodies are crystalline precipitates of oxidised haemoglobin that occur with oxidant-induced damage. Causes of Heinz body anaemia are shown in **Table 7.1**.
- Schistocytes are erythrocyte fragments with pointed margins, which are seen most commonly in microangiopathic anaemia due to disseminated intravascular coagulation (DIC), iron-deficiency anaemia, myelofibrosis, haemangiosarcoma, heart failure, glomerulonephritis and dirofilariasis.
- Acanthocytes (or spur cells) are erythrocytes with irregularly spaced spicule-like projections (in contrast to echinocytes, where the spicules are evenly spaced) and are usually seen in animals with liver disorders or disease that causes erythrocyte fragmentation.

Table 7.1 Causes of Heinz body anaemia in dogs

Onion and garlic ingestion
Zinc toxicity
Copper toxicity
Naphthalene toxicity
Drug therapy

- Acetaminophen
- Methylene blue
- Benzocaine
- Vitamin K
- Phenylhydrazine

Oxidant heavy metals

Biochemistry

- An azotaemia is present with a disproportionate raise in urea (about 4 times the upper reference interval) compared with creatinine (just over the upper reference interval). Due to the proximal tubular resorption of urea, dehydration and delivery of excessive amounts of nitrogenous waste from gastrointestinal haemorrhage may provoke a disproportionate rise in urea. These should be differentiated from renal azotaemia and contemporaneous interpretation of urine SG is recommended.
- There is a mild increase in phosphate, which may be due to decreased renal excretion, excessive absorption from the GI tract, shifts across body fluid compartments (e.g. from intracellular to extracellular fluid) or metabolic acidosis.
- The bilirubin is markedly elevated. Hyperbilirubinaemia may be pre-hepatic, hepatic or post-hepatic. In the absence of no elevations in hepatic transaminases and in combination with the anaemia and haemolysed supernatant on the blood sample, a pre-hepatic jaundice is most likely.
- A very mild raise in CK of debateable significance is present.

2. **How would you interpret these findings in light of the patient's history and physical examination findings? How would you investigate this patient further?**
   - The first steps in investigating anaemia is any animal are to
     - Determine the severity of the anaemia.
     - Determine whether the anaemia is regenerative or non-regenerative.
     - Determine the clinical impact of the anaemia on the patient to determine whether any immediate action needs to be taken.
   - In this patient the anaemia is very severe and it is regenerative. It is difficult to tell, with in the limitations of physical examination possible in this aggressive patient, what, if any, clinical impact of anaemia there is. The heart rate is perhaps slightly higher than we might expect of a dog of this breed type (which often have bradydysrhythmia due to increased vagal tone) but could be simply due to excitement/aggression and there is no alteration in pulse quality. It is usually safest in such circumstances to operate under the assumption that some degree of decompensation may be present but not clinically detectable.
   - The patient has pallor and icteric mucous membranes, which are likely to reflect the anaemia and hyperbilirubinaemia.

- There is a soft systolic heart murmur over the left basilar region. Murmurs may be acquired due to structural or functional heart disease or due to altered blood viscosity or high output cardiac states. The most common acquired cardiac disease causing a left-sided systolic murmur is myxomatous mitral valve disease in which the murmur is harsh in quality rather than soft and is apical rather than basilar. These findings are suggestive of a haemic murmur.
- There appears to be at least two mechanisms by which anaemia may have developed:
  - Haemolysis (detectable in the colour of the serum and the hyperbilirubinaemia), which can be further characterised as being accompanied by increased numbers of Heinz bodies, suggesting oxidative injury.
  - Iron deficiency anaemia, detectable due to the presence of hypochromasia and low reticulocyte haemoglobin. The most common cause of iron deficiency is protracted external blood loss, usually via the gastrointestinal tract. The history of black tarry faeces also supports this.
- The patient is azotaemic and this may be multifactorial in nature, and the azotaemia
  - May be pre renal due to fluid loss secondary to recent vomiting.
  - May be, particularly in light of the disproportionate rise in urea and history of black tarry faeces, contributed to by gastrointestinal blood loss.
  - May be pre-renal due to effects of whole blood loss in addition to vomiting.
- Further investigation might therefore include:
  - Assessment of urinalysis to allow for further interpretation of the azotaemia in the light of urine specific gravity.
  - Assessment of serum iron and ferritin to characterise iron status.
  - Diagnostic imaging of the gastrointestinal tract by radiography and ultrasound to attempt to determine a structural cause/site of blood loss, which might cause iron deficiency and this may also both help evaluate for potential causes of the vomiting and be used to assess for metallic foreign bodies, which may be a cause of Heinz body haemolytic anaemia. Zinc-containing coins are not usually encountered in the UK (compared with the USA) but other metallic foreign bodies which might act as oxidants are found.
  - Potentially evaluation by endoscopy might be indicated, both to evaluate gastrointestinal blood loss and for possible foreign body retrieval dependent on the results of imaging tests.

Transfusion 'triggers'

In this patient, consideration needs to be given as to whether blood product support is indicated. Whilst there is no particular haematocrit at which a transfusion is 'triggered', a case-by-case assessment of the physiological impact of and predicted rate of decrease in haematocrit needs to inform decision making. For example, dogs with chronic anaemias may tolerate slow declines to very low haematocrits whilst animals with acutely decreasing haematocrits may require transfusion of blood when their haematocrit reaches 0.20–0.25 l/l. In this patient assessment based on physical examination is difficult but one could anticipate that both haemolysis and blood loss are entities that have potential to worsen rapidly, even though the evidence of iron deficiency suggests that chronic blood loss may have been occurring.

Findings that might suggest that transfusion support is physiologically necessary may include development of tachycardia, tachypnoea, weakness or profound lethargy, evidence of organ dysfunction that might be reasonably attributed to hypoxia or development of high-output cardiac failure. Practical/premonitory considerations may also dictate whether transfusion should be given, such as the situation where physiological compensation is currently present, but the recorded rate of decline of haematocrit is so rapid that it could be anticipated that it may continue to a life-threatening degree in advance of reasonable expectation of any treatment response.

- It should also be considered that the azotaemia is likely to, at least in part, reflect diminished renal blood flow and that fluid therapy is likely indicated. It could be rationalised that were transfusion to be given, the delivery of whole blood, which would provide both oxygen-carrying capacity in the form of transfused erythrocytes and also plasma, would be the ideal blood product to give.

Diagnosis

This patient was extremely challenging due to temperament and bit two experienced veterinary staff during assessment. Euthanasia was advised, as the owner could also only handle the dog wearing gauntlets and had herself been bitten on several occasions, but declined. Investigation had to therefore proceed along pragmatic/expedient lines. The dog was blood typed as DEA 1.1 negative and, under sedation, radiography and ultrasound of the abdomen were performed, and a transfusion of 450 ml of DEA 1.1 negative fresh whole blood was begun.

Radiography (**Figure 7.2**) demonstrated a 1.5 × 3.3 cm metallic foreign body to be present in the lumen of the fundus. The small intestine was diffusely gas-filled and tubular in shape, but measured within normal limits in diameter, and these changes were felt to be compatible with functional ileus. Visible portions of the hepatic, splenic and renal silhouettes were unremarkable. An incidental small amount of spondylosis ventral to L4/5 was noted.

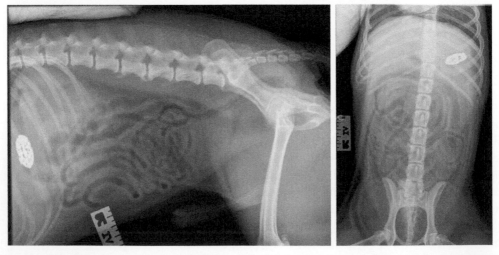

Figure 7.2 Right lateral (overcollimated) and dorsoventral abdominal view showing a metallic foreign body in the fundus of the stomach.

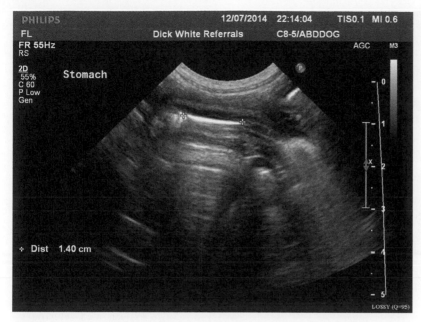

Figure 7.3 Abdominal ultrasound demonstrating foreign body in stomach.

On abdominal ultrasound (**Figure 7.3**) the gastric wall was uniformly thickened (7 mm) keeping a normal multi-layered pattern and was moderately distended with fluid and gas. A foreign object creating a 'comet-tail' artefact was identified, corresponding to the previously reported metallic object in radiographs. Both kidneys were within normal limits for size but show ill-defined corticomedullary distinction, though otherwise normal architecture and remaining examination including the rest of the gastrointestinal tract, pancreas, liver, bladder and lymph nodes was normal.

It was suspected that the cause of the Heinz body haemolytic anaemia, the vomiting and the iron-deficiency was the metallic foreign body and under brief general anaesthesia upper gastrointestinal endoscopy was performed. The object, which appeared disc-like with serrated projections around the circumference, was found within the fundus (**Figure 7.4**) and the surrounding gastric mucosa was ulcerated and markedly irregular. Evaluation of the pylorus and the proximal duodenum demonstrated no more distal lesions. Using a basket forceps the object was retrieved without event and was seen to be a badge from a ski school. The badge was subsequently sent for X-ray fluorescence analysis (**Table 7.2**) and was found to be comprised largely of zinc and copper, either or both of which may have provoked the Heinz body anaemia.

After completion of transfusion and recovery, the patient became unexaminable without unacceptable risk to staff safety, though a post-transfusion PCV was 27%. As soon as considered practical and safe the dog was discharged home to receive omeprazole 20 mg p/o SID and ferrous sulphate 200 mg p/o SID, both for 4 weeks. Regular verbal follow-up was performed as further blood sampling was not possible without both chemical restraint and a dog-catcher. The dog continued to return to a normal level of energy and the owner was able to report normal colour to the oral mucous membranes and return to normal stool colour. The dog remains clinically normal 1 year after diagnosis.

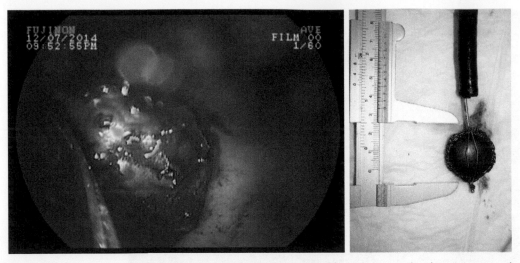

Figure 7.4 Endoscopic view of foreign body in situ and after retrieval from the stomach, where it is grasped within a set of basket forceps.

Table 7.2 X-ray fluorescence analysis of the foreign body

Aluminium oxide	0.6%
Calcium oxide	0.3%
Chloride	3.8%
Copper oxide	**54%**
Potassium oxide	0.1%
Magnesium oxide	0.2%
Nickel oxide	0.08%
Phosphorus pentoxide	0.4%
Lead oxide	0.02%
Silicon dioxide	0.2%
Sulphur trioxide	1.0%
Zinc oxide	**39%**
Selenium (IV) oxide	0.5%

Discussion

As with all anaemic patients, the initial goals of diagnosis should be to establish the severity of the anaemia, whether it is regenerative or non-regenerative and to try and establish the clinical consequences of the anaemia at the time of presentation. The differential diagnosis for a regenerative anaemia was rapidly expedited in this case by examination of the blood film and by integrating the haematological and biochemical findings with the clinical history. The usefulness of the blood smear evaluation cannot be overemphasised and whilst bench-top haematology analysers can proffer highly useful information, it is absolutely essential that these are not relied on as the sole means of haematological evaluation and examination of a fresh blood smear as a competent clinician is always needed. In non-emergency cases, whilst the appeal of an in-house analyser is immediacy and commercial imperative, employing the services of a professional clinical pathology laboratory (provided that such a service has a suitably qualified veterinary clinical pathologist, or similarly experienced individual, reviewing a blood smear from every patient) is invaluable. Veterinary surgeons should always acquaintance themselves with just what the level of scrutiny of blood samples is by a qualified individual before considering any commercial laboratory.

Further reading

Bexfield, N., Archer, J. & Herrtage, M. (2007) Heinz body haemolytic anaemia in a dog secondary to ingestion of a zinc toy: a case report. *Vet J* **174**, 414–417

Hammond, G.M., Loewen, M.E. & Blakley, B.R. (2004) Diagnosis and treatment of zinc poisoning in a dog. *Vet Hum Toxicol* **46**, 272–275

Houston, D.M. & Myers, S.L. (1993) A review of Heinz-body anemia in the dog induced by toxins. *Vet Hum Toxicol* **35**, 158–161

Clinical presentation

A 5 year 8 month-old male-neutered Labrador (**Figure 8.1**) is presented with a 48-hour history of lethargy and of limping on the left foreleg, which has become noticeably swollen to the owner. On examination the dog is depressed, his mucous membranes are very pale and there is blood oozing from his gum margins bilaterally. The left foreleg is diffusely swollen centred on the carpal joint, which appears to be effused but not warm or particularly painful on manipulation. Other joints appear normal. Resting respiratory rate is 36/min with a normal respiratory effort and no adventitial lung sounds. Heart rate is 140/min with a normal rhythm and peripheral pulses are hyperdynamic. A soft, grade II/VI systolic heart murmur is auscultable on the left side midway between the cardiac apex and base. Abdominal palpation demonstrates mild but reproducible discomfort dorsally in the sublumbar region but no obvious palpable structural abnormalities are detected and no lymphadenomegaly is found. Rectal temperature is 38.5 °C and a small amount of fresh blood is noted on the rectal thermometer afterwards. The patient has not travelled outside the United Kingdom, is not receiving any veterinary-prescribed medications and has an unremarkable previous medical history.

Questions

1. What is the problem list identified from the history and physical examination?
2. What differential diagnoses would you consider?
3. What would your initial investigative plan be?

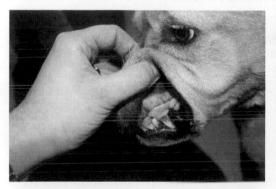
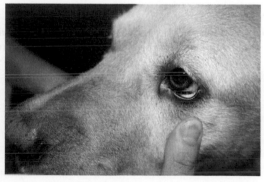
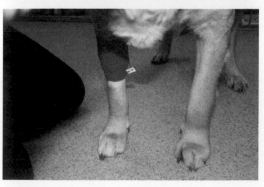

Figure 8.1 The patient at presentation.

Canine Internal Medicine: What's Your Diagnosis? First Edition. Jon Wray.
© 2018 John Wiley & Sons Ltd. Published 2018 by John Wiley & Sons Ltd.

Answers

1. What is the problem list identified from the history and physical examination?

Some of the potential problems that one might include in a problem list are either so broad/common to many pathologies that they are unsuitable to problem-solve based on them or are very likely to be the consequence of illness rather than a primary problem in themselves. It is important when constructing a problem list to think 'physiologically' and to apply judicious clinical common-sense in marshalling the order of problems according to clinical importance rather than, say, weighting each equally (**Table 8.1**). Affording greater emphasis to 'pivotal' problems in this way (see Case 3, page 33), greatly helps deductive problem-solving.

Table 8.1 Problem list for Case 8

A problem list for this patient might include

- Mucous membrane pallor.
- Ooze of blood from gum margins and fresh blood in the lower gastrointestinal tract.
- Swelling of the left carpal region associated with lameness and without obvious heat or tenderness of the joint.
- Palpable discomfort in the sublumbar region.
- Soft heart murmur which is systolic, left-sided and has a point of maximal intensity between the base and apex.

To this we can add problems that are likely to be broad or secondary in nature:

- Lethargy.
- Hyperdynamic peripheral pulse quality associated with a heart rate of 140/min (this heart rate is not necessarily abnormal and heart rates in dogs in the veterinary clinic will commonly be between 60 and 160/min. It should be interpreted in the context of the animal's clinical status and demeanour).

Initial considerations in bleeding patients

When bleeding is present one should firstly consider whether this may be due to local/traumatic bleeding injury or whether the distribution of bleeding sites is incompatible with this. The latter would suggest a more generalised bleeding disorder (sometimes referred to as a 'bleeding diathesis' or 'tendency'). One should consider that a bleeding diathesis may be due to a problem in any or a combination of the three main steps in formation of, and subsequent remodelling of, a stable blood clot namely:

- Primary haemostasis, which results in formation of a primary platelet plug.
- Secondary haemostasis, which results in stabilisation of the primary plug with cross-linked fibrin.
- The fibrinolytic system by which the clot is remodelled.

Lastly, one should also remember that bleeding tendencies can occur through generalised vascular disorders such as vasculitis. A summary is shown in **Figure 8.2**.

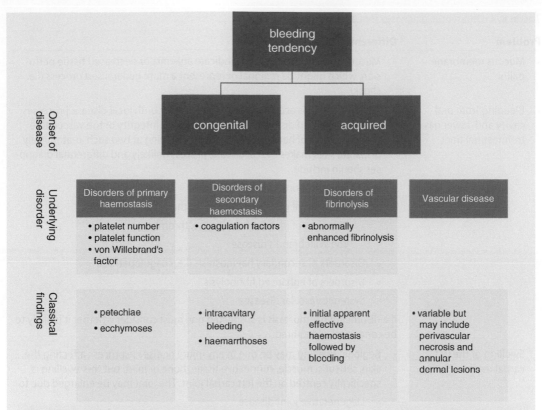

Figure 8.2 Initial considerations in patients with a possible bleeding tendency. Note that bleeding within some areas that are particularly well supplied with blood vessels such as intraocular and gastrointestinal bleeding and epistaxis are commonly seen with both primary and secondary haemostatic defects.

2. What differential diagnoses would you consider?

The following differential diagnoses might be constructed with the more 'pivotal' clinical problems considered first (**Table 8.2**).

Anaemia versus shock

Integrating this problem list and differential diagnoses, the presence of pallor with hyperdynamic pulses, rather than reduced pulse quality as might be expected in shock, is suggestive of anaemia and this too might be relevant to the soft systolic heart murmur. Presence of bleeding might implicate a cause of the anaemia.

Single joint swellings are uncommon with inflammatory joint diseases such as erosive and non-erosive arthropathies (which usually cause polyarthritis) and whilst monoarticular joint swelling is more common with septic arthritis, the lack of pain, heat or fever are all inconsistent with this. In the presence of bleeding from other sites it would therefore be sensible to consider that haemarthrosis would be the most likely cause.

Table 8.2 Differential diagnoses for Case 8

Problem	Differential diagnoses
• Mucous membrane pallor	• Mucous membrane pallor may indicate anaemia or decreased tissue perfusion, which might be regional or represent a more generalised process (i.e. shock).

• Bleeding from oral cavity and lower gastrointestinal tract	• When bleeding is occurring one must consider both local disease processes and a generalised disorder affecting either the integrity of the vasculature or mechanisms of haemostasis (or both). Bleeding at two such anatomically disparate sites makes a local disease process unlikely and differential diagnoses should include
	
	   ○ Disorders of primary haemostasis
	      - Disorders of platelet number (e.g. thrombocytopenia)
	      - Disorders of platelet function (i.e. thrombocytopathia)
	      - Von Willebrand's disease
	   ○ Disorders of secondary haemostasis (i.e. coagulopathies)
	   ○ Disorders of enhanced fibrinolysis
	   ○ Systemic vascular diseases
	
	If a disorder of haemostasis is suspected one must consider whether it is likely to be congenital or acquired.

• Swelling of the left carpal region	• Regional swelling may be due to any injury or disease process affecting the skin, subcutis, muscle, connective tissue, bone or joint, but this swelling is specifically centred on the left carpal joint. The joint may be enlarged due to
	
	   ○ Degenerative joint disease
	   ○ Inflammatory joint disease
	      - Sterile inflammation
	      - Septic inflammation
	   ○ Blood (i.e. haemarthosis)
	   ○ Malformation/cyst
	   ○ Tumour

• Palpable discomfort in the sublumbar region	• Structures of the sublumbar region which may give rise to discomfort on palpation include
	
	   ○ The kidneys
	   ○ The adrenal glands
	   ○ The local lymph nodes (lumbar, medial iliac)
	   ○ The aorta and caudal vena cava
	   ○ The lumbar lymphatic trunk and cisterna chyli
	   ○ The retroperitoneal space
	
	and of course discomfort may arise from the lumbar bony spine, spinal cord, meninges or local musculature.

• Soft heart murmur	• A soft heart murmur in this location may be due to
	
	   ○ Alteration in blood viscosity
	      - Anaemia
	      - Polycythaemia
	   ○ Fever
	   ○ Hypertension

Problem	Differential diagnoses
	∘ An ejection murmur arising within the left ventricular outflow tract (though this would not commonly have a timbre of being 'soft')
	∘ Murmurs associated with stenosis of the left ventricular outflow tract, aortic valve, pulmonic valve or a murmur of relative pulmonic stenosis due to atrial septal defect. However, all of these murmurs would be expected to be more intense at the cardiac base.
• Lethargy	• Lethargy is a rather non-specific clinical sign with a very broad differential diagnosis and although is a definite 'problem' it is not generally useful for the purposes of clinical problem solving.
• Hyperdynamic peripheral pulse	• Hyperdynamic pulses may be detected
	∘ With excitement
	∘ With high cardiac output states such as in anaemia or fever/sepsis
	∘ With disorders that increase the difference between systolic and diastolic pressure such as patent ductus arteriosus or severe aortic regurgitation, neither of which are likely here due to the characteristics of the described murmur.

3. What would your initial investigative plan be?

Having determined that anaemia and bleeding are likely to be present, it is sensible before anything else to

(a) Establish a thorough clinical history from the owners.

(b) Determine whether this patient has a clinical status that requires immediate therapeutic intervention.

In considering (b) the clinician should decide upon how well the patient is clinically 'coping' with the current situation and the time-frame over which any deterioration has been noted to occur (extrapolation of which might suggest that a currently compensating patient may not do so for much longer). It is important that any emergency therapeutic action is taken with due consideration to obtaining relevant samples before these are rendered obsolete, e.g. by blood transfusion. The owners should be questioned about:

• Whether the illness is acute in onset or is occurring in the setting of longer-term concerns that the dog is unwell.

• Vaccination, medication, travel and worming history as well as previous medical history.

• History of any previous unexplained haemorrhage, prolonged bleeding after surgery*, melaena, or excessive bruising.

• Potential for exposure to
  ∘ Anticoagulant rodenticides.
  ∘ Molluscan intermediate hosts of *Angiostrongylus vasorum*.

> **Remember that inadequate haemostasis is *the* most common reason for post-surgical bleeding**
>
> *Some caution should be undertaken in interpretation of this. In the author's experience veterinary surgeons are often tempted to suspect a haemostatic defect as a cause of post-operative bleeding, especially after ovariohysterectomy, rather than consider inadequately performed surgical haemostasis!

First diagnostic steps

- A PCV and evaluation of a fresh blood smear or performance of a complete blood count (which should *always* include performance of a fresh blood smear evaluation) to establish
  - ○ Is the patient anaemic and if so how anaemic?
  - ○ Is there evidence of regeneration consistent with blood loss or haemolysis?
  - ○ Are there adequate platelet numbers to suggest that thrombocytopenia is not a cause of the observed bleeding? Dogs with thrombocytopenia generally need to have a platelet count <50 x 109/l before a spontaneous bleeding tendency occurs. It should be remembered that platelet numbers will commonly temporarily decrease due to consumption during acute whole blood loss, to then rebound to an elevated number. Platelet numbers are also decreased commonly in disseminated intravascular coagulation (DIC).

Watch the proteins!

Assessment of total plasma/serum proteins, bearing in mind that this should be interpreted in the light of hydration of the patient, is useful in determining the likelihood of acute haemorrhage versus, for example, haemolysis. A decreased PCV accompanied by a fall in plasma proteins is suggestive of whole blood loss in the acute setting.

In this case, although a systemic haemostatic disorder appears likely, there are no cardinal signs of thrombocytopenia such as petechiation. Furthermore, if the joint swelling is haemorrhagic in origin, then haemarthroses are considered a sign seen most often in secondary haemostatic defects. The patient is an adult dog with no previous medical history, which suggests that if a haemostatic defect is present it is likely to be acquired rather than being congenital. Therefore, assuming platelet numbers are found to be adequate, assessment of secondary coagulation should be undertaken.

- ○ Assessment of secondary haemostasis may be undertaken:
  - - By performance of a prothrombin time (PT) and activated partial thromboplastin time (APTT) on a citrated plasma sample taken with a clean/atraumatic needle stick (bear in mind the possibility of prolonged bleeding and choose a site and apply prolonged pressure judiciously). This assesses intrinsic, extrinsic and common coagulation pathways
    - -- At a commercial reference laboratory.
    - -- Using a bench-top 'stat' analyser.
  - - By performing an activated clotting time (ACT) *but*
    - -- This only assesses common and intrinsic pathways.
    - -- This requires a specific collection tube containing a siliceous activator and maintaining tubes at 37 °C during assessment – many veterinary surgeons confuse ACT with looking at whole blood clotting time (below).
  - - By evaluating whole blood clotting time (WBCT)
    - -- This is extremely crude and time to clot formation of samples merely placed in glass tubes is hugely variable in dogs and commonly times are longer than many veterinary surgeons expect, being often 6–7 minutes in normal dogs.
  - - By assessment of a global test of haemostasis such as thromboelastography (TEG).

Assess platelet count before a buccal mucosal bleeding time

Although a popular test, buccal mucosal bleeding times (BMBTs) are a fairly crude assessment of *primary* haemostasis. However, they should not be undertaken before a platelet count is assessed, if platelet numbers are low (since the BMBT will definitely be abnormal in this setting) or where secondary coagulation problems are suspected as in this case. In the latter two situations, prolonged bleeding may be produced from a test that was not clinically necessary.

Second diagnostic steps

The most likely causes of acquired secondary coagulopathy are shown in **Table 8.3**.

- Assessment for *A.vasorum* may be undertaken most rapidly and with greatest sensitivity by performing a cage-side ELISA 'snap' test for *A. vasorum* antigen (Angiodetect™, Idexx).
  - Evidence of L1 larvae may be seen after microscopic examination of faeces, sputum, vomitus or BAL samples, but these methods lack sensitivity and organism identification may be difficult.
  - Practically, prior to receipt of diagnostic test results it is sensible to treat dogs with acquired secondary coagulopathy in endemic areas with appropriate antiparasitic therapy with urgency.
- Anticoagulant rodenticide toxicity is most commonly diagnosed presumptively based on
  - Exposure and
  - Demonstration of a secondary haemostatic defect that resolves with administration of vitamin K.
  - Specific testing for vitamin K antagonism can be undertaken (see below) but is not always highly sensitive due to the time lapse between exposure and testing.
- DIC is a clinical diagnosis made with supportive clinical pathological evidence. A consensus on diagnosis of DIC in veterinary medicine does not exist (reflecting the dynamic nature of this state, which precludes basing a diagnosis on static variables) though several reasonable proposals have been made. The finding of a combination of
  - An inciting disease state
  - Evidence of procoagulation
  - Evidence of fibrinolysis
  - Evidence of consumption of coagulation inhibitors

  has been proposed to make a diagnosis of DIC. In reality, tests commonly used to demonstrate evidence of fibrinolysis (such as D-dimer, fibrin degradation products) commonly suffer from methodological concerns and poor specificity in diagnosis of DIC.

Table 8.3 Common causes of secondary acquired coagulopathy

- Anticoagulant rodenticide exposure
- Disseminated intravascular coagulation resulting from
  - *Angiostrongylus vasorum* infestation
  - Neoplasia
  - Systemic inflammatory/infectious disease processes
  - Snake bite envenomation
- Liver disease

- Evidence of hepatic disease that may lead to acquired coagulopathy might include
  - Finding of abnormalities of liver function implied by
    - Abnormal serum pre- and/or post-prandial bile acids
    - Subnormal serum urea, cholesterol, glucose and albumin.
  - Biochemical and diagnostic imaging evidence of biliary obstruction, since vitamin K required for activation of some serine protease anticoagulant factors (II, VII, IX, X) is fat-soluble and intestinal absorption requires the presence of bile.

In this case the joint swelling and the sublumbar pain may be relevant and require further evaluation (e.g. by considering radiographic assessment of the left carpus and arthrocentesis, diagnostic imaging of the sublumbar region) but these areas could represent simply further sites of bleeding rather than representing a site of causative pathology.

Diagnosis and treatment

In this case the dog had no prior medical history of bleeding, was not on any medication and had not been systemically unwell. The onset of clinical signs was acute and the owners felt that the dog had notably worsened between the referral appointment being made and presentation. The owners recalled that they had recently placed a rodenticide on part of their property, which was subsequently found to be diphenacoum.

- A complete blood count and examination of a blood smear on admission demonstrated:

Haematology

Parameter	Value	Units	Range
RBC	**1.88**	$\times 10^{12}$/l	(5.5–8.5)
Haemoglobin	**4.9**	g/dl	(12.0–18.0)
Haematocrit	**0.14**	l/l	(0.37–0.55)
Mean cell volume	75.4	fl	(60–77)
Mean cell haemoglobin concentration	34.5	g/dl	(30.0–38.0)
Mean cell haemoglobin	**26**	pg	(19.5–25.5)
Total white cell count	14.44	$\times 10^9$/l	(6.0–15.0)
Neutrophils	11.67	$\times 10^9$/l	(3.0–11.5)
Lymphocytes	1.89	$\times 10^9$/l	(1.0–4.8)
Monocytes	0.69	$\times 10^9$/l	(0.2–1.4)
Eosinophils	0.04	$\times 10^9$/l	(0.1–1.2)
Basophils	0.02	$\times 10^9$/l	(0.0–0.1)
Platelets	**78**	$\times 10^9$/l	(200–500)
Film comment:	White cell morphology: unremarkable		
	Red cell morphology: mild to moderate anisocytosis with mild polychromasia		
	Platelet morphology: platelets are consistent with analyser count; no clumping seen		

Parameter	Value	Units	Range
Total protein	35	g/l	(54–77)
Albumin	13	g/l	(25–40)
Globulin	22	g/l	(23–45)

The platelet count, though markedly reduced, was not felt to be low enough to explain the clinical signs of bleeding and a test of secondary coagulation was performed:

Parameter	Value	Units	Range
Prothrombin time (PT)	>30	seconds	(7.0–12.0)
Activated partial thromboplastin time (APTT)	>200	seconds	(15.0–25.0)

- A test for *Angiostrongylus vasorum* antigen (Angio-detect SNAP, Idexx) was negative and a faecal sample was negative for lungworm larvae.
- A test for D-dimer was <250 ng/ml (0–250).

A diagnosis was made of acquired secondary haemostatic disorder with severe anaemia accompanied by evidence of regeneration (anisocytosis and polychromasia) and panhypoproteinaemia, consistent with a blood-loss anaemia. Thrombocytopenia was considered to probably be consumptive and in combination with the prolongation of PT and APTT a further consideration was that DIC may be present. Given the environmental presence of diphenacoum, secondary acquired coagulopathy was favoured.

- Samples were submitted to a reference laboratory for vitamin K and vitamin K epoxide levels and for detection of Warfarin derivatives by mass spectrometry.
- The dog was blood-typed and found to be DEA 1.1 positive. A 450 ml unit of fresh whole blood from a healthy donor dog was transfused over 4 hours without event. Post-transfusion the heart murmur was not auscultable and the peripheral pulse quality was normal, the heart rate decreased to 112/min and mucous membrane colour improved.
- Vitamin K1 therapy was instituted (immediately after collection of blood samples) at a dose of 2.5 mg/kg s/c q12 hours for 24 hours, followed by 2.5 mg/kg p/o SID continuously thereafter.
- The left carpal swelling resolved overnight on the first night of hospitalisation and was not seen to recur; a presumptive diagnosis of resolving haemarthrosis due to secondary haemostatic defect was made.
- Haematology and PT/APTT the day following admission was:

Parameter	Value	Units	Range
RBC	3.94	× 10¹²/l	(5.5–8.5)
Haemoglobin	10.0	g/dl	(12.0–18.0)
Haematocrit	0.30	l/l	(0.37–0.55)
Mean cell volume	75.5	fl	(60–77)
Mean cell haemoglobin concentration	33.6	g/dl	(30.0–38.0)
Mean cell haemoglobin	25.3	pg	(19.5–25.5)
Total white cell count	15.89	× 10⁹/l	(6.0–15.0)

(Continued)

Parameter	Value	Units	Range
Neutrophils	11.23	$\times 10^9/l$	(3.0–11.5)
Lymphocytes	2.04	$\times 10^9/l$	(1.0–4.8)
Monocytes	0.73	$\times 10^9/l$	(0.2–1.4)
Eosinophils	0.58	$\times 10^9/l$	(0.1–1.2)
Basophils	0.00	$\times 10^9/l$	(0.0–0.1)
Platelets	**134**	$\times 10^9/l$	(200–500)
Film comment:	White cell morphology: unremarkable		
	Red cell morphology: mild anisocytosis with moderate polychromasia		
	Platelet morphology: platelets are consistent with analyser count; no clumping seen		
Reticulocyte count 128.5	**128.5**	$\times 109/l$	(0–80)

Parameter	Value	Units	Range
Prothrombin time (PT)	8.5	seconds	(7.0–12.0)
Activated partial thromboplastin time (APTT)	19.5	seconds	(15.0–25.0)

- Biochemical evaluation of total bilirubin, hepatic transaminases and bile acids were within reference limits.
- The improvement in haematocrit and coagulation parameters may have been due to the blood transfusion alone and could not be taken as an indication that the therapeutic presumption of vitamin K antagonism was correct.
- Due to the possibility of DIC, and due to the finding of sublumbar pain, an ultrasound examination of the abdomen was undertaken (**Figure 8.3**). This demonstrated the following findings:

- Liver, spleen, kidney, adrenals, pancreas, bladder, GIT unremarkable.
- There is a tiny amount of free fluid in the peritoneal cavity, seen close to the bladder; however this is otherwise unremarkable. There is a similar tiny amount seen in the caudal pleural cavity.
- The retroperitoneal space is enlarged, particularly on the left, although a small amount of change is also seen on the right. There are a few areas with hypoechoic fluidy material spreading between the fascial planes, but this is mostly solid echogenic material, similar in echogenicity to the spleen, which does not 'swirl' or have any Doppler signal.

Conclusions

- No parenchymal/viscous abnormality was identified.
- Abnormal retroperitoneal space – enlarged with solid looking tissue conforming around the left kidney approximately 5 cm x 3 cm x 2.5 cm – ddx haemorrhage (with clotting, although this is not a typical appearance of a resolving/organising haematoma) versus solid tissue of another cause, ddx neoplastic or inflammatory tissue.

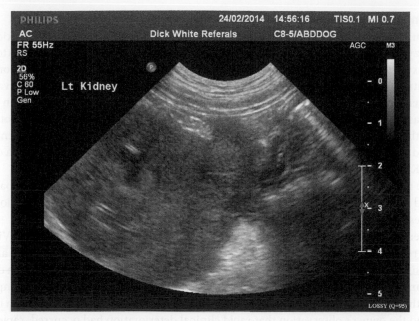

Figure 8.3 Ultrasound examination of retroperitoneal space on the second day of admission showing tissue mass conforming around the left kidney.

- Collection of ultrasound-guided fine needle aspiration cytology from the conforming soft tissue was considered. However, in the light of clinical improvement and a strong possibility that this might simply represent a resolving area of previous haemorrhage, it was decided to defer sampling until this was proven to be persistent on a stage ultrasound scan after 48 hours. At this scan was reported:

- The retroperitoneal space contains a small amount of anechoic fluid, as well as heterogeneous hyperechoic fat.
- A small pocket of cellular fluid remains visible adjacent to the caudal pole of the left kidney (1.5 cm x 1.5cm).

Conclusion
- Resolving retroperitoneal haemorrhage.

- Continuing to make a full clinical recovery, the dog was maintained on oral vitamin K1 therapy at 2.5 mg/kg p/o SID.
- A complete blood count, assessment of serum proteins and PT/APTT after a further 48 hours demonstrated all findings to be within reference limits and the patient was discharged home to continue with oral vitamin K1 for a further 4 weeks.
- HCt and PT/APTT were assessed after a further week, and again 48 hours after discontinuation of oral vitamin K1 therapy, and were found to be normal at each time-point.
- Vitamin K levels were mildly reduced and vitamin K epoxide mildly increased, findings consistent with vitamin K antagonism. Mass spectrometry for warfarin derivatives was negative.

Discussion

Hydroxycoumarin rodenticides (warfarin derivatives) act by inhibiting vitamin K epoxide reductase, an enzyme that recycles vitamin K production from vitamin K epoxide. The latter results from carboxylation of glutamyl residues of certain anticoagulant serine proteases (factors II, VII, IX, X) by vitamin K to form their active form. The result of this inhibition is lack of activated anticoagulant serine proteases. Since, of these, factor VII has the shortest half-life (6 hours in the dog), laboratory assessment most commonly demonstrates an initial prolongation in the prothrombin time since this assesses the extrinsic pathway, though in most cases by the time of identification both PT and APTT are prolonged. Prolongation of APTT with normal PT would make a diagnosis of vitamin K antagonism unlikely.

In acute rodenticide poisoning, induction of emesis and provision of charcoal adsorbant would be indicated but given that clinical exposure had likely occurred in excess of 48 hours prior to presentation these measures would not have been helpful.

The severity of the anaemia was felt to be enough to cause a haemic heart murmur. Vitamin-K antagonist rodenticide toxicity was strongly suspected though DIC, hepatic disease and *Angiostrongyliasis* could not be absolutely excluded. Thrombocytopenia has been reported in dogs with anticoagulant rodenticide toxicity (Lewis et al. 1997) and is thought to be due to consumption.

Due to the severity of the anaemia in this case, the physical examination findings of a high-output state and the owner's observation that rapid clinical deterioration had occurred, rapid decompensation was anticipated and blood-product treatment was given.

It would have also been a suitable choice to administer fresh frozen plasma and a DEA 1.1 positive packed red blood cell transfusion or fresh frozen plasma and bovine haemoglobin-glutamer (Oxyglobin) since both coagulation factors and oxygen carrying cells/haemoglobin-glutamer are clinically indicated. In a clinically stable patient in which further immediate deterioration was not anticipated, watchful regular reassessment after institution of vitamin K therapy would be an appropriate course of action, or administration of coagulation factors via plasma without haemoglobin transfusion.

Intracavitary and intraparenchymal bleeding and subsequent resolution can appear confusing and caution is urged when interpreting diagnostic imaging findings in patients with coagulopathy. In particular, the author has seen several cases where mural haemorrhage within the gastrointestinal tract and bladder has created an appearance on ultrasound indistinguishable from infiltrative mass lesions and serial evaluation for resolution is required to make this distinction. Haemarthroses, tracheal haemorrhage, haemoptysis and epistaxis are also commonly reported.

Vitamin K1 treatment is effective but the duration of treatment is dictated by the generation of hydroxycoumarin ingested. Treatment for 2 weeks is probably sufficient for first generation hydroxycoumarins, such as warfarin, dicoumarin and fumarin, but at least 4 weeks' therapy is recommended for second generation products, such as diphenacoum, brodifacoum and bromadiolone. It is recommended that prothrombin time is assessed 48 hours after discontinuation of therapy and if any prolongation is seen then treatment is reinstituted for a further month.

Where vitamin K antagonism has occurred, non-reduced vitamin K epoxide is expected to accumulate. Tests such as the PIVKA test (proteins induced by vitamin K absence or antagonism), which is really a variation of the PT test, have fallen out of favour and are not specific for vitamin K antagonism. In this case the lack of finding of warfarin derivatives on mass spectrometry was unexpected but might reflect the lapse of time since exposure, leading to levels waning to undetectable amounts.

Reference

Lewis, D.C., Bruyette, D.S., Kellerman, D.L. & Smith, S.A. (1997) Thrombocytopenia in dogs with anticoagulant rodenticide-induced hemorrhage: eight cases (1990–1995). *J Am Anim Hosp Assoc* **33**, 417–422

Further reading

DuVall, M.D., Murphy, M.J., Ray, A.C. & Reagor, J.C. (1989) Case studies on second-generation anticoagulant rodenticide toxicities in nontarget species. *J Vet Diagn Invest* **1**, 66–68

Petterino, C., Paolo, B. & Tristo, G. (2004) Clinical and pathological features of anticoagulant rodenticide intoxications in dogs. *Vet Hum Toxicol* **46**, 70–75

Sheafor, S.E. & Couto, C.G. (1999) Anticoagulant rodenticide toxicity in 21 dogs. *J Am Anim Hosp Assoc* **35**, 38–46

Waddell, L.S., Poppenga, R.H. & Drobatz, K.J. (2013) Anticoagulant rodenticide screening in dogs: 123 cases (1996–2003). *J Am Vet Med Assoc* **242**, 516–521

Clinical presentation

A 2 year-old female-neutered Labrador crossbreed (**Figure 9.1**) is presented for investigation of lameness and profound lethargy. The owner reports that in the last 2 weeks the dog has become progressively more 'stilted' in her gait and they have noticed lameness of the left forelimb, and both hindlimbs at different times. They feel that she is uncomfortable when trying to lie down and to stand, and seems increasingly reluctant to climb stairs. The dog has not travelled outside the United Kingdom.

Clinical examination demonstrates a bright dog in normal body condition. No abnormalities of hydration, pulse or respiratory rate or on cardiothoracic auscultation are noted and abdominal palpation is normal. Rectal temperature is elevated at 39.7 °C and joint effusions with some moderate pain on flexion is noted of both stifles and tarsi. Neurological examination is normal.

Questions

1. What is the problem list for this dog?
2. What are the differential diagnoses of multiple joint effusions in the dog?
3. How would you investigate this case further?

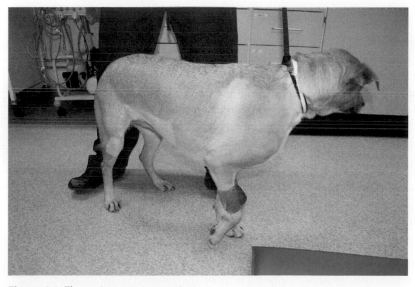

Figure 9.1 The patient at presentation.

Canine Internal Medicine: What's Your Diagnosis? First Edition. Jon Wray.
© 2018 John Wiley & Sons Ltd. Published 2018 by John Wiley & Sons Ltd.

Answers

1. What is the problem list for this dog?

An appropriate problem list might be:

- Shifting lameness
- Joint effusions (stifles, tarsi)
- Pyrexia
- Lethargy

2. What are the differential diagnoses for multiple joint effusions in the dog?

Polyarthropathies

Multiple joint effusions are most commonly detected in polyarthropathies, of which immune-mediated polyarthropathies predominate. Terminology may be confusing as in human arthrology, strictly speaking involvement of four or less joints is termed pauciarticular or oligoarticular and polyarthropathies involve five or more joints. In veterinary medicine polyarthropathy is usually accepted to mean pathology affecting multiple joints without well-defined criteria of how many are affected.

Joint effusions may also be seen due to traumatic injuries and septic arthritis though such disorders commonly affect just one joint (monoarticular). Exceptions may occur in dogs with a source of circulating bacteraemia, such as bacterial endocarditis and in puppies with omphalophlebitis that may sometimes develop multiple joint infections. Haemarthroses may occur in dogs with congenital or acquired disorders of secondary haemostasis.

Canine polyarthropathies are defined as being erosive or non-erosive and in order to distinguish between these radiographic assessment of joints needs to be performed (**Table 9.1**).

Rheumatoid factor (RF) and antinuclear antibodies (ANA)

Erosive polyarthropathies are very rare, accounting for <1% of canine polyarthropathies. Rheumatoid arthritis is rare and diagnostic criteria must be adhered to for secure diagnosis, which include the presence of erosive changes, a positive rheumatoid factor in serum, inflammatory joint fluid, extra-articular signs such as lymphadenomegaly and histological changes on synovial membrane biopsy. Similarly, systemic lupus erythematosus (SLE) is frequently overdiagnosed and strict diagnostic criteria of demonstration of polysystemic immune-mediated diseases associated with a positive antinuclear antibody (ANA) test needs to be performed. Note that ANA and RF antibodies are frequently present in patients with inflammatory disorders other than rheumatoid arthritis and systemic lupus erythematosus and the finding of positive serology results does not imply a diagnosis of these.

Table 9.1 Classification and differential diagnoses of polyarthropathies

Erosive polyarthropathies	Rheumatoid arthritis
	Felty's syndrome (rheumatoid arthritis, neutropenia and splenomegaly)
	Erosive polyarthritis of greyhounds
Non-erosive polyarthropathies	Immune-mediated polyarthritis
	• Type I (idiopathic/primary)
	• Type II (reactive/infection-associated)
	• Type III (gastrointestinal disease-associated)
	• Type IV (neoplasia-associated)
	Polyarthritis associated with arthropathic systemic infections
	• *Borrelia burgdorferi* (Lyme disease)
	• *Leishmania infantum**
	• Canine monocytotropic Ehrlichiosis (*Ehrlichia canis*)*
	• Canine granulocytotropic Ehrlichiosis (*Ehrlichia ewingii*)*
	• Canine granulocytotropic anaplasmosis (*Anaplasma phagocytophilum*)
	• Bartonellosis
	• *Mycoplasma* spp.
	• Bacterial polyarthritis secondary to valvular endocarditis
	Associated with multi-systemic immune-mediated disease
	• Systemic lupus erythematosus
	• Polyarthritis/polymyositis syndrome
	• Steroid-responsive meningitis-arteritis/immune-mediated polyarthritis syndrome
	Drug and vaccine associated, especially Trimethoprim-sulphonamide in Dobermann pinschers
	Miscellaneous and breed-associated polyarthropathies
	• Juvenile polyarthropathy of Akitas
	• Shar-pei fever
	• Polyarteritis nodosa

*Not known to be endemic in the United Kingdom.

3. How would you investigate this case further?

- Confirmation of multiple joint effusions and discrimination between erosive and non-erosive polyarthropathies by
  - Orthogonal radiographs of affected joints (with consideration to survey cavitary radiography at the same time).
  - Synoviocentesis of multiple joints.

Number of joints to sample

Conventionally at least three joints should be sampled and shown to demonstrate compatible cytological changes before a diagnosis of polyarthritis is made. It is important to note that development of erosive changes may be delayed for many days or even weeks after development of clinical signs. For a discussion of synoviocentesis technique see Johnson and Mackin (2012a, 2012b).

- Diagnostic testing to exclude non-erosive systemic infectious arthropathies and immune-mediated polyarthropathy secondary to other systemic disease. Note that in the United Kingdom where infectious causes are relatively rare, such investigation may be costly and of relatively low diagnostic yield and it is sensible to warn pet owners of this in advance. Worldwide prevalence of infectious causes may differ from country to country and application of local knowledge of infectious diseases is recommended. Investigation might include:
  ○ Assessment of haematology, biochemistry and urinalysis. Note that hyperglobulinaemia with concurrent acute-phase decrease in serum albumin is common in most inflammatory disorders. Dogs with immune-mediated polyarthritis very frequently have evidence of concurrent protein-losing nephropathy and this is presumably due to glomerulonephropathy secondary to immune-complex deposition. Resolution is often seen with therapy of the underlying condition in the authors' experience (though should not be presumed, and convalescent re-assessment of this is advised).
  ○ Serological testing/PCR for
    - *Borrelia burgdorferi*
    - *E.canis*
    - *A.phagocytophilum*
    - *Bartonella* spp.
  ○ Assessment of serum antinuclear antibodies (ANA) if non-erosive and rheumatoid factor (RF) if erosive polyarthropathy but see caveat above that positive titres of both of these are very frequently seen in animals with a variety of inflammatory disorders.
  ○ Consider survey radiographs of the thorax and abdomen and abdominal ultrasound examination. Although most cases of polyarthritis in the UK are primary immune-mediated polyarthritis (IMPA), IMPA secondary to focal or generalised inflammatory or neoplastic lesions or primary gastrointestinal pathology occurs uncommonly. Whilst typically dogs with endocarditis will have heart murmurs detectable on presentation, in one study of 71 dogs with endocarditis a heart murmur was detected in only 41 of these and it is sensible to evaluate the heart valves by echocardiography, if possible, in dogs with fever and shifting lameness.

Joint fluid analysis

Synoviocentesis samples should be assessed for gross appearance, viscosity, cell count, cytology and protein. Normal cell counts are historically reported as <3000/μl, though most recent consensus uses <1000/μl to be normal and protein 20–45 g/l. The predominant cell types in normal joints should be lymphocytes and mononuclear cells, with immune-mediated and septic inflammation causing marked elevations in cell counts with >12% of those cells being neutrophils. The neutrophil morphology (non-degenerate in immune-mediated conditions versus degenerate in septic arthritis) may be helpful to differentiate these conditions.

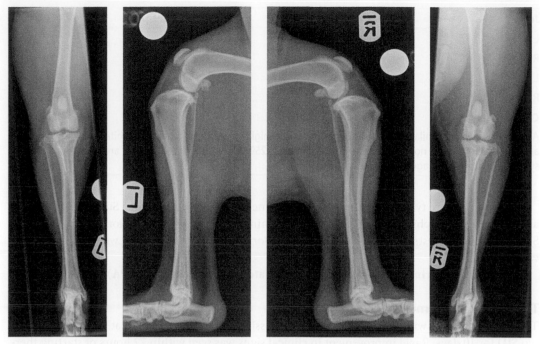

Figure 9.2 (left to right) Cranial-caudal left stifle and tarsal joint, lateral left stifle and tarsal joint, lateral right stifle and tarsal joint, cranial-caudal right stifle and tarsal joint.

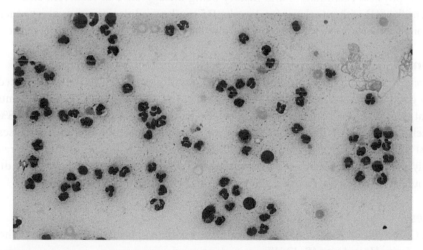

Figure 9.3 Photomicrograph of synoviocentesis sample from the patient (Wright-Giemsa ×50).

Diagnosis

In this case joint radiographs demonstrated multiple joint effusions without erosive changes present (**Figure 9.2**).

Haematology and biochemistry were normal and urinalysis demonstrated no proteinuria. Multiple synoviocentesis samples were taken and a representative photomicrograph is displayed (**Figure 9.3**) along with results summarised below.

Joint	Gross appearance	White cell count/µl	Protein
L elbow	Cloudy pink	17 780	55
R elbow	Cloudy pink	1123	56
L stifle	Cloudy pink	5800	55
R stifle	Cloudy pink	12 280	57

Cytology

All samples showed similar appearance of moderately to highly increased numbers of white cells, of which approximately 75% are non-degenerate neutrophils with 25% mononuclear cells (which are a mixture of synoviocytes, macrophages and lymphocytes).

These results are typical of a non-erosive immune-mediated polyarthritis. Survey thoracic and abdominal radiographs were normal and an abdominal ultrasound examination was also normal. Serology and PCR tests for *Ehrlichia*, *Anaplasma*, *Borrelia* and *Bartonella* spp. were negative. ANA was negative.

A diagnosis of **primary (type I) immune-mediated polyarthritis (1° IMPA)** was made.

Treatment/outcome

The dog was treated with an initial immunosuppressive dose of prednisolone at a dose of 2 mg/kg p/o SID for 10 days. Rapid improvement in clinical signs was seen within 72 hours of starting therapy and lameness resolved completely. On re-examination after a further week, joint effusions had resolved and the prednisolone dosage was subsequently gradually reduced by 25% every 3 weeks contingent on physical examination and history being unsuggestive of recurrent effusion. After a dose of 0.5 mg/kg SID without relapse for 3 weeks, 0.5 mg/kg prednisolone once every other day was instituted for a further 2 months before discontinuation of therapy. No subsequent relapse was seen.

Discussion

The prognosis with most non-erosive polyarthritis caused by primary immune-mediated disease is generally good and in one study 56% of dogs were cured after a single course of immunomodulatory treatment and 13% relapsed but were subsequently cured. In the same study 18% of dogs required lifelong therapy. In the author's experience, as in most immune-mediated diseases, relapse occurs most commonly when the veterinary surgeon or owner reduces immunosuppression too precipitously, and both impatience and over-reaction to side effects due to lack of careful discussion of these should be assiduously guarded against.

References

Johnson, K.C. & Mackin, A. (2012a) Canine immune-mediated polyarthritis: Part 1: Pathophysiology. *J Am Anim Hosp Assoc* **48**, 12–17

Johnson, K.C. & Mackin, A. (2012b) Canine immune-mediated polyarthritis: Part 2: Diagnosis and treatment. *J Am Anim Hosp Assoc* **48**, 71–82

Further reading

Clements, D.N., Gear, R.N., Tattersall, J., Carmichael, S. & Bennett, D. (2004) Type I immune-mediated polyarthritis in dogs: 39 cases (1997–2002). *J Am Vet Med Assoc* **224**, 1323–1327

Dunn, K.J. & Dunn, J.K. (1998) Diagnostic investigations in 101 dogs with pyrexia of unknown origin. *J Small Anim Pract* **39**, 574–580

Hepatobiliary Disease

Canine Internal Medicine: What's Your Diagnosis? First Edition. Jon Wray.
© 2018 John Wiley & Sons Ltd. Published 2018 by John Wiley & Sons Ltd.

Clinical presentation

A 10 year-old male-neutered Shetland Sheepdog (**Figure 10.1**) weighing 10.8 kg is presented for investigation of frequent episodes of what appear to be transient abdominal pain over the last month. The owner reports that the dog will refuse to eat for up to 48 hours at a time and during this period appears to stretch frequently and adopt a 'prayer' position. The dog also appears to be uncomfortable lying down during these episodes. No ataxia or proprioceptive loss has been noted and vomiting and diarrhoea have not been features. The dog has previously been treated with glucocorticoids (methylprednisolone 2 mg p/o every other day) for the past year for pruritic skin disease considered to be atopic dermatitis.

On physical examination the dog is bright and in a somewhat overweight body condition (body condition score 3.5/5). Heart rate is 96/min with normal rhythm, respiratory rate is 24/min with normal effort and rectal temperature is 38.9 °C. Mucous membranes are pink, moist and with a normal capillary refill of <2 seconds. Thoracic auscultation is normal. Abdominal palpation yields intermittent guarding/boarding of the abdominal musculature on palpation of the cranioventral abdomen. Remaining examination is normal.

Pancreatitis is suspected and a haematology, biochemistry and canine specific PLI sample is assessed and an abdominal ultrasound performed.

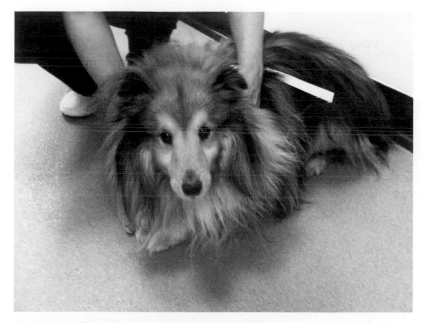

Figure 10.1 The patient at presentation.

Canine Internal Medicine: What's Your Diagnosis? First Edition. Jon Wray.
© 2018 John Wiley & Sons Ltd. Published 2018 by John Wiley & Sons Ltd.

Haematology

Parameter	Value	Units	Range
RBC	**5.14**	× 10^{12}/l	(5.5–8.5)
Haemoglobin	**11.9**	g/dl	(12.0–18.0)
Haematocrit	**0.35**	l/l	(0.37–0.55)
Mean cell volume	67.9	fl	(60–77)
Mean cell haemoglobin Conc	34.1	g/dl	(30.0–38.0)
Mean cell haemoglobin	23.1	pg	(19.5–25.5)
Total white cell count	**16.91**	× 10^9/l	(6.0–15.0)
Neutrophils	**15.6**	× 10^9/l	(3.0–11.5)
Lymphocytes	**0.85**	× 10^9/l	(1.0–4.8)
Monocytes	0.43	× 10^9/l	(0.2–1.4)
Eosinophils	**0.03**	× 10^9/l	(0.1–1.2)
Basophils	0.0	× 10^9/l	(0.0–0.1)
Platelets	332	× 10^9/l	(200–500)
Film comment:		No abnormalities detected	

Biochemistry

Parameter	Value	Units	Range
Total protein	54	g/l	(54–77)
Albumin	25	g/l	(25–40)
Globulin	29	g/l	(23–45)
Urea	4.9	mmol/l	(2.5–7.4)
Creatinine	81	µmol/l	(40–145)
Potassium	5.4	mmol/l	(3.4–5.6)
Sodium	145	mmol/l	(139–154)
Chloride	105	mmol/l	(105–122)
Calcium	2.4	mmol/l	(2.1–2.8)
Magnesium	0.76	mmol/l	(0.62–0.90)
Inorganic phosphate	1.2	mmol/l	(0.60–1.40)
Glucose	5.5	mmol/l	(3.3–5.8)
ALT	62	IU/l	(13–88)
AST	17	IU/l	(13–60)
ALKP	**835**	IU/l	(14–105)
GGT	4	IU/l	(0–10)
Bilirubin	2	µmol/l	(0–16)
Cholesterol	**9.9**	mmol/l	(3.8–7.0)

Parameter	Value	Units	Range
Triglyceride	**1.3**	mmol/l	(0.56–1.14)
Creatine kinase	114	IU/l	(0–190)
Amylase	819	IU/L	(400–1250)
Lipase	97	IU/L	(8–120)
Canine Spec PLI	309	µg/l	<200 normal, >400 consistent with pancreatitis

On ultrasound examination the pancreas could be visualised well and had a normal appearance to the left limb, right limb and body. The gall bladder appeared abnormal and a representative still image is shown in **Figure 10.2**. The hyperechoic material within the gall bladder was not gravity-dependent and the appearance did not alter with position. Remaining ultrasound findings were normal and both adrenal glands were visualised and normal in size, shape and echotexture.

Questions

1. What is the abnormality shown in Figure 10.2?
2. What is(are) the mechanism(s) by which this abnormality may develop and what may have led to the abnormality in this case?
3. Do the clinical findings explain the given medical history? What therapy would you recommend?

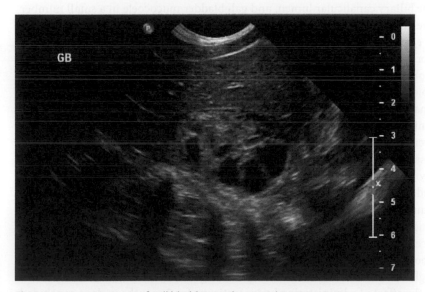

Figure 10.2 Appearance of gall bladder on ultrasound examination.

Answers

1. What is the abnormality shown in Figure 10.2?

The ultrasonographic appearance has all the hallmarks of a gall bladder mucocoele. Classically these are characterised by granular, hyperechoic and centralised non-gravity-dependent gall bladder contents, which do not change with agitation or patient position. Mucocoeles often have what is described as a 'stellate' (as here) or 'kiwi-fruit' appearance (reviewed by Besso et al. 2000).

Gall bladder mucocoele is a pathological accumulation of inspissated bile and/or mucus in the distended gallbladder and is commonly accompanied by cystic mucosal hyperplasia of the gall bladder wall.

2. What is(are) the mechanism(s) by which this abnormality may develop and what may have led to the abnormality in this case?

Essentially the cause of gallbladder mucocoele is incompletely understood. Inspissation of material within the gall bladder may result from incomplete gall bladder emptying and although cystic mucosal hyperplasia of the gall bladder wall is commonly detected histopathologically it is not known whether this is causal or simply an epiphenomenon. A breed predisposition has been reported in Shetland sheepdogs and also in Miniature Schnauzers, Pomeranians and Cocker Spaniels. Presence of hyperlipidaemia is associated with an increased odds ratio of nearly 3 for developing mucocoele (Kutsonai et al. 2014) and mucocoele is frequently diagnosed in animals with concurrent disease, especially endocrinopathies. The odds of mucocoele in dogs with hyperadrenocorticism are 29 times those without hyperadrenocorticism and an increased risk in patients with hypothyroidism but not diabetes mellitus is reported (Mesich et al. 2009). An initial association was reported between mutations in the ABCB4 gene, which encodes for a membrane phospholipid transporter and is integral to transport of phophatidyl choline from the hepatocyte to the biliary canalicular lumen, and gall bladder mucocoele in a small number of dogs, but the same group has since, with a larger cohort of dogs and in contrast, reported no association (Mealey et al. 2010; Cullen et al. 2014). A proportion of dogs with gall bladder mucocoele have been reported to have concurrent bacterial cholecystitis, though again whether this is cause or effect of cholestasis is unknown.

In this patient biochemical findings include a hyperlipidaemia and isolated elevation in ALKP and the haematology demonstrates a leukogram of stress or glucocorticoid excess. A familial hyperlipidaemia has been reported in the Shetland Sheepdog breed (Sato et al. 2000; Mori et al. 2000) but hyperlipidaemia is commonly also seen in endocrinopathies and in iatrogenic glucocorticoid excess. Pancreatitis may also cause hyperlipidaemia and though there is overlap in the clinical symptomology of pancreatitis and gall bladder mucocoele, and pancreatitis should not be excluded as a possibility on the basis of diagnostic tests since the sensitivity of serum amylase, serum DGGR lipase, canine specific PLI and pancreatic ultrasound is less than 100%; nonetheless, neither is there any supportive evidence for pancreatitis in this patient. This patient has been receiving methylprednisolone chronically and such administration might be expected to cause both hyperlipidaemia and hyperphosphatasaemia. Whilst it is not known whether iatrogenic glucocorticoid excess is a risk factor for gall bladder mucocoele formation, one study assessing the effect of administering hydrocortisone for 3 months in dogs concluded that this neither led to an increased rate of formation of ultrasonographically detectable gall bladder 'sludge' nor in composition of constituents of bile commonly implicated in gall bladder 'sludge' formation.

Comorbidities in mucocoele patients

It is prudent in animals with gall bladder mucocoele to

- Assess for the presence of hyperlipidaemia and if detected to explore diagnostically the possibilities of
  - Hypothyroidism
  - Hyperadrenocorticism
  - Diabetes mellitus
  - Pancreatitis
  - Protein-losing nephropathy
  - Cholestasis
- Consider entities that may result in biliary stasis
- Consider concurrent bacterial cholecystitis

In this patient, because exogenous glucocorticoids have been given for some time, assessment for naturally occurring hyperadrenocorticism is likely to be severely limited (though the normal appearance to both adrenal glands makes a functional adrenal gland tumour extremely unlikely).

3. Do the clinical findings explain the given medical history? What therapy would you recommend?

(Apparent) abdominal pain is a common clinical presentation in internal medicine and the causes can be many and varied. A typical differential diagnosis is shown in **Table 10.1**. Note that thoracolumbar spinal pain is commonly misidentified as abdominal pain and careful spinal palpation and neurological examination should be performed in all patients with apparent abdominal pain.

Anorexia and abdominal pain are commonly reported in case series of dogs with gall bladder mucocoele and in a total of 112 dogs described in five case series, approximately 45% presented with abdominal pain and 53% with anorexia (see References and Further reading). Vomiting and jaundice are also commonly reported. However, gall bladder mucocoele is often also detected as an incidental finding during abdominal ultrasound evaluation and assessment of the significance of it can also be confounded by the presence of other diseases that may cause abdominal pain, especially pancreatitis. Furthermore, unexplained rises in cholestatic liver enzymes, which may be strongly associated with the presence of gall bladder mucocoele, are also commonly seen in many disorders concurrently diagnosed with it, such as hyperadrenocorticism and pancreatitis.

Therapy may be medical or surgical. Traditionally surgery (cholecystectomy) has been recommended, primarily based on the risk of gall bladder rupture and subsequent peritonitis. The impact of peritonitis due to gall bladder rupture is enormously variable, ranging from focal sterile bile peritonitis, which is quickly contained spontaneously by local adhesion formation (and patients are seen infrequently in which at the time of celiotomy for other problems, the gall bladder fossa is found to contain no gall bladder but focal adhesions from a historical gall bladder rupture), to fulminant bacterial peritonitis primarily in those cases in which concurrent bacterial cholecystitis exists. However, one study showed no association between the presence of

Table 10.1 Differential diagnosis of abdominal pain

Differential diagnosis of abdominal pain

D (Degenerative)

- Spinal pain due to intervertebral disc disease mimicking abdominal pain

A (Anomalous, Anatomical)

- Gastrointestinal foreign body, intussusception
- Obstructive cholelithiasis
- Torsion of
  - Liver lobes
  - Spleen
  - Mesentery
  - Colon
- Gastrointestinal ileus (structural or functional)
- Upper and lower urinary tract obstruction especially due to urolithiasis

M (Metabolic)

- Hypoadrenocorticism

N (Neoplastic, Nutritional)

- Intra-abdominal neoplasia, especially carcinomatosis, mast cell tumour
- Dietary indiscretion, dietary intolerance

I (Infectious, Inflammatory, Immune-mediated)

- Pancreatitis
- Pansteatitis
- Cholecystitis
- Gall bladder mucocoele
- Gastritis
- Enteritis
- Colitis
- Necrosis, ulceration, rupture or perforation of the gastrointestinal tract
- Peritonitis
- Abscessation of the liver, pancreas, spleen, mesentery or kidneys

T (Traumatic, Toxic)

- Gastrointestinal irritant toxin ingestion

V (Vascular)

Thrombosis of

- Mesenteric vessels
- Portal vein
- Hepatic vessels

positive bile culture in cases of gall bladder rupture and survival. Approximately 3–12% of bacterial cultures of bile or gall bladder wall taken from dogs with gall bladder mucocoele are positive (Pike et al. 2004; Worley et al. 2004; Crews et al. 2009; Malek et al. 2013). Between 16% and 47% of dogs with gall bladder mucocoele explored surgically have been reported to have gall bladder rupture found at celiotomy and up to 50% of patients have been found to have focal peritonitis adjacent to the gall bladder (Pike et al. 2004; Worley et al. 2004; Crews et al. 2009; Malek at al. 2013). The sensitivity of abdominal ultrasound, even when performed by experienced diagnostic imaging specialists, in determining that gall bladder rupture has occurred is disappointing and reported between 20% and 86%. Thus it could be argued that surgical intervention should be perhaps considered 'sooner rather than later' upon identification of a gall bladder mucocoele and should not necessarily be precluded by negative findings (other than that of mucocoele) on ultrasound evaluation. The perioperative mortality rate for dogs with gall bladder mucocoele has been variably reported between 7% and 31% in dogs with mucocoele and in dogs with gall bladder disease including mucocoele with no apparent difference in mortality between patients with and without mucocoele, rupture or positive culture results (Pike et al. 2004; Worley et al. 2004; Crews et al. 2009; Malek et al. 2013). Reported contributory factors to mortality include pancreatitis, cholangitis, thromboembolic disease, peritonitis and hypotension.

Successful resolution of gall bladder mucocoele with medical therapy comprising ursodeoxycholic acid and thyroid hormone supplementation in hypothyroid dogs has been reported in a limited number of cases (Walter et al. 2008) and, given the not-insignificant peri-operative mortality rates reported with cholecystectomy, non-surgical management may be considered on a case-by-case basis (though it is prudent to keep any decision not to perform surgery constantly under very proactive review).

In this patient, the lack of convincing explanations for the presenting clinical signs of anorexia and abdominal pain other than the gall bladder mucocoele might dictate that surgical intervention is appropriate.

Diagnosis

In this patient assessment of thyroid status by measurement of total T4 and serum TSH was normal and measurement of the urine protein:creatinine ratio was also normal. A prothrombin time and activated partial thromboplastin time were performed in anticipation of surgical exploration and were normal.

An exploratory celiotomy was performed and the gall bladder found to be turgid and non-compressible (**Figure 10.3**).

The pancreas was found to be normal in appearance, with the liver enlarged with rounded edges and a somewhat pale and friable appearance/texture. Both adrenal glands were inspected and were grossly normal. A cholecystectomy was performed and liver biopsies obtained. The gall bladder was sectioned; bile was submitted for cytology and the bile and gall bladder wall were submitted for an aerobic/anaerobic culture (which were negative). Histopathology of the gall bladder demonstrated abundant luminal inspissated mucinous material with large amounts of bright yellow granular pigment. The lining epithelium was thrown into numerous variably tall thin folds and occasionally formed dilated cystic structures, supported by small amounts of collagenous stroma. These cystic structures surrounded aggregates of mucin. The lining epithelium was well organised, tall columnar with extensive vacuolation of the cytoplasm. Scattered lymphocytes and plasma cells were present within the lamina propria. The liver biopsies demonstrated well-organised hepatic parenchyma with marked diffuse cloudy swelling of the hepatocytes and mild biliary hyperplasia. Scant evidence of any inflammation was present and subsequent periodic acid schiff (PAS) staining confirmed the accumulation of large amounts of glycogen.

The dog recovered uneventfully from surgery and clinical signs resolved. It was considered possible that the isolated hyperphosphatasaemia, hepatic glycogen accumulation and hyperlipidaemia might be due to naturally occurring pituitary-dependent hyperadrenocorticism or due to

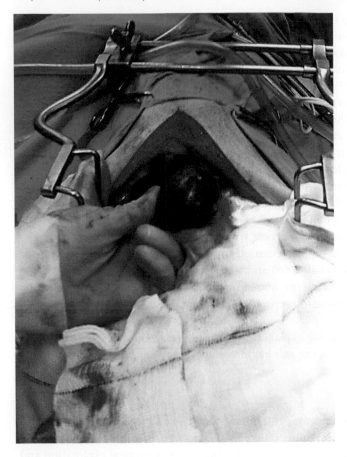

Figure 10.3 Intraoperative picture with exteriorisation of a turgid gall bladder.

the combined effects of gall bladder mucocoele and chronic methylprednisolone administration. Serial monitoring of the ALKP was therefore undertaken after discontinuation of the methylprednisolone and control of the atopy with ciclosporin and this was found to return to normal over a 3 month period, suggesting that this was not due to hyperadrenocorticism.

Discussion

Gall bladder mucocoele is an increasingly commonly recognised clinical entity in canine practice and this may be due to a combination of increased availability, resolution and clinical experience with ultrasound, as well as an increased awareness of the condition. Care needs to be taken not to overinterpret results of hepatobiliary ultrasound examination, as the presence of biliary sludge within the gall bladder as well as large numbers of anatomical variants, which may conspire to confuse the inexperienced/occasional ultrasonographer, is often confused with gall bladder mucocoele. Decision making as to the correct course of action in treating mucocoele can be difficult as even in the hands of experienced professional surgical specialists, peri-operative morbidity and mortality can be significant and any surgery must be undertaken with a clear understanding and communication of these risks. Nonetheless, the high rate of gall bladder rupture, which may not always be ultrasonographically apparent, has led to the common recommendation for cholecystectomy to be performed in the majority of cases.

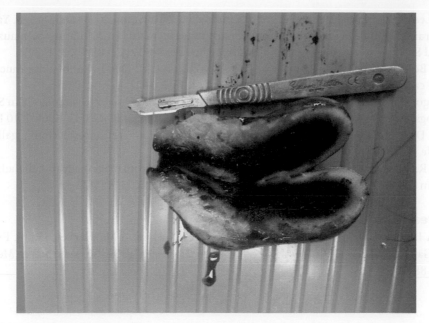

Figure 10.4 Gall bladder mucocoele after surgical removal. Note the relatively well-organised inspissated contents. Courtesy of Jackie Demetriou.

The aetiopathogenesis of this interesting condition has yet to be fully elucidated and it is striking the variation in spectrum of disease severity of the gall bladder in these patients. In some a turgid and pathologically 'quiet' gall bladder (see **Figure 10.4**) is found; in others extensive gall bladder wall necrosis and rupture quickly develops and the difference between these ultrasonographically is not always distinct.

References

Besso, J.G., Wrigley, R.H., Gliatto, J.M. & Webster, C.R. (2000) Ultrasonographic appearance and clinical findings in 14 dogs with gallbladder mucocele. *Vet Radiol Ultrasound* **41**, 261–271

Crews, L.J., Feeney, D.A., Jessen, C.R., Rose, N.D. & Matise, I. (2009) Clinical, ultrasonographic, and laboratory findings associated with gallbladder disease and rupture in dogs: 45 cases (1997–2007). *J Am Vet Med Assoc* **234**, 359–366

Cullen, J.M., Willson, C.J., Minch, J.D., Kimbrough, C.L. & Mealey, K.L. (2014) Lack of association of ABCB4 insertion mutation with gallbladder mucoceles in dogs. *J Vet Diagn Invest* **26**, 434–436

Kutsunai, M., Kanemoto, H., Fukushima, K., Fujino, Y., Ohno, K. & Tsujimoto, H. (2014) The association between gall bladder mucoceles and hyperlipidaemia in dogs: a retrospective case control study. *Vet J* **199**, 76–79

Malek, S., Sinclair, E., Hosgood, G., Moens, N.M., Baily, T. & Boston, S.E. (2013) Clinical findings and prognostic factors for dogs undergoing cholecystectomy for gall bladder mucocele. *Vet Surg* **42**, 418–426

Mealey, K.L., Minch, J.D., White, S.N., Snekvik, K.R. & Mattoon, J.S. (2010) An insertion mutation in ABCB4 is associated with gallbladder mucocele formation in dogs. *Comp Hepatol* **9**, 6

Mesich, M.L., Mayhew, P.D., Paek, M., Holt, D.E. & Brown, D.C. (2009) Gall bladder mucoceles and their association with endocrinopathies in dogs: a retrospective case-control study. *J Small Anim Pract* **50**, 630–635

Mori, N., Lee, P., Muranaka, S., Sagara, F., Takemitsu, H., Nishiyama, Y., Yamamoto, I., Yagishita, M. & Arai, T. (2010) Predisposition for primary hyperlipidemia in Miniature Schnauzers and Shetland Sheepdogs as compared to other canine breeds. *Res Vet Sci* **88** (3), 394–399

Pike, F.S., Berg, J., King, N.W., Penninck, D.G. & Webster, C.R. (2004) Gallbladder mucocele in dogs: 30 cases (2000–2002). *J Am Vet Med Assoc* **224**, 1615–1622

Sato, K., Agoh, H., Kaneshige, T., Hikasa, Y. & Kagota, K. (2000) Hypercholesterolemia in Shetland Sheepdogs. *J Vet Med Sci* **62** (12), 1297–1301. doi: 10.1016/j.rvsc.2009.12.003. Epub 2010 Jan 12

Walter, R., Dunn, M.E., d'Anjou, M.A. & Lecuyer, M. (2008) Nonsurgical resolution of gallbladder mucocele in two dogs. *J Am Vet Med Assoc* **232**, 1688–1693

Worley, D.R., Hottinger, H.A. & Lawrence, H.J. (2004) Surgical management of gallbladder mucoceles in dogs: 22 cases (1999–2003). *J Am Vet Med Assoc* **225**, 1418–1422

Further reading

Aguirre, A.L., Center, S.A., Randolph, J.F., Yeager, A.E., Keegan, A.M., Harvey, H.J. & Erb, H.N. (2007) Gallbladder disease in Shetland Sheepdogs: 38 cases (1995–2005). *J Am Vet Med Assoc* **231**, 79–88

Clinical presentation

A 4-year-old male-neutered Wirehaired Fox Terrier weighing 7.7 kg (**Figure 11.1**) is presented with a recent history of dullness, mental confusion and aimless wandering. He has previously been diagnosed with a congenital cerebellar ataxia and has always had a hypermetric gait in all four limbs. The owners also report that he has suffered from intermittent and self-limiting but frequent (once monthly) gastrointestinal upsets comprising vomiting and small intestinal diarrhoea. These have always resolved with symptomatic management of starvation and a bland diet.

Four weeks ago they introduced another dog into the household and fed both the dogs a new diet, which is a complete wet maintenance diet for adult dogs; the new dog is healthy.

In the last four days the owners have noted that the Wirehaired Fox Terrier has become progressively dull, sleepy and at times difficult to rouse and has taken to aimlessly wandering about the house with his head down and nose nearly touching the ground. Frequently they have found him appearing 'glazed' and staring into space.

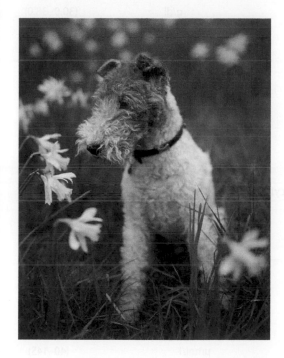

Figure 11.1 The patient (owner's photograph).

Canine Internal Medicine: What's Your Diagnosis? First Edition. Jon Wray.
© 2018 John Wiley & Sons Ltd. Published 2018 by John Wiley & Sons Ltd.

Physical examination demonstrates a very quiet dog in normal body condition. The dog is interactive when stimulated but the remaining time appears dull and disinterested but is standing and ambulatory. Mucous membrane colour, capillary refill and hydration are normal. Heart rate is 92/min with equal and synchronous pulses of normal quality, respiratory rate is 16/min and rectal temperature 38.4 °C. No abnormalities are detected on thoracic auscultation, abdominal palpation, evaluation of the skin and external lymph nodes. When walking the dog has a hypermetric gait, which is symmetrical and worse in the forelimbs than the hindlimbs; this is reported always to have been present since he was a puppy by the owners.

A haematology and biochemistry sample were taken and the following results obtained:

Haematology

Parameter	Value	Units	Range
RBC	14.2	$\times 10^{12}/l$	(5.5–8.5)
Haemoglobin	7.64	g/dl	(12.0–18.0)
Haematocrit	0.41	l/l	(0.37–0.55)
Mean cell volume	**54**	fl	(60–77)
Mean cell haemoglobin Conc	34.4	g/dl	(30.0–38.0)
Mean cell haemoglobin	**18.6**	pg	(19.5–25.5)
Total white cell count	10.18	$\times 10^{9}/l$	(6.0–15.0)
Neutrophils	6.88	$\times 10^{9}/l$	(3.0–11.5)
Lymphocytes	2.78	$\times 10^{9}/l$	(1.0–4.8)
Monocytes	0.4	$\times 10^{9}/l$	(0.2–1.4)
Eosinophils	0.1	$\times 10^{9}/l$	(0.1–1.2)
Basophils	0.02	$\times 10^{9}/l$	(0.0–0.1)
Platelets	224	$\times 10^{9}/l$	(200–500)
Film comment:	A microcytosis is present on the blood film		

Biochemistry

Parameter	Value	Units	Range
Total protein	50	g/l	(54–77)
Albumin	**22**	g/l	(25–40)
Globulin	28	g/l	(23–45)
Urea	**2.4**	mmol/l	(2.5–7.4)
Creatinine	74	µmol/l	(40–145)
Potassium	4.5	mmol/l	(3.4–5.6)
Sodium	147	mmol/l	(139–154)
Chloride	118	mmol/l	(105–122)
Calcium	2.4	mmol/l	(2.1–2.8)
Magnesium	0.79	mmol/l	(0.62–0.90)
Inorganic phosphate	1.2	mmol/l	(0.60–1.40)

Parameter	Value	Units	Range
Glucose	5.5	mmol/l	(3.3–5.8)
ALT	**169**	IU/l	(13–88)
AST	**126**	IU/l	(13–60)
ALKP	77	IU/l	(14–105)
GGT	3	IU/l	(0–10)
Bilirubin	5	µmol/l	(0–16)
Cholesterol	**3.5**	mmol/l	(3.8–7.0)
Triglyceride	0.58	mmol/l	(0.56–1.14)
Creatine kinase	112	IU/l	(0–190)

Questions

1. Interpret the laboratory findings. How are these likely to relate to the dog's clinical signs?
2. What diagnostic test is indicated next in this patient?
3. How can the principle diagnostic suspicion be verified in this dog?

Answers

1. Interpret the laboratory findings. How are these likely to relate to the dog's clinical signs?

- Haematology
  - Principle finding is microcytosis. Microcytosis may be seen in
    - Iron-deficient anaemia, especially resulting from external blood loss such as chronic gastrointestinal haemorrhage.
    - Portosystemic shunting.
    - Hepatic dysfunction.
    - As a breed-related finding in the Shiba Inu and Japanese Akita.
- Biochemistry
  - A mild hypoalbuminaemia is present. Common causes include
    - As a 'negative acute-phase' shift in presence of inflammatory conditions.
    - Protein-losing nephropathy.
    - Protein-losing enteropathy.
    - Hepatic dysfunction.
    - Portosystemic shunting.
    - Malabsorption.
    - Third-space loss.
  - Decrease in urea is present. This is an uncommon finding in dogs and causes include
    - Hepatic dysfunction.
    - Portosystemic shunting.
    - Glucosuria.
    - Central or nephrogenic diabetes insipidus.
    - Urea cycle enzyme deficiency (very rare).
  - Mild elevations (<3–4 times the upper reference interval) in ALT and AST are seen. ALT is an enzyme found in the hepatic cytosol and AST is found in hepatic cytosol and skeletal muscle. Both are generally elevated in the presence of hepatocellular damage but at low increases do not distinguish between primary hepatocellular injury and 'reactive' or 'secondary' hepatopathy.

- ◦ Hypocholesterolaemia is present, which may be seen in
  - Hepatic dysfunction.
  - Portosystemic shunting.
  - Protein-losing enteropathy.
  - Hypoadrenocorticism.

The dog presented here has exhibited changes in mentation. Specifically both the level of consciousness (difficulty in rousing) and the 'content' of the consciousness have been altered. This is suggestive of a diffuse forebrain problem (although an altered level of consciousness may also be seen in brainstem disorders) and, taken with the microcytosis and biochemical findings, may implicate hepatic encephalopathy due to impaired hepatic function, portosystemic shunting (either congenital or acquired) or a combination of these may be underlying.

The changes in hepatic transaminases are very modest, and although one should be wary that some dogs with fulminant hepatic failure and reduced functional hepatic mass may not have marked elevations in hepatic transaminases due to lack of cellular release of cytosolic enzymes, it is more common for dogs with portosystemic shunts to have minimal or no elevation in hepatic transaminases than it is for dogs with other severe generalised liver disease.

2. **What diagnostic test is indicated next in this patient?**

The most appropriate test would be to assess hepatic function in this patient. Remember that assessment of hepatic transaminases does not evaluate hepatic function.

Bear in mind that portosystemic shunting may be detected in adult dogs as well as in puppies and that it may be congenital or acquired, in the latter case multiple portosystemic collaterals usually arise secondary to development of portal hypertension.

Tests of liver function

Liver function may be assessed by

- Assessment of fasting bile acid.
- Assessment of a bile acid stimulation test.
- Assessment of fasting ammonia.
- Assessment of ammonia before and after stimulation, with either an oral ammonia tolerance test or by assessing pre- and post-prandial ammonia.
- Evaluation of analytes that are reduced as a result of hepatic dysfunction and so may offer corroborative evidence for hepatic dysfunction. These include
  - ◦ Albumin
  - ◦ Urea
  - ◦ Cholesterol
  - ◦ Glucose

However, note that it is very common for these last to be maintained within a reference interval even in the face of severe hepatic dysfunction and decrease may be seen only relatively late in the course of hepatic failure.

Of these, assessment of bile acids is most commonly performed; where ammonia is evaluated it is important to note that the analyte is unstable at room temperature and immediate cooling to 4 °C in an ice bath and analysis within 4 hours is recommended. Whilst a resting bile acid result that is very high is abnormal, the sensitivity of using bile acids to assess liver function is significantly enhanced by measuring serum bile acids after a 12 hour fast, then 2 hours after being fed a meal containing both fat and protein to stimulate gall bladder emptying.

In theory bile acid elevations are seen when there is

- Decreased bile acid clearance from portal blood due to
  ○ Diffuse hepatocellular disease resulting in loss of hepatic function.
  ○ Decreased functional hepatic mass.
  ○ Portosystemic venous shunting, either a congenital (usually single) or multiple acquired shunting vessels.
- Decreased bile acid excretion in bile due to
  ○ Obstructive cholestasis
    - Hepatic
    - Post-hepatic
  ○ Functional cholestasis (which is often sepsis-associated).

Problems with interpretation of serum bile acids

Commonly reported laboratory reference intervals are a value of up to approximately 15 μmol/l for fasting bile acids and up to 25 μmol/l for post-prandial bile acids. Studies have shown high sensitivity for bile acids in detecting hepatic dysfunction and portosystemic shunts and where a threshold of 25 μmol/l is used for a post-prandial sample, the reported specificity is high. However, clinical experience suggests that many animals that do not have identifiable hepatic disease or evidence of cholestasis or portosystemic shunting may have pre- and/or post-prandial bile acid levels that fall above the reference interval reported by many laboratories. Furthermore, many bench-top analysers report bile acids in a semi-quantitative way, with an upper limit of detection of approximately 30 μmol/l. There exists a substantial 'grey area' of bile acids, between about 25 and 70 μmol/l where many ill animals will fall and which, whilst abnormal compared with reference intervals, does not seem to correlate well with clinical findings of hepatic disease, cholestasis or portosystemic shunting. This is important to recognise as diagnostic tests (see below) to differentiate these may at least be associated with incurring additional expense for the owner and, in the cases of liver biopsy and portovenography, involve some risk of adverse consequences, including some that are potentially life-threatening for the patient. There is therefore somewhat of a 'disconnect' between the 'decision threshold' to take further diagnostic action based on diagnostic sensitivity when weighed up against clinical specificity and patient risk. For unclear reasons it seems to be common that clinicians strongly associated elevated bile acids with hepatic dysfunction and portosystemic shunting and less so with cholestasis, whilst the latter is a common feature of many hepatic and post-hepatic (especially pancreatitis) disorders that occur frequently in veterinary medicine. It is recommended that conscious effort is maintained to keep this in mind when evaluating bile acids in clinical patients.

The pattern of bile acid stimulation test can sometimes be helpful:

- Very high (100–400 µmol/l) pre- *and* post-prandial bile acid results are most commonly seen in the presence of portosystemic shunting, but are not specific for this and nor do they differentiate between congenital and acquired, single and multiple shunts.
- Moderately (70–150 µmol/l) raised pre- and post-prandial bile acids are commonly seen in hepatic dysfunction.
- A normal fasting bile acid and markedly abnormal (>70 µmol/l) post-prandial bile acid is seen very commonly in animals with portal vein hypoplasia/microvascular dysplasia.

Raised fasting ammonia levels are detected in fulminant hepatic failure but are most commonly detected in congenital or acquired portosystemic shunts. Note that Irish Wolfhound puppies develop a moderate hyperammonaemia at 6–7 weeks of age, which subsequently resolves; this is due to reduced urea cycle enzyme activity. The sensitivity of ammonia measurement can be increased by performing an ammonia measurement 2–6 hours after a meal (as for bile acid stimulation, but in some animals ammonia appears to take about 6 hours to peak) or by performing an 'ammonia tolerance test' (ATT). The ATT is more popular in some countries than others and involves the administration of ammonium chloride either orally (0.1 g/kg but no more than 2 ml/kg in 20–50 ml of water) or per-rectum (2 ml/kg of a 5% ammonium chloride solution) with samples collected for ammonia measurement before and 30 minutes after oral administration or 20 + 40 minutes after rectal administration. Hepatic encephalopathy may be precipitated by administration but appears rare and is reported to be more uncommon with rectal administration.

3. **How can the principle diagnostic suspicion be verified in this dog?**

Portosystemic shunting in dogs may be identified by diagnostic imaging tests, which demonstrate the presence of shunting of blood from portal to systemic circulation, which show good anatomical resolution for surgical planning, or both. Conventional radiography is not used to diagnose the presence or absence of portosystemic shunting but radiographic signs that may be supportive of congenital portosystemic shunts include small liver size, bilateral renomegaly and possibly the presence of urocystoliths (though bear in mind that ammonium urate uroliths have low radiodensity and may not be seen with conventional plain radiography). Most commonly used methods for portosystemic shunt identification include

- Abdominal vascular ultrasonography.
- Computed tomography (CT) angiography.
- Scintigraphy.
- Portovenography.

Advantages and disadvantages of each of these are listed in **Table 11.1**.

Additionally, transit of agitate saline injected into the splenic pulp and followed ultrasonographically may help determine portosystemic shunting if identified within the systemic circulation (since it should normally be removed by the hepatic microcirculation) and can, in some cases, provide additional anatomical detail.

Diagnosis

In this patient a bile acid stimulation test was performed and pre- and post-prandial bile acids were unequivocally elevated at 224 µmol/l and 341 µmol/l respectively.

Table 11.1 Comparison of different methods for diagnosing portosystemic shunts

Diagnostic test method	Advantages	Disadvantages
Abdominal vascular ultrasonography (**Figure 11.2**)	• Relatively inexpensive compared with other tests • Reasonably high sensitivity (dependent on level of experience of operator) • Large and anatomically simple shunts, and particularly left divisional intrahepatic portosystemic shunts can often be identified by relatively inexperienced individuals • Does not require anaesthesia or surgery • May provide anatomically useful information for surgical planning • Contemporaneous assessment of hepatic vascularity, size, concurrent pathology and presence of urolithiasis	• Detection is highly operator-dependent and extensive experience with vascular ultrasound is advantageous. False negative findings common with inexperienced operators and occasionally even with very experienced ultrasonographers • May be technically limited in large or obese patients or those with large amounts of intestinal ingesta or gas • Acquired portosystemic collaterals take some experience to identify • Many complex shunts are anatomically challenging and studies may not define anatomy sufficiently for surgical planning • Insufficient anatomical detail to plan endovascular closure of intrahepatic shunts

CT angiography* (**Figure 11.3**)	• Exquisite detail of anatomy of most portosystemic shunts
	
	• Sufficient anatomical detail for
	  ° Surgical planning
	  ° Planning of endovascular closure of intrahepatic shunts
		• Equipment investment very expensive
		
		• Much increased expense compared with ultrasound
		
		• Requires general anaesthesia

Scintigraphy* (**Figure 11.4**) (two principle techniques are per-rectal technetium scintigraphy and per-splenic technetium scintigraphy)	• Is the only currently available means of directly quantifying the shunting fraction • When per-splenic scintigraphy is used, some anatomical information about the shunt is gained • Is helpful in answering the question 'shunt or no shunt?'	• Equipment investment is expensive and expertise limited to relatively few institutions • Acquisition and use of radio-isotopes requires special handling facilities, licensing and isolation of the patient (less so with per-splenic than per-rectal) • Per-rectal scintigraphy has variable absorption and up to 25% studies may be non-diagnostic • generally very poor anatomical resolution • Increased personnel exposure to ionising radiation
Portovenography* (**Figure 11.5**)	• Allows direct assessment of shunt anatomy • Allows direct assessment of results of temporary or permanent attenuation, at the time of surgery	• Requires general anaesthesia and celiotomy is thus performed at the time of surgical attenuation • Small risk of subsequent mesenteric or portal thrombosis

(Continued)

Diagnostic test method	Advantages	Disadvantages
	• Equipment costs are low if being performed with radiography rather than fluoroscopy • Surgical skills required to perform are widely held • Can be combined with surgical attenuation of portosystemic shunt and biopsy of the liver	• If performed with fluoroscopy (ideal) 　○ Equipment investment is expensive 　○ Increased personnel exposure to ionising radiation

*Note that studies such as CT angiography, scintigraphy and portovenography should be performed by the centre that is to be performing any surgical or interventional closure of a portosystemic shunt. It is diagnostically inappropriate to perform such studies without the requisite surgical or interventional skills and aftercare needed for optimal treatment of such patients.

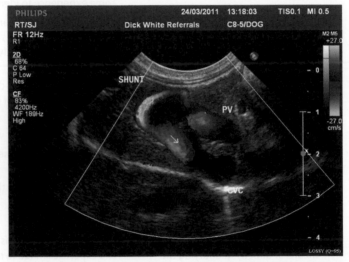

Figure 11.2 Transverse ultrasound view of liver with colour-flow Doppler showing a congenital right-divisional intrahepatic portosystemic shunt (PV = portal vein, CVC = caudal vena cava).

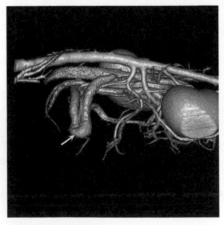 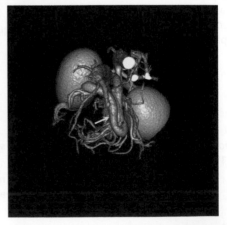

Figure 11.3 Lateral and cranial-caudal CT angiogram 3D reconstruction of an extrahepatic portocaval shunt (arrows). Courtesy of Anna Adrian.

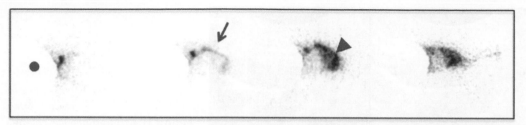

Figure 11.4 Scintigraphy of a portosystemic shunt (patient is seen in lateral position with head to the right of the images). Technetium has been injected into the spleen which is masked (red dot). In successive images (from left to right) the isotope can be seen to opacify the shunting vessel (in this instance a portoazygos shunt, arrowed) and then the heart (arrowhead) without the hepatic parenchyma being opacified first. Courtesy of Andrew Holloway.

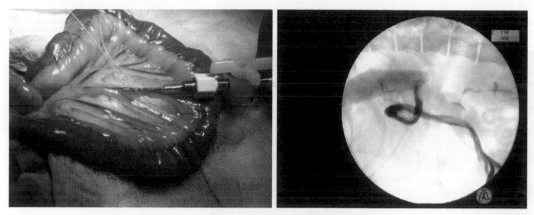

Figure 11.5 Intraoperative cannulation of a jejunal mesenteric tributary to perform a fluoroscopic portovenogram.

Abdominal ultrasound examination demonstrated microhepatica, the presence of a single extrahepatic portocaval (spleno-caval) shunt (**Figure 11.6**) and cystourolithiasis without evidence of urinary obstruction (**Figure 11.7**).

Urinalysis (via cystocentesis) demonstrated a urine pH of 6.0, SG of 1.023 and occasional urate crystals. A subsequent urine culture was negative.

The dog was treated with amoxicillin 20 mg/kg p/o TID, lactulose 5 ml p/o TID (adjusted upwards or downwards to effect loose but not liquid stools) and placed on a commercial hepatic support diet. Resolution of the somnolence, aimless wandering and behavioural changes were seen. After 4 weeks of medical therapy it was recommended that surgical attenuation of the shunt was performed and after performance of a portovenogram (**Figure 11.8**, left panel) the shunting vessel was banded with cellophane. Post-banding portovenography demonstrated good 'arborisation' of hepatic portal tributaries (**Figure 11.8**, right panel). An uneventful surgical recovery ensued and medical and dietary management was continued for a further 4 weeks, following which staged discontinuation every 4 weeks of antibiotics, lactulose, then diet was performed. An abdominal ultrasound examination 2 months after cellophane banding demonstrated no residual flow though the shunting vessel and fasting and post-prandial bile acids 4 months after surgery were 0.8 μmol/l (0–15) and 32 μmol/l (<25) respectively. A repeat ultrasound examination 6 weeks after surgery showed dissolution of the bladder uroliths and no residual shunting through the abnormal vessel. The dog continues to be clinically normal, with the exception of the continued hypermetria, 3 years after surgery.

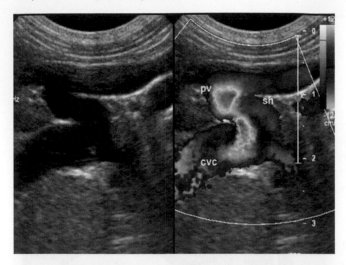

Figure 11.6 Ultrasound view of the portocaval shunt vessel without (left panel) and with (right panel) colour-flow Doppler imaging: pv = portal vein, sh = shunt, cvc = caudal vena cava. Specifically this is a splenocaval shunt, flow from the splenic vein being seen encoded in red towards the bottom right of the image.

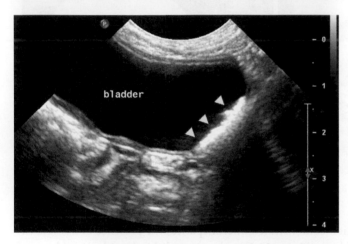

Figure 11.7 Sagittal ultrasound of urinary bladder showing a number of echodense structures (arrowheads) with distal acoustic shadowing within the dependent portion of the bladder, and being consistent with uroliths.

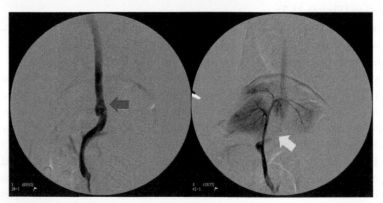

Figure 11.8 Ventrodorsal intraoperative mesenteric portovenogram before (left panel) and after (right panel) cellophane banding of the portocaval shunt. The shunting vessel can be seen to enter the caudal vena cava in the midline at the area of the blue arrow. The site of shunt attenuation by the cellophane band is indicated by the yellow arrow. Note that in contrast with the left image, in which no flow into hepatic portal tributaries can be seen, in the right image, tree-like 'arborisation' of the hepatic portal tributaries is occurring.

Discussion

Portosystemic shunts can be congenital or acquired with congenital PSS commonly comprising a single communicating vessel between the portal venous circulation and the systemic circulation via the caudal vena cava or azygos vein. Of congenital shunts, 66–75% are extrahepatic. Intrahepatic portosystemic shunts are most commonly identified in larger breeds of dog (though we have also seen a number of terriers with intrahepatic shunts through our clinic). Whilst the overwhelming majority of dogs and cats with portosystemic shunts present at <1 year of age with signs consistent with hepatic encephalopathy consequences of portosystemic shunting (depression, confusion, visual disturbances, somnolence, seizures, hypersalivation in cats) a substantial minority of dogs are diagnosed when adults. Reasons for this may be multifactorial but commonly dogs with more subtle signs of encephalopathy may have these signs dismissed as behavioural idiosyncrasies, and it is possible that such patients have smaller portosystemic shunts, shunts in to the azygos or phrenic vessels, and lower 'shunt fractions' than dogs presenting at an earlier age. It is common for such patients to have, in retrospect, a history of recurrent and self-limiting gastrointestinal upsets. Sometimes obstructive urolithiasis in male dogs with ammonium urate uroliths may precipitate recognition of a congenital shunt. Dogs with portal vein hypoplasia (PVH, previously known as microvascular dysplasia) are commonly identified when they are showing no clinical signs of encephalopathy but when abnormal bile acids are identified serendipitously on a biochemical 'panel' of tests. Yorkshire Terriers, Maltese Terriers, Lhasa Apsos and Miniature Schnauzers are overrepresented with congenital extrahepatic portosystemic shunts. More than one shunting vessel may be seen in some dogs.

Acquired portosystemic shunts

Acquired portosystemic shunts (**Figure 11.9**) usually develop secondary to portal venous hypertension and most commonly are due to vasculo-obstructive liver disease such as hepatic fibrosis and cirrhosis. The most common site of these is the left splenogonadal shunting system. Smaller acquired portal collaterals known as varices may also develop, usually in the paraoesophageal area, left gastric vein, biliary, omental, duodenal or colonic.

Most congenital extrahepatic portosystemic shunts are single though there are cases where more than one congenital portosystemic shunt or where both congenital and acquired portosystemic shunts coexist. The majority of single congenital extrahepatic shunts are splenocaval (as here), splenophrenic, splenoazygos, gastric-caval or gastric-azygos. Clinical signs appear to be more consistently severe in animals with vena-caval insertion of the shunt rather than azygos and if the shunt insertion is caudal to the liver. Surgical management of single congenital extrahepatic portosystemic shunts results in significant improvement in survival and lower frequency of ongoing signs than medical management and is the recommended treatment option. Methods of shunt attenuation that result in gradual shunt occlusion (cellophane banding, placement of an Ameroid constrictor, hydraulic occlusion devices) have become the most popular method due to the advantages of gradual occlusion on reduction of the development of signs of portal hypertension after acute attenuation, and results in an excellent outcome in 80–85% of cases. Pre-operative medical management for 3 weeks with a combination of antimicrobial, lactulose and dietary therapy is recommended since the rate of peri-operative seizure complications seems unacceptably high when

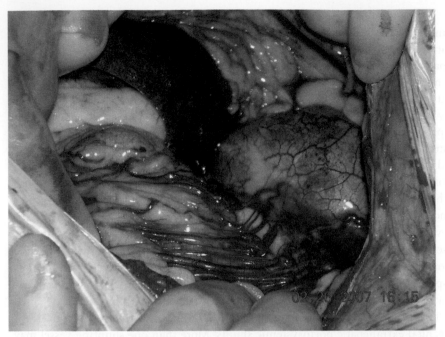

Figure 11.9 Left splenogonadal acquired portosystemic shunts in a dog with portal hypertension.

attenuation is performed without prior medical management. Although the mechanisms by which this should be the case is unclear, a substantial body of experience of surgical management of these cases exists to support this strategy. Ammonium urate uroliths may be elected to be removed concurrently at the time of shunt surgery, particularly in male dogs where more of a risk of urethral obstruction exists; however, shunt attenuation and treatment of any concurrent urinary tract infection results in rapid dissolution of ammonium urate uroliths.

Further reading

Berent, A.C. & Tobias, K.M. (2009) Portosystemic vascular anomalies *Vet Clin North Am Small Anim Pract* **39**, 513–541

Bertolini, G. (2010) Acquired portal collateral circulation in the dog and cat. *Vet Radiol Ultrasound* **51**, 25–33

Buob, S., Johnston, A.N. & Webster, C.R. (2011) Portal hypertension: pathophysiology, diagnosis, and treatment. *J Vet Intern Med* **25**, 169–186

Daniel, G.B. (2009) Scintigraphic diagnosis of portosystemic shunts. *Vet Clin North Am Small Anim Pract* **39**, 793–810

D'Anjou, M.A. (2007) The sonographic search for portosystemic shunts. *Clin Tech Small Anim Pract* **22**, 104–114

Eh, G.C., Phillips, H., Underwood, L. & Selmic, L.E. (2015) Risk factors for urolithiasis in dogs with congenital extrahepatic portosystemic shunts: 95 cases (1999–2013). *J Am Vet Med Assoc* **246**, 530–536

Greenhalgh, S.N., Reeve, J.A., Johnstone, T., Goodfellow, M.R., Dunning, M.D., O'Neill, E.J., Hall, E.J., Watson, P.J. & Jeffery, N.D. (2014) Long-term survival and quality of life in dogs with clinical signs associated with a congenital portosystemic shunt after surgical or medical treatment. *J Am Vet Med Assoc* **245**, 527–533

Kim, S.E., Giglio, R.F., Reese, D.J., Reese, S.L., Bacon, N.J. & Ellison, G.W. (2013) Comparison of computed tomographic angiography and ultrasonography for the detection and characterization of portosystemic shunts in dogs. *Vet Radiol Ultrasound* **54**, 569–574

Kraun, M.B., Nelson, L.L., Hauptman, J.G. & Nelson, N.C. (2014) Analysis of the relationship of extrahepatic portosystemic shunt morphology with clinical variables in dogs: 53 cases (2009–2012). *J Am Vet Med Assoc* **245**, 540–549

Mankin, K.M. (2015) Current concepts in congenital portosystemic shunts. *Vet Clin North Am Small Anim Pract* **45**, 477–487

Nelson, N.C. & Nelson, L.L. (2011) Anatomy of extrahepatic portosystemic shunts in dogs as determined by computed tomography angiography. *Vet Radiol Ultrasound* **52**, 498–506

van den Bossche, L., van Steenbeek, F.G., Favier, R.P., Kummeling, A., Leegwater, P.A. & Rothuizen, J. (2012) Distribution of extrahepatic congenital portosystemic shunt morphology in predisposed dog breeds. *BMC Vet Res* **8**, 112

van Straten, G., Spee, B., Rothuizen, J., van Straten, M. & Favier, R. P. (2015) Diagnostic value of the rectal ammonia tolerance test, fasting plasma ammonia and fasting plasma bile acids for canine portosystemic shunting. *Vet J* **204**, 282–286

Zwingenberger, A. (2009) CT diagnosis of portosystemic shunts. *Vet Clin North Am Small Anim Pract* **39**, 783–792

Clinical presentation

An 8 year-old female-neutered Labrador (**Figure 12.1**) weighing 28 kg is presented with a history of visible icterus and reduced appetite for 4 days. No vomiting or diarrhoea has been reported. The dog is regularly vaccinated against distemper virus, infectious canine hepatitis, parvovirus, parainfluenzavirus and leptospirosis (*L. canicola, L. icterohaemorrhagiae*), has no history of travel outside the United Kingdom and has had no previous medical problems, known access to intoxicants or any prescription medications.

Physical examination demonstrates a bright dog in normal body condition but with visible icterus of the sclera, conjunctiva, oral mucous membranes, inner ear pinnae and skin. The dog is apparently well hydrated and physical examination is otherwise normal including a normal rectal temperature of 38.3 °C.

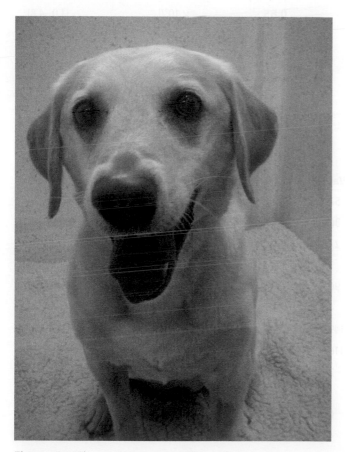

Figure 12.1 The patient at presentation.

Canine Internal Medicine: What's Your Diagnosis? First Edition. Jon Wray.
© 2018 John Wiley & Sons Ltd. Published 2018 by John Wiley & Sons Ltd.

A blood sample and urinalysis taken from the dog demonstrates the following:

Haematology

Parameter	Value	Units	Range
RBC	7.3	$\times 10^{12}/l$	(5.5–8.5)
Haemoglobin	16.9	g/dl	(12.0–18.0)
Haematocrit	0.50	l/l	(0.37–0.55)
Mean cell volume	68.5	fl	(60–77)
Mean cell haemoglobin concentration	33.7	g/dl	(30.0–38.0)
Mean cell haemoglobin	23.1	pg	(19.5–25.5)
Total white cell count	6.78	$\times 10^9/l$	(6.0–15.0)
Neutrophils	5.27	$\times 10^9/l$	(3.0–11.5)
Lymphocytes	**0.85**	$\times 10^9/l$	(1.0–4.8)
Monocytes	0.23	$\times 10^9/l$	(0.2–1.4)
Eosinophils	0.42	$\times 10^9/l$	(0.1–1.2)
Basophils	0.01	$\times 10^9/l$	(0.0–0.1)
Platelets	225	$\times 10^9/l$	(200–500)
Film comment:		Some platelet clumping on film	

Biochemistry

Parameter	Value	Units	Range
Total protein	57	g/l	(54–77)
Albumin	30	g/l	(25–40)
Globulin	27	g/l	(23–45)
Urea	3.2	mmol/l	(2.5–7.4)
Creatinine	90	µmol/l	(40–145)
Potassium	4.9	mmol/l	(3.4–5.6)
Sodium	149	mmol/l	(139–154)
Chloride	116	mmol/l	(105–122)
Calcium	2.4	mmol/l	(2.1–2.8)
Magnesium	–	mmol/l	(0.62–0.90)
Inorganic phosphate	0.90	mmol/l	(0.60–1.40)
Glucose	4.4	mmol/l	(3.3–5.8)
ALT	**961**	IU/l	(13–88)
AST	**203**	IU/l	(13–60)
ALKP	**461**	IU/l	(14–105)

Parameter	Value	Units	Range
GGT	**39**	IU/l	(0–10)
Bilirubin	**307**	μmol/l	(0–16)
Cholesterol	5	mmol/l	(3.8–7.0)
Triglyceride	1.1	mmol/l	(0.56–1.14)
Creatine kinase	145	IU/l	(0–190)

Urinalysis (cystocentesis sample)

Parameter	Value	Units	Range
Appearance	Icteric		
Chemistry			
Specific gravity	1.032		
pH	6.5		
Protein	–		
Nitrite	–		
Blood/Hb	+		
Glucose	–		
Ketones	–		
Bilirubin	+++		
Urobilinogen	+		
Cytology			
Red cells	2	/hpf	(0–2)
White cells	0	/hpf	(0–2)
Epithelial cells	0	/hpf	(0–5)
Casts	0		
Crystals	0		
Bacteria	0		
Other	–		

Questions

1. How would you interpret these results?
2. What differential diagnoses would you consider?
3. What further investigation would you perform for this dog and what considerations need to be taken?

Answers

1. How would you interpret these results?

Haematology demonstrated mild lymphopenia. Lymphopenia is commonly seen in acute inflammation including acute bacterial and viral infections and endotoxaemia, as part of a stress leukogram in response to endogenous glucocorticoids, due to exogenous glucocorticoids and less commonly due to depletion or hypoplasia.

Serum biochemistry demonstrates elevations in ALT, AST, ALKP and GGT (collectively colloquially termed 'liver enzymes') and of total bilirubin.

Assessment of 'liver enzymes'

Assessment of liver enzyme elevations should take into account knowledge of their site and aetiology of production/elevation, interpretation of the magnitude of elevation and rate of elimination.

- ALT (alanine (amino)transferase) is found predominantly within hepatocyte cytosol and in the dog has a half-life of 45–60 hours. Minimal amounts are also found within skeletal myocytes. It is considered predominantly a marker of hepatocellular injury.
- AST (aspartate transaminase) is found within hepatocyte cytosol and mitochondria as well as within skeletal muscle. The half-life in the dog is approximately 12 hours. It is considered predominantly a marker of hepatocellular and skeletal muscular injury and in the former it is often considered (due to the short half-life and mitochondrial location) that significant elevations may indicate a more severe hepatocellular injury.
- ALKP (alkaline phosphatase) is found in cell membranes of hepatocytes and especially biliary epithelium and increases are most commonly associated with cholestasis. The half-life in the dog is 60 hours. Tissue non-specific ALKP is also produced by osteoblasts. An isoform of ALKP, C-ALKP, is produced by hepatocytes when stimulated by glucocorticoids (either exogenous or endogenous).
- GGT (gamma-glutamyltransferase) is also a membrane-associated enzyme considered a marker of cholestasis. Elevations closely parallel ALKP though the magnitude of increases is usually much less and it is a poorly sensitive marker of cholestasis in the dog, though is quite specific. Some mild glucocorticoid and barbiturate induction can occur.

As a rule-of-thumb, many clinicians will evaluate elevations in liver enzymes above 3 × the upper reference limit (URL) to be significant since it is very common to find canine patients with enzyme levels that fall outside reference intervals due to non-specific elevation in enzyme activity and due to 'reactive' or 'secondary' hepatopathy. This commonly occurs due to pathology (especially inflammatory) that occurs within the anatomical vicinity of the liver (for instance in acute enteritis), in the presence of hepatic hypoxaemia or congestion and due to systemic diseases, especially endocrinopathies. It is important to ascertain the possibility of exposure to exogenous glucocorticoids (including in topical products) before assessing the significance of elevations in liver enzymes.

In this case significant elevations in enzymes signifying hepatocellular damage (ALT approximately 11 × URL, AST approximately 3 × URL) and cholestasis (ALKP approximately 4 ×

URL, GGT approximately 4 × URL) are present with a 'pattern' of elevation that suggests hepatocellular injury predominating compared with cholestasis. It is important to note that

- The magnitude of elevation cannot be used to determine the aetiology, prognosis or likelihood/rate of recovery from hepatocellular injury and
- These enzymes do not indicate liver *function*.

Liver function can be assessed more directly by provocative testing (such as bile acid stimulation test – see below) and inferred indirectly, though with poor sensitivity (i.e. such changes are only likely to occur relatively late in the course of hepatic dysfunction) by decreases in albumin, urea, glucose and cholesterol (hypoglycaemia being a very late finding).

Hyperbilirubinaemia is present. At levels of bilirubin >30 μmol/l clinical yellowing of mucous membranes and plasma known as jaundice or icterus (the two terms are interchangeable and merely describe yellowish discolouration) may be detected.

- Bilirubin is produced from the degradation of heme from effete erythrocytes and circulates bound to albumin.
- It is removed from plasma by conjugation within hepatocytes or via renal excretion.
- The rate limiting step in bilirubin excretion is energy-dependent transport of conjugated bilirubin from the hepatocytes into bile canaliculi and thence into the intestine.

Icterus/jaundice is defined as given in **Table 12.1**.

Although both unconjugated (Bu) and conjugated bilirubin (Bc) can be measured separately (and theoretically, post-hepatic icterus will result in a greater proportion of Bc:Bu whilst pre-hepatic shows the reverse pattern), in reality there may be considerable overlap between these, not least due to accumulation of subfractions over time and this is not, clinically, a reliable method to determine between aetiologies of icterus. Practically, distinction between these is undertaken by

(a) Interpretation of a concurrent haematocrit for anaemia, which may indicate pre-hepatic jaundice. Note, however, that where haemolysis and concurrent haemoconcentration occur, hyperbilirubinaemia may be pre-hepatic but a normal haematocrit may be seen and conversely anaemia and concurrent hyperbilirubinaemia may be seen in those disorders where hepatic disease and bleeding or bone marrow disease are occurring together.
(b) Observing the relative magnitude of changes in enzyme markers of hepatocellular damage versus cholestasis.
(c) Performing diagnostic imaging, especially ultrasound, to determine if extrahepatic bile duct obstruction is occurring.

Table 12.1 The three major types of jaundice

Pre-hepatic jaundice	Due to release of heme by haemolysis of red blood cells that overwhelms the hepatic elimination capacity of bilirubin (birirubin uptake or excretion of conjugated bilirubin)
Hepatic jaundice	Due to • Decreased functional hepatic mass • Decreased bilirubin conjugation
Post-hepatic jaundice	Decreased conjugated bilirubin excretion due to obstructive cholestasis of the biliary tract. In dogs the most common cause of this is extrahepatic bile duct obstruction (EHBDO) by pancreatitis

The bilirubinuria is a reflection of the hyperbilirubinaemia. Urobilinogen is not felt to be of clinical value in the dog. The scant hematuria is likely to reflect the sampling method, though pathological causes cannot be discounted. Repetition of assessment on a free-catch sample taken some time after cystocentesis may help to distinguish it.

2. What differential diagnoses would you consider?

Here the clinical pathology results indicate a combination of both hepatocellular injury and cholestasis; no inference can be made as to liver function only that *insufficient dysfunction* exists to affect those secondary markers of function such as serum albumin, urea, glucose and cholesterol. Icterus/jaundice is also present and in a well-hydrated animal with normal haematocrit, practically, pre-hepatic icterus/jaundice can be excluded. Thus our differential diagnosis may initially start, broadly, with

- Hepatic icterus/jaundice.
- Post-hepatic icterus/jaundice.

In the latter situation we would logically expect that perhaps markers of cholestasis (bilirubin, ALKP, GGT and cholesterol) would become elevated to a greater magnitude proportionally than those markers of hepatocellular injury. In this case, the opposite is true so whilst post-hepatic icterus/jaundice should certainly not be discounted, it is the less likely situation.

World Small Animal Veterinary Association (WSAVA) liver standardisation

The WSAVA Liver Standardisation Group classifies disorders of the liver and biliary tract under the following subdivisions (which are clinical, rather than being exclusively either anatomical or aetiological):

1. Circulatory disorders of the liver
2. Biliary disorders
3. Hepatic parenchymal disorders
4. Neoplastic disorders

Of these circulatory disorders, at least primary ones can be discounted since they do not generally result in jaundice or marked elevations of hepatic transaminases (not because of age of the patient). Note, however, that it is certainly possible for secondary acquired vascular disorders (acquired portosystemic shunts) to occur in the setting of these abnormalities. Differential diagnoses within the other subdivisions that should be considered are given in **Tables 12.2, 12.3 and 12.4**.

Lack of diagnostic specificity of liver enzymes

It can be seen from the above that whilst hepatocellular and cholestatic markers are sensitive for detecting hepatic pathology, they are not generally specific for a particular disorder and the differential diagnostic possibilities are very broad. It is therefore extremely important to keep an open mind and to appreciate the breadth of possible aetiologies when considering liver enzyme abnormalities.

Table 12.2 Differential diagnosis of biliary disorders

Biliary cystic disease	Poorly characterised in veterinary medicine and proposed classification based on human 'fibropolycystic' liver disease include
	• Congenital polycystic disease
	• Adult polycystic disease
	• Dilated bile duct cysts (Caroli's disease)
	• Choledochal cysts
	• Microhamartoma
	Depending on the site, these may have predominantly space-occupying pathophysiology, cholangitis or be associated with portal hypertension if hepatic fibrosis co-exists
Biliary atresia	
Cholestasis (diminished or absent bile flow)	Intrahepatic cholestasis
	• Associated with a wide variety of parenchymal liver diseases (see below) with cholestasis occurring secondarily due to local effects on intrahepatic biliary tracts
	Extrahepatic cholestasis
	• Intraluminal obstruction of the biliary tract
	○ Obstructive choleliths
	○ Obstructive mucinous debris
	• Mural/luminal constriction of the biliary tract
	○ Inflammation
	○ Neoplasia
	• Extraluminal obstruction of the terminal common bile duct
	○ Pancreatitis
	○ Inflammatory and space-occupying disease of the duodenum at the major duodenal papilla
Cholangitis (inflammation of bile-conducting structures)	• Neutrophilic cholangitis (usually associated with ascending bacterial infections)
	• Lymphocytic cholangitis
	• Destructive cholangitis (usually associated with drugs or viral infection)
	• Cholangitis associated with liver flukes
Gall bladder disease	• Cystic mucinous hyperplasia/mucocoele
	• Bacterial cholecystitis
	• Gall bladder infarction

Table 12.3 Differential diagnosis of hepatic parenchymal disease (based on WSAVA classification)

Congenital and genetic metabolic liver diseases	• Glycogen storage diseases
	• Hepatic amyloidosis
Acquired metabolic liver diseases	• Hepatic amyloidosis
	• Hepatic steatosis

(Continued)

Acute, reversible hepatocytic injury	• Cloudy swelling (hydropic degeneration) • Corticosteroid-induced glycogen accumulation • Hepatocellular steatosis (lipidosis, fatty change) Note that these appear to be histologically similar and periodic acid Schiff (PAS) staining is useful to determine glycogen presence and Oil Red O or Sudan black for lipid

Hepatocellular death and necrosis	This is really a histological classification rather than an aetiological one. It may represent part of a continuum of increasing severity of damage from un-resolved acute, potentially reversible hepatocyte injury, or may be caused by
	
	• Toxins (especially aflatoxicosis, amanita mushroom spp. toxicity, blue-green algae, Sago palms, xylitol, heavy metals, hydrocarbons
	• Drugs (especially amiodarone, azathioprine, azole antifungals, carpro-fen, diazepam, lomustine, methimazole, paracetamol, phenobarbitone, sulphonamides)
	• Hypoxia, liver lobe torsion, ischaemia, thrombosis, congestion
	• Due to concurrent pancreatitis
	• Infectious diseases of which the most common associated with acute hepatocellular death and necrosis are
	   ◦ Canine adenovirus I (infectious canine hepatitis)
	   ◦ Canine herpesvirus
	   ◦ *Toxplasma gondii*
	   ◦ *Clostridium piliforme*

Acute and chronic hepatitis (may or may not have con-current fibrosis ± cirrhosis present)	Non-granulomatous infectious causes of acute and chronic hepatitis • *Leptospira* spp. • Canine adenovirus 1 • Acidophil cell hepatitis • *Clostridium piliforme* • *Toxoplasma gondii* • *Hepatozoon canis** • *Ehrlichia canis** • *Rickettsia rickettsiae** • *Leishmania infantum** • *Babesia canis, Babesia gibsoni** Granulomatous acute and chronic hepatitis • *Bartonella henselae* and *clarridgeiae* • *Mycobacterium* spp. • Fungal hepatitis especially *Histoplasma capsulatum*, Coccidioides immitis*, Blastomyces dermatitidis** • *Echinococcus multilocularis** • *Prototheca* spp. Copper-associated hepatitis • Bedlington Terrier

- West Highland White Terrier
- Skye Terrier
- Dobermann Pinscher
- Dalmatian
- Labrador Retriever

Autoimmune-hepatitis
- Dobermann Pinscher?

Idiopathic hepatitis
- Any breed but especially
  - Cocker Spaniel
  - English Springer Spaniel
  - West Highland White Terrier
  - Labrador Retriever
  - German Shepherd

Alpha-1-antitrypsin associated?
- Cocker Spaniel

Lobular dissecting hepatitis

Drug and toxin associated (see above)

Eosinophilic hepatitis

Hepatic abscesses and focal granulomata	Usually spontaneous, bacterial and without underlying predisposing cause identified in most cases

* = diseases not currently thought to be endemic to the United Kingdom (caution should be applied since increased free animal movement within Europe and increased geographical range of some arthropods makes this status precarious).

Table 12.4 Differential diagnoses for hepatic neoplasia

Descriptors of hepatic neoplasia	
	By nature
	• Primary hepatic neoplasia
	• Secondary (metastatic) hepatic neoplasia
	By distribution
	• Massive (focal, large, single lobe)
	• Nodular
	• Diffuse
	By anatomic/cellular origin
	• Hepatocellular
	• Cholangiocellular
	• Vascular/mesenchymal
	• Carcinoid
	• Haematopoietic

(Continued)

Common forms of primary hepatic neoplasia

Hepatocellular neoplasia
- Benign nodular hyperplasia
- Hepatocellular adenoma
- Hepatocellular carcinoma

Cholangiocellular neoplasia
- Biliary adenoma
- Biliary carcinoma

Vascular/mesenchymal neoplasia
- Haemangiosarcoma
- Fibrosarcoma
- Leiomyoma
- Leiomyosarcoma
- Osteosarcoma
- Rhabdomyosarcoma

Hepatic carcinoid and hepatoblastoma

Haematopoietic neoplasia
- Lymphoma
- Malignant histiocytosis
- Mast cell tumour
- Plasma cell tumour

3. What further investigation would you perform for this dog and what considerations need to be taken?

Before considering further investigation it should be borne in mind that

- The ability of hepatocytes to recover from finite insults is prodigious and in many circumstances acute hepatocellular disease may spontaneously recover without the need for investigation or provision of specific or supportive therapy. The decision to investigate should be based on
  - Severity of clinical signs.
  - Persistence of clinical signs/abnormalities.
  - Significant pre-test probability of diagnostic testing yielding therapeutically useful information.
  - Serial re-evaluation of hepatocellular and cholestatic markers is a rational means of informing clinical decision making in pursuing a definitive diagnosis by attempting to answer the question 'is this process persisting/worsening or improving?', *provided* that one bears in mind that occasionally animals with fulminant hepatic failure and rapidly decreasing functional hepatic mass may have falling liver enzymes, which represent lack of functional liver tissue releasing them, rather than a clinical improvement.

Match the frequency of assessment to the half-life of the analyte in question

The frequency of re-evaluation is *appropriate to the half-life of the analytes* concerned and the clinical status of the animal, that is assessment of these more frequently than once or twice a week in a clinically stable animal is unlikely to be diagnostically helpful and represents injudicious use of client resources as well as exposing patients to overly intrusive veterinary attention

- The differential diagnosis for such signs is lengthy and investigation may be expensive; coupled with this, relatively few of the differential diagnoses have specific treatments that differ from each other and there is a reasonable argument for watchful re-evaluation or empirical/supportive therapy in some cases.
- Some forms of investigation, especially those involving liver biopsy, must be undertaken with some degree of caution since
  - It is very unlikely that repeated biopsy would be either permitted or advisable and thus meticulous planning of what 'clinical questions' need to be answered by material obtained needs to be performed by the clinician well ahead of taking any biopsies.
  - Biopsy includes a low but significant risk to the patient, including in the worst-case scenario, risk of death.

  Further investigation might include the following.

Laboratory tests
- Assessment of liver function
  - This is unlikely to help distinguish between differential diagnoses other than that abnormalities of function are more likely to indicate a more diffuse disease process.
  - This may be useful for
    - Prognostication.
    - Therapeutic and perioperative planning.
  - Assessment of bile acids is the most commonly performed means of assessing this (see **Case 11**) but it should be borne in mind that disorders causing cholestasis will automatically elevate bile acid levels since these are excreted via the biliary tract.
- Assessment of coagulation status
  - The activated vitamin-K-dependent serine proteases factors II, VII, IX, X may be depleted in the presence of cholestasis since vitamin K absorption is a fat-dependent process, itself requiring the presence of bile acids and cholesterol to form micelles. Furthermore, most coagulation factors (with the exception of von Willebrand's factor) are produced within the liver and hepatic dysfunction may lead to depletion of these and thus coagulopathy.
  - This is unlikely to help distinguish between differential diagnoses other than that abnormalities of function are more likely to indicate a more diffuse disease process.
  - However, assessment of platelet count and of prothrombin time/activated partial thromboplastin time prior to any liver biopsy procedure is recommended.
- Specific testing for systemic infectious diseases associated with hepatitis. In the United Kingdom this might most rationally involve

- ○ Serological testing for *Leptospira* spp. since vaccination in many cases may offer protection to the serovars *L. canicola* and *L. icterohaemorrhagiae* only and duration of immunity appears quite variable.
  - The microscopic agglutination test (MAT) which measures IgM and some IgG is classically held to be positive at titres >1:800 or where a fourfold increase in titre is seen. However, cross-reactivity with vaccinal serovars and some disprorportionate elevation in MAT for *L. autumnalis and L. bratislava* may be seen in patients vaccinated with quadrivalent vaccines.
  - PCR testing is also available though cannot readily distinguish between serovars.
  - A disadvantage of both methods is that subclinical carriers shed organisms and that PCRs may detect non-pathogenic serovars.
- ○ Possibly serology or PCR testing for *Bartonella* spp.
- ○ *Toxoplasma gondii* serology.
- ○ Serological testing for canine adenovirus 1 in unvaccinated animals.

Diagnostic imaging

Whilst radiography may detect gross hepatomegaly or microhepatica, or deformation of the liver margin or shift in position of organs caudal to it due to mass lesions, it is relatively insensitive in the diagnosis of hepatobiliary diseases.

Cross-sectional imaging techniques such as computed tomography (CT) may provide good anatomical detail and CT has become the diagnostic imaging test of choice for anatomical determination of vascular liver disease and abdominal evaluation in very obese canine patients. However, it is limited by increased cost, lack of availability and the need for general anaesthesia.

Systematic ultrasound evaluation of the hepatobiliary tract

Diagnostic ultrasound has become the diagnostic imaging test of choice in most hepatobiliary diseases, combining good anatomical detail, subjective parenchymal textural assessment, evaluation of the biliary tract and local extrahepatic organs and being both cost-effective and safe without the need for general anaesthesia. Ultrasound-guided sampling of hepatobiliary structures can also be performed. Systematic evaluation of the hepatobiliary tract involves

- Evaluation of liver size.
- Evaluation of the liver's anatomical associations.
- Evaluation of the hepatic parenchyma for echogenicity, homogeneity of architecture and presence or absence of localised changes.
- Evaluation of the gall bladder, common bile duct (both intrahepatic and extrahepatic) and intrahepatic bile ducts.
- Changes in vascularity.
- Presence or absence of free abdominal fluid or gas.

Direct sampling of the hepatobiliary tract

Several methods exist to obtain diagnostic material from the hepatobiliary tract but it is essential to plan a material collection method based on the differential diagnosis and the anticipated diagnostic fate/use of specimens obtained. A comparison of diagnostic utility of different specimens is shown in **Table 12.5** and these considerations should take place *before* any hepatobiliary sampling technique.

Table 12.5 Diagnostic utility of different liver specimens

Diagnostic utility	Sample material	Notes
Cytology of liver parenchyma or nodular lesion	Fine needle aspirate (FNA)	For parenchymal liver diseases agreement between FNA and histological diagnosis is at best very modest. It is poorly sensitive for diagnosis of inflammatory liver disorders and may result in diagnostic bias towards vacuolar hepatopathies including steatosis. Clinicians should be wary that misclassification of mixed disorders in which some vacuolar change is present, is commonplace with this method
		In focal liver lesions, cytology has good specificity and positive predictive value for neoplasia, but has quite poor sensitivity of only 52%
Histopathology of liver tissue	Liver tissue, fixed in formalin, obtained by • Surgical wedge biopsy at celiotomy • Laparoscopic biopsy • Core biopsy taken with spring-loaded device (e.g. Tru-Cut), Menghini needle or other, with or without ultrasound guidance	***See discussion below*** For needle biopsies, 14G sample size is recommended by the WSAVA liver standardisation group with 16G samples reserved for smaller patients
Microbiological assessment of tissue (for bacterial, fungal or mycobacterial culture)	Liver tissue obtained as above submitted unfixed	Whole tissue should be submitted (collected into a sterile sample pot and kept moist with sterile moistened gauze) without delay to the laboratory. Bacteriological swabs from tissue are not recommended
Assessment of liver copper	Liver tissue obtained by • Surgical wedge biopsy at celiotomy • Laparoscopic biopsy • Core biopsy	Semi-quantitative assessment for copper accumulation may be performed by special staining (rubeanic acid or rhodanine stain) and the distribution of copper may also be assessed by histological examination of relatively small biopsies. However, quantification of copper usually requires larger (surgical or laparoscopic) biopsies
Cytology of bile	Bile aspirated • At celiotomy • During laparoscopy • By ultrasound-guided cholecystocentesis	
Microbiological assessment of bile (for bacterial, fungal or mycobacterial culture)	Bile aspirated • At celiotomy • During laparoscopy • By ultrasound-guided cholecystocentesis	

There are pros and cons to each of the three major methods of liver biopsy (core biopsy, laparoscopic and surgical) and these are summarised below in **Table 12.6**. In the author's opinion, currently laparoscopic biopsy may offer the best combination of safety, generation of diagnostically useful and accurate sample size, gross evaluation of extrahepatic structures and palatability to owners.

Ensuring safe biopsy sampling

Regardless of the technique it is important to assess coagulation status beforehand and to have a contingency plan of proactive assessment for post-biopsy haemorrhage in the hours following biopsy. The overall rate of minor complications in dogs undergoing ultrasound-guided needle core liver biopsy is 18.5% and for major complications (mainly life-threatening haemorrhage) is 4.2%. Consideration of the risk/benefit ratio and owner counselling as to risk and contingency planning is mandatory in all cases.

Table 12.6 Comparison between liver biopsy methods

Method	Pros	Cons	Number of portal triads/ specimen reported	Overall level of agreement with final diagnosis reported
Needle core biopsy	• Minimally invasive/uncommon client resistance • Least costly • Allows sampling of any depth when performed with ultrasound guidance • Bile for cytology and culture may also be collected • Allows focussed targeting of nodular lesions within parenchyma • Widely available • Rapid recovery time	• 17% inadequate for diagnosis • Number of portal triads and overall level of agreement with final diagnosis in studies is low • Samples usually inadequate for quantification of copper • Risk of complications, especially unwitnessed haemorrhage is higher than for other techniques • Minimal invasiveness commonly leads clinicians to underestimate risk	2.9	48–67%
Laparoscopic biopsy	• Minimally invasive/uncommon client resistance • Allows gross inspection of liver and extrahepatic structures	• Relatively expensive • Less widely available equipment and skill required	8–13	60–86%

Method	Pros	Cons	Number of portal triads/specimen reported	Overall level of agreement with final diagnosis reported
	• Allows relatively large biopsy size to be taken with few inadequate biopsies • Samples adequate for histopathology, culture and for copper quantification • Bile for cytology and culture may also be collected • Some haemostasis may be achieved by crushing edge of sample • Visual Inspection for haemorrhage at time of biopsy and immediately after achieved • Can be converted to celiotomy with minimal delay if surgical haemostasis required • Rapid recovery time	• Peripheral areas of liver lobes only sampled – deep intraparenchymal lesions may be missed and peripheral fibrosis may not be representative		
Surgical wedge biopsy	• Allows gross inspection of liver and extrahepatic structures • Allows large biopsy size to be taken • Bile for cytology and culture may also be collected • Some haemostasis may be achieved by crushing edge of sample • Visual inspection for haemorrhage at time of biopsy and immediately after achieved and surgical control of haemorrhage may be performed at time • Samples adequate for histopathology, culture and for copper quantification	• Invasive/frequent client resistance • More prolonged recovery time • Expensive	20–30	Not reported

Diagnosis

- PT and APTT in this patient were within reference intervals.
- cPLI, amylase and lipase were within reference intervals.
- Pre- and post-prandial bile acids were 2.9 µmol/l (0–10) and 36 µmol/l (0–15). The latter was determined as a mild rise within the interpretive 'grey zone'.
- MAT for *Leptospira* spp. was <1:200, both initially and a convalescent result 3 weeks later.
- A PCR for *Bartonella* spp. was negative.
- An abdominal ultrasound examination (**Figure 12.2**) demonstrated the following:
  - Liver: smaller size than normal. Moderately hypoechoic parenchyma, with irregular caudal edges. Heterogeneous (mildly) echotexture and echogenicity. No evidence of the presence of a hepatic mass. Gall bladder: NAD. Cystic duct and CBD not seen.
  - Spleen: NAD.
  - Kidneys and urinary bladder: NAD.
  - Intra-abdominal lymph nodes: NAD.
  - Adrenal glands: within normal limits.
  - Pancreas: NAD.

Pending the results of infectious disease laboratory tests, the patient was treated supportively with ursodeoxycholic acid at a dose of 10 mg/kg p/o SID and a weight-appropriate s-Adenosyl-methionine/sylibin/vitamin E combination product. Retesting of serum liver enzymes after a further 6 days, during which time the dog remained bright and still ate daily, albeit small amounts of food, demonstrated little progression or improvement in these.

Laparoscopic liver biopsy was performed and cholecystocentesis performed for cytology and culture. The liver biopsy material was submitted for histopathology including copper staining, copper quantification and bacterial culture.

At laparoscopy (**Figure 12.3**) the liver appeared slightly small and areas of the margins of some hepatic lobes appeared slightly pale and irregular though overall the lobes appeared

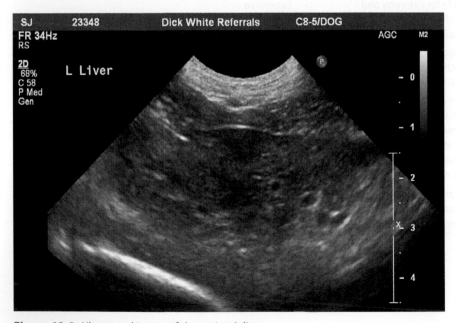

Figure 12.2 Ultrasound image of the patient's liver.

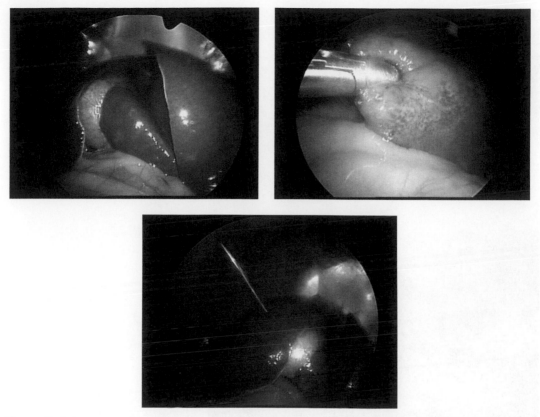

Figure 12.3 Laparoscopic images: (top) gross appearance of liver, (middle) biopsy being collected and (bottom) needle centesis of gall bladder.

well-defined and these changes were subtle. The gall bladder was aspirated trans-hepatically. No apparent haemorrhage or leakage of bile was noted during laparoscopy and initial recovery was uneventful.

Post-operatively the pulse rate and quality, mucous membrane colour and respiratory rate were monitored hourly for 8 hours and a PCV and total protein assessment was made after 4 hours. The heart rate remained between 96 and 108 bpm for 8 hours and peripheral pulse quality remained good. An area of peri-umbilical subcutaneous haemorrhage ('Cullen's sign' *sic*), indicative of intra-abdominal bleeding, was noted 4 hours post-laparoscopy (**Figure 12.4**) and assessment of PCV and total protein at this time was 45% and 60 g/l. An abdominal FAST[3] ('Focussed Abdominal Sonography for Trauma, Triage and Tracking') ultrasound scan demonstrated scant fluid at the cystocolic and hepatosplenic views only (sic) and was repeated after 10 hours, which showed little change. The dog remained cardiovascularly stable and monitoring of cardiovascular parameters was performed at progressively longer intervals over the following 24 hours with no apparent deterioration in cardiovascular status. A small and non-progressive post-biopsy haemorrhage was suspected.

Bile cytology and culture was normal/negative. Histopathology findings from the liver were as below:

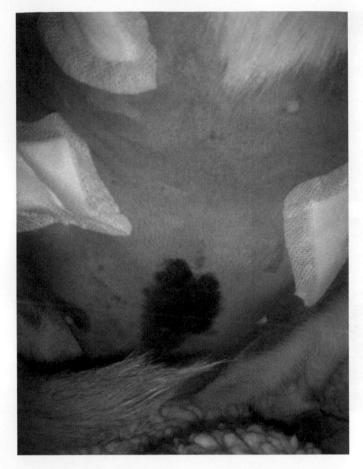

Figure 12.4 Cullen's sign after laparoscopic biopsy.

Microscopic description

Liver (four sections). The sample consists of multiple sections of liver. These liver sections have a moderately undulating capsule and are expanded by a mild to moderate increase in fibrous tissue and inflammation. Often the portal triads in these liver sections are expanded by an elevated amount of fibrous connective tissue with lesser amounts of biliary hyperplasia. These areas of fibrosis and biliary hyperplasia are often distorting the standard portal–centrilobular architecture of the liver. Often areas of fibrosis do appear to extend into the parenchyma and entrap clusters of hepatocytes. These areas of fibrosis often contain low to moderate numbers of neutrophils, small lymphocytes and frequent plasma cells. Often in the periportal to mid-zonal regions are moderate density clusters of gold pigment laden macrophages. Aggregates of macrophages and inflammatory cells often appear to obscure the portal interface. Along the portal interface, occasional hepatocytes are disassociated and fewer hepatocytes appear to be individually necrotic. With the often mild inflammation in these sections, a reactive hepatitis was carefully considered. However, the disruption of the portal interface by the areas of fibrosis and inflammation, the overall disruption of the normal portal architecture in these liver sections and obscuring of the interface by inflammatory cells would all be more suggestive of an interface hepatitis.

Histological diagnosis

Hepatitis, interface, neutrophilic-lymphocytic and histiocytic, chronic, multifocal, moderate with fibrosis, moderate, liver.

Addendum

A copper stain is performed in these sections. Frequent aggregations of hepatocytes (20–40% of hepatocytes in HPF areas and often in the periportal regions) contain mild to occasionally moderate amounts of cytoplasmic copper positive granules (black granules). These findings would be indicative of excessive copper accumulation. In addition, the copper-containing hepatocytes are often in periportal areas, which may be suggestive of secondary hepatocellular copper accumulation.

Specialist tests

Quantitative hepatic copper is 1346 µg/g dry weight.

A diagnosis of **interface hepatitis with moderate copper accumulation** was made. In this case it was unknown whether copper accumulation was primary or secondary though the predominantly peri-portal distribution of copper accumulation is more typical of secondary accumulation (in primary copper-associated hepatitis, copper is found predominantly in a centrolobular/zone 3 location).

Treatment and outcome

Pending results of *Leptospira* spp. serology, *Bartonella* spp. PCR and bacterial cultures of bile and liver tissue, the dog was treated with clavulanate-amoxycillin 20 mg/kg p/o BID and doxycycline 10 mg/kg p/o SID. These were discontinued after 7 days when all results were returned. Ursodeoxycholic acid and s-Adenosylmethionine/silybin/vitamin E were given during this time and continually thereafter. The dog recovered well from biopsy but remained with reduced appetite and visible icterus.

On receipt of the biopsy results D-penicillamine was administered at an approximate dose of 13 mg/kg p/o q12 hours continuously and prednisolone was also given at 0.5 mg/kg p/o q24 hours for 4 weeks and then reduced to 0.5 mg/kg p/o q48 hours. Appetite steadily improved over several days and icterus reduced. At this stage a diet low in copper and high in zinc (Royal Canin Hepatic Support) was introduced successfully and fed continuously.

Serial, initially two-weekly, assessment of biochemistry showed a reduction in bilirubin, ALT and ALKP (see **Table 12.7**).

Table 12.7 Serial evaluation of ALT, ALKP and bilirubin

Time from institution of treatment	Initial	2 weeks	4 weeks	10 weeks	6 months	13 months	Reference range
ALT	**961**	**658**	**122**	60	47	59	13–88
ALKP	**461**	**233**	**524**	389	353	386	14–105
Total bilirubin	**307**	**19**	5	11	3	3	0–16

ALT and bilirubin continued to return to normal and icterus resolved. ALKP remained modestly elevated having initially reduced due to the superimposed effects of corticosteroids iso-enzyme induction.

Though it was planned to repeat assessment of hepatic copper by ultrasound-guided core tissue biopsy of the liver after 12 months, this was precluded on cost grounds by the dog's owners. However, given the continued clinical remission and biochemical normalisation of ALT, at this time D-penicillamine was stopped and treatment continued with zinc sulphate at a dose of 1 mg/kg elemental zinc p/o q24 hours; 22 months after diagnosis the dog is still asymptomatic.

Discussion

Chronic hepatitis in dogs is commonly diagnosed but the aetiological cause is ill-defined compared with the situation in human beings in which viral, metabolic and alcohol-induced syndromes predominate and are well defined. Well-known breed predispositions are seen in Dobermann Pinschers, Bedlington Terriers, West Highland White and Skye Terriers, Dalmatians, Cocker Spaniels and Labrador Retrievers with an association with abnormalities of copper accumulation reported in many of these. In Cocker Spaniels the cause is not well defined and in the Dobermann both copper-associated and immune-mediated aetiologies (the latter of which may be the predominant cause in other breeds) have been proposed. Copper-associated hepatitis has been reported in both European and North American families of Labrador Retrievers but, in contrast to this case, the site of copper accumulation in such cases tends to be centrolobular (zone 3) and copper accumulation may occur in peri-portal regions as a consequence of hepatic dysfunction rather than as a cause of it.

Therapy of chronic hepatitis associated with accumulation of copper (whether cause or effect) comprises therapies that may be divided into those aimed at reducing inflammation and fibrosis, those to reduce hepatic copper accumulation and those aimed at supporting/ameliorating deleterious consequences of hepatocellular dysfunction.

Corticosteroid therapy with prednisolone is usually advocated for both anti-inflammatory and antifibrotic effects. Additional immunomodulatory drugs in the form of azathioprine, ciclosporin or chlorambucil are favoured by some clinicians but there is currently little data to support their use in this setting. Similarly, additional antifibrotic agents such as colchicine are frequently advocated without clinical controlled studies supporting their use and caution is recommended when using colchicine due to an unfavourable array of potential side effects including bone marrow toxicity.

The use of D-penicillamine as a copper chelator, in combination with diets that are low in copper, have been shown to be successful in reducing hepatic copper concentration on sequential biopsy specimens. Zinc supplementation may also be used and in practice is often introduced after penicillamine has been given for 6–12 months in substitution for it.

Ursodeoxycholic acid is a hydrophilic bile acid with choleretic, anti-inflammatory and immunomodulatory properties and may act as an antifibrotic agent and antioxidant. Whilst clinical studies in dogs are lacking and restricted to case reports, evidence in humans with biliary cirrhosis is positive and other antioxidants, when evaluated in dogs with liver disease, have shown equally supportive evidence. Of these S-adenosylmethionine (SAMe) has been shown to increase hepatic glutathione concentration/reduce glutathione depletion in a variety of canine and feline hepatopathies. This nutraceutical is often combined with vitamin E and silybin, the active component of milk thistle, which, whilst commonly advocated for its antioxidant effects has a less sound evidence base for use in dogs than SAME.

The prognosis for chronic hepatitis in Labradors is extremely variable and there are few studies evaluating significant numbers of dogs with similar stages of hepatic disease. In one study of

24 client-owned Labradors with hepatitis, the median age of diagnosis was 9.3 years (range 3.9–14 years) and median survival time was 374 days. However, a huge range in survival time from 1 to 2645 days was reported, with patients in which prothrombin time increase or thrombocytopenia were seen as being associated with a survival <2 months.

Further reading

Boomkens, S.Y., Penning, L.C., Egberink, H.F., van den Ingh, T.S. & Rothuizen, J. (2004) Hepatitis with special reference to dogs. A review on the pathogenesis and infectious etiologies, including unpublished results of recent own studies. *Vet Q* **26**, 107–114

Fieten, H., Biourge, V.C., Watson, A.L., Leegwater, P.A., van den Ingh, T.S. & Rothuizen, J. (2014) Nutritional management of inherited copper-associated hepatitis in the Labrador retriever. *Vet J* **199**, 429–433

Fieten, H., Biourge, V.C., Watson, A.L., Leegwater, P.A., van den Ingh, T.S. & Rothuizen, J. (2015) Dietary management of labrador retrievers with subclinical hepatic copper accumulation. *J Vet Intern Med* **29**, 822–827

Fieten, H., Dirksen, K., van den Ingh, T.S., Winter, E.A., Watson, A.L., Leegwater, P.A. & Rothuizen, J. (2013) D-penicillamine treatment of copper-associated hepatitis in Labrador retrievers. *Vet J* **196**, 522–527

Hoffmann, G., Jones, P.G., Biourge, V., van den Ingh, T.S., Mesu, S.J., Bode, P. & Rothuizen, J. (2009) Dietary management of hepatic copper accumulation in Labrador Retrievers. *J Vet Intern Med* **23**, 957–963

Hoffmann, G., van den Ingh, T.S., Bode, P. & Rothuizen, J. (2006) Copper-associated chronic hepatitis in Labrador Retrievers. *J Vet Intern Med* **20**, 856–861

Honeckman, A. (2003) Current concepts in the treatment of canine chronic hepatitis. *Clin Tech Small Anim Pract* **18**, 239–244

Johnston, A.N., Center, S.A., McDonough, S.P., Wakshlag, J.J. & Warner, K.L. (2013) Hepatic copper concentrations in Labrador Retrievers with and without chronic hepatitis: 72 cases (1980–2010). *J Am Vet Med Assoc* **242**, 372–380

Kemp, S.D., Zimmerman, K.L., Panciera, D.L., Monroe, W.E., Lcib, M.S. & Lanz, O.I. (2015) A comparison of liver sampling techniques in dogs. *J Vet Intern Med* **29**, 51–57

Petre, S.L., McClaran, J.K., Bergman, P.J. & Monette, S. (2012) Safety and efficacy of laparoscopic hepatic biopsy in dogs: 80 cases (2004–2009). *J Am Vet Med Assoc* **240**, 181–185

Poldervaart, J.H., Favier, R.P., Penning, L.C., van den Ingh, T.S. & Rothuizen, J. (2009) Primary hepatitis in dogs: a retrospective review (2002–2006). *J Vet Intern Med* **23**, 72–80

Rawlings, C.A. & Howerth, E.W. (2004) Obtaining quality biopsies of the liver and kidney. *J Am Anim Hosp Assoc* **40**, 352–358

Rothuizen, J. & Twedt, D.C. (2009) Liver biopsy techniques. *Vet Clin North Am Small Anim Pract* **39**, 469–480

Shih, J.L., Keating, J.H., Freeman, L.M. & Webster, C.R. (2007) Chronic hepatitis in Labrador Retrievers: clinical presentation and prognostic factors. *J Vet Intern Med* **21**, 33–39

Smedley, R., Mullaney, T. & Rumbeiha, W. (2009) Copper-associated hepatitis in Labrador Retrievers. *Vet Pathol* **46**, 484–490

Vasanjee, S.C., Bubenik, L.J., Hosgood, G. & Bauer, R. (2006) Evaluation of hemorrhage, sample size, and collateral damage for five hepatic biopsy methods in dogs. *Vet Surg* **35**, 86–93

Gastroenterology

Pocket Tutor Gastroenterology, First Edition. Ian Wurie.
© 2018 John Wiley & Sons Ltd. Published 2018 by John Wiley & Sons Ltd.

Clinical presentation

An 8 year-old male-neutered Beagle (**Figure 13.1**) is presented with a history of weakness, depression and abdominal distension. His owners report that recently he has lost weight and that his stools have occasionally been loose but without dyschezia, urgency or loss of faecal continence. When loose his stools are light-tan in colour and of a soupy consistency. He has lost weight and in the last 4 days the owners have noted his abdomen becoming distended. He has continued to eat but they describe coarse generalised tremors developing in the preceding four days and within the previous 48 hours the dog has experienced two seizure-like events which the owners have captured on their mobile phone video facility. These episodes comprise involuntary lateral recumbency with extensor rigidity developing in all four limbs, accompanied by coarse generalised tremor, which becomes more pronounced until tonic-clonic motor activity in all four limbs is noted. Episodes have lasted about 1 minute and spontaneous and complete recovery has ensued afterwards.

The dog is vaccinated yearly and wormed every 6 months with febantel/praziquantel/pyrantel. It has never travelled outside the United Kingdom, is fed a complete commercial dry dog food and has no prior medical history except for some small intestinal diarrhoea 2 months ago which resolved with dietary manipulation within one week.

On physical examination the dog is quiet but interactive and in a thin body condition (BCS 2/5). There is obvious symmetrical abdominal distension and intermittent coarse generalised tremor of head and trunk. Rectal temperature is 38.6 °C, pulse rate 120/min and respiratory rate 16/min. Peripheral pulse quality is poor and distal limbs, ears and oral cavity are cool to the touch. Mucous membrane colour is pink, membranes are moist, capillary refill is 2.5 s. Cardiothoracic auscultation is normal. Abdominal palpation demonstrates a palpable fluid ballottement but no other abnormalities can be discerned. There is generalised muscle wastage.

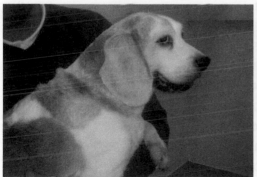 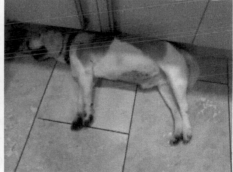

Figure 13.1 The patient at presentation and still image from video footage of a seizure episode.

Canine Internal Medicine: What's Your Diagnosis? First Edition. Jon Wray.
© 2018 John Wiley & Sons Ltd. Published 2018 by John Wiley & Sons Ltd.

The following laboratory results were obtained from this patient at the time of presentation:

Haematology

Parameter	Value	Units	Range
RBC	8.40	$\times 10^{12}/l$	(5.5–8.5)
Haemoglobin	**18.1**	g/dl	(12.0–18.0)
Haematocrit	**0.56**	l/l	(0.37–0.55)
Mean cell volume	67.1	fl	(60–77)
Mean cell haemoglobin concentration	32.1	g/dl	(30.0–38.0)
Mean cell haemoglobin	21.5	pg	(19.5–25.5)
Total white cell count	**20.2**	$\times 10^9/l$	(6.0–15.0)
Neutrophils	**16.66**	$\times 10^9/l$	(3.0–11.5)
Lymphocytes	1.75	$\times 10^9/l$	(1.0–4.8)
Monocytes	**1.58**	$\times 10^9/l$	(0.2–1.4)
Eosinophils	0.15	$\times 10^9/l$	(0.1–1.2)
Basophils	0.05	$\times 10^9/l$	(0.0–0.1)
Platelets	479	$\times 10^9/l$	(200–500)
Film comment:	Red cells: unremarkable morphology		
	White cells: unremarkable morphology		

Biochemistry

Parameter	Value	Units	Range
Total protein	**34**	g/l	(54–77)
Albumin	**11**	g/l	(25–40)
Globulin	23	g/l	(23–45)
Urea	5.6	mmol/l	(2.5–7.4)
Creatinine	48	µmol/l	(40–145)
Potassium	4.4	mmol/l	(3.4–5.6)
Sodium	150	mmol/l	(139–154)
Chloride	**124**	mmol/l	(105–122)
Calcium	**1.1**	mmol/l	(2.1–2.8)
Magnesium	**0.53**	mmol/l	(0.62–0.90)
Inorganic phosphate	1.38	mmol/l	(0.60–1.40)
Glucose	4.9	mmol/l	(3.3–5.8)
ALT	**112**	IU/l	(13–88)
AST	**82**	IU/l	(13–60)
ALKP	54	IU/l	(14–105)
GGT	2	IU/l	(0–10)
Bilirubin	2	µmol/l	(0–16)

Parameter	Value	Units	Range
Cholesterol	**1.9**	mmol/l	(3.8–7.0)
Triglyceride	0.8	mmol/l	(0.56–1.14)
Creatine kinase	185	IU/l	(0–190)

Questions

1. What is your problem list for this dog based on the history and physical examination?
2. What is your interpretation of the laboratory findings?
3. What are the differential diagnoses for the abdominal fluid and which of these is most likely given the laboratory results?
4. What is the most likely cause of this dog's seizures and what is the most likely mechanism by which this has developed?
5. How would you investigate this dog's problems further?

Answers

1. What is your problem list for this dog based on the history and physical examination?

The diarrhoea is pale and voluminous and is accompanied by weight loss and not by dyschezia or urgency. The clinical problem list for this dog is

- Weakness
- Depression
- Ascites
- Weight loss
- Small intestinal diarrhoea (see Case 15, Table 15.1)
- Coarse generalised tremor
- Seizure
- Hypovolaemia

2. What is your interpretation of the laboratory findings?

The haematology shows a marginal increase in haematocrit and haemoglobin without a rise in red blood cell count. Although this marginal elevation is unlikely to be significant, it may by the same token reflect early/mild polycythaemia, which may in turn be 'relative' (due to dehydration) or 'absolute'. If absolute this may be an appropriate response to physiological need (erythropoietin-stimulated in setting of hypoxaemia) or inappropriate, though the latter is very unlikely to be responsible at this marginal level.

The neutrophilia together with monocytosis are likely to represent a chronic inflammatory response.

The most striking biochemical abnormalities are profound hypoalbuminaemia (accompanied by normal globulin), severe hypocalcaemia and hypocholesterolaemia. The increases in the hepatic transaminases ALT and AST are so mild that they are of debateable significance.

Hypoalbuminaemia

Severe hypoalbuminaemia (<20 g/l) most commonly arises due to protein-losing nephropathy (PLN), protein-losing enteropathy (PLE) or failure of hepatic production in patients with severe functional liver disease. Probably the most common cause of hypoalbuminaemia in veterinary small animal patients is a reduction seen accompanying chronic or inflammatory illnesses as a 'negative acute phase' response; however, in this situation the hypoalbuminaemia is almost always very mild and seldom <20 g/l. The hypoalbuminaemia of PLE is often, but not exclusively, accompanied by hypoglobulinaemia (i.e. as a panhypoproteinaemia), but in some patients with PLE albumin loss either predominates or precedes development of hypoglobulinaemia, or globulin levels remain normal due to the off-setting of any loss by inflammation within the gastrointestinal tract. Protein-losing nephropathy should never be excluded on the basis of normal urea and creatinine as severe dysfunction in glomerular permselectivity may occur without these being elevated. Severe hepatic dysfunction may also result in subnormal urea, cholesterol and glucose and may also be accompanied by increases in hepatocellular and cholestatic markers, though these do not in themselves indicate hepatic function or lack thereof.

Hypocalcaemia may be seen accompanying hypoalbuminaemia, due to decreased PTH activity, acute pancreatitis, puerperal tetany, hypovitaminosis D, ethylene glycol toxicity and disorders that result in excess urinary excretion, complexing of Ca^{2+} with anions or with acute myopathy or tumour lysis (see Case 2). Spurious hypocalcaemia may also be seen, especially with EDTA contamination of samples. Of these puerperal tetany can be immediately discounted in this patient.

Hypocholesterolaemia is uncommon and seen most frequently with decreased production due to portosystemic shunts, in the presence of protein-losing enteropathies and with hypoadrenocorticism.

Hypomagnesaemia may be seen due to decreased plasma protein binding, inadequate intestinal absorption or increased urinary excretion.

3. What are the differential diagnoses for the abdominal fluid and which of these is most likely given the laboratory results?

Differential diagnoses for an abdominal fluid type are shown in **Table 13.1**.

Their differentiation and characteristics are tabulated below in **Table 13.2**. Note that the distinction between 'pure' and 'modified' transudate is a somewhat artificial one and not based on mechanistic determinants of fluid production. Some authorities argue, with some justification, against such a distinction but it has become a commonly used classification.

In a patient with such a low serum albumin, a pure transudate is the most likely fluid.

4. What is the most likely cause of this dog's seizures and what is the most likely mechanism by which this has developed?

Table 13.1 Differential diagnosis for abdominal fluid

Types of abdominal fluid
• Pure transudate
• Modified transudate
• Exudate
• Blood
• Urine
• Bile
• Chyle

Table 13.2 Distinguishing features of common fluid types

	Pure transudate	Modified transudate	Exudate	Other
Pathogenesis	Extravasation of low-protein fluid due to decreased vascular colloid oncotic pressure (usually in hypoalbuminaemic states). Occasionally pure transudates may occur in early stages of right-sided congestive heart failure, though modified transudate is more common. Pure transudates also occur in the setting of portal venous hypertension, the mechanism of production being complex and not simply due to extravasation of fluid due to increased hydrostatic pressure in post-sinusoidal vessels	Extravasation of fluid principally from increased hydrostatic pressure in vessels due to right-sided congestive heart failure or tamponade. However, modified transudates may also be neoplastic in origin or represent local fluid production from organ torsion	The most common cause is inflammation, which may be septic or non-septic. The most common cause of septic effusion is penetration/rupture of the gastrointestinal tract. Non-septic exudates may also be neoplastic in origin or represent local fluid production from organ torsion	Other considerations are: • Chyle • Blood • Bile • Urine Specific analysis of fluid including cytology, triglyceride content compared with serum (chyloabdomen), total bilirubin compared with serum (bilioabdomen), creatinine concentration compared with serum (uroabdomen)
Fluid protein	<20 g/l	20–50 g/l	>30 g/l	Chyle is typically rich in small lymphocytes and has a triglyceride content greater than that of plasma; over time chylous effusion becomes steadily more neutrophil-rich. Chylous effusions may be classified as modified transudates or exudates depending on cellularity
Fluid nucleated cell count	<1500/μl	<5000/μl	>5000/μl	
Nucleated cell type	Variable but low in number	Mostly neutrophils, macrophages and reactive mesothelial cells	Neutrophils and macrophages. Degenerative neutrophils and possible intracellular bacteria are hallmarks of septic exudates	
Common aetiologies	Severe hypoalbuminaemia Portal hypertension	Commonly right-sided congestive heart failure and cardiac tamponade	Septic peritonitis, pancreatitis, neoplasia, after surgery	

Seizure classification

Seizure classification is complicated by many different terminologies and fluidity of their use. Current classifications may include

- Primary/genetic/idiopathic seizures.
- Structural/secondary/symptomatic seizures (due to structural CNS disease).
- Reactive seizures (due to systemic disease, metabolic derangements or intoxication).
- Unknown/cryptogenic (seizure in absence of, or prior to, investigative efforts).

In this case a profound hypocalcaemia of 1.1 mmol/l is a very plausible cause of reactive seizures. Clinical signs (predominantly neurological) are seen in hypocalcaemic patients typically with total calcium (tCa^{2+}) <1.6 mmol/l and free calcium (fCa^{2+}) <0.8 mmol/l.

Although total calcium (tCa^{2+}) may decrease in the setting of hypoalbuminaemia, since only 35% of total calcium is protein-bound, a level of 1.1 mmol/l is very unlikely to develop through hypoalbuminaemia alone, and furthermore hypoalbuminaemia does not affect free calcium levels. The most likely differential diagnoses for such a profoundly low total calcium in a symptomatic seizuring patient would be of lack of PTH (hypoparathyroidism) or due to hypovitaminosis D. Since the latter most often accompanies severe protein-losing enteropathy, whereas serum proteins should be normal in the setting of hypoparathyroidism, this is the most likely cause.

5. **How would you investigate this dog's problems further?**

Further assessment should, if possible, include

- Abdominal paracentesis and fluid collection/analysis for protein, total nucleated cell count and cytological evaluation.
- Urinalysis, specifically including the urine protein:creatinine ratio to exclude protein-losing nephropathy as a cause of the hypoalbuminaemia.
- Assessment of pre- and post-prandial bile acids to assess hepatic function.
- Assessment of serum free calcium (often referred to as 'ionised' calcium).
- Assessment for acute pancreatitis by both canine pancreatic lipase immunoreactivity and ultrasound examination.
- Provided that free calcium is also abnormally low *and on a concurrent blood sample so that the result can be interpreted in the light of a known hypocalcaemia*:
  ○ Assessment of PTH (note that specific handling requirements exist for this analyte and communication with the reference laboratory beforehand is recommended).
  ○ Assessment of 25 hydroxy-vitamin D.
- Investigation of causes and consequences of the small intestinal diarrhoea which may include
  ○ Assessment of TLI, folate and cobalamin.
  ○ Diagnostic imaging of the small intestine and local abdominal contents.
  ○ Assessment of faecal parasitology and cultures for pathogenic organisms.
  ○ Histopathological assessment of the small intestine by either of
    - Endoscopy or
    - Surgical full-thickness biopsy.
  ○ See also Case 2 for discussion of calcium metabolism and assessment

There are pros and cons to both endoscopic and surgical means of obtaining biopsies and these are summarised in **Table 13.3**.

Table 13.3 Endoscopic versus surgical intestinal biopsies

	Endoscopic biopsies	**Full-thickness surgical biopsies**
Pros	• No surgical recovery time • Biopsy sites heal rapidly as not full-thickness • Allows visualisation of mucosal surface from lumen for both diagnostic evaluation and targeted collection of biopsies • Very many biopsies may be taken without a significant increase in risk • Gastrostomy and/or jejunostomy feeding tube may be placed at the same time	• Biopsies sufficiently large to include all relevant layers of gut wall and to give good architectural information • Lymphangiectasia and lymphoma may be better diagnosed by this method • The entire small intestine can be visualised and biopsies taken from anywhere in it • Biopsies less likely to be affected by oedema or crush artefact • Extraintestinal organs can be evaluated at the same time and should a surgically amenable problem be determined, the procedure may be both diagnostic and therapeutic • Gastrostomy and/or Jejunostomy feeding tube may be placed at the same time
Cons	• Technically demanding – many veterinary surgeons perform non-diagnostic procedure through an inability to intubate the small intestine • Collection of small intestinal biopsies limited to proximal small intestine and distal only with well-prepared colonoscopy and ileoscopy (except with double-balloon enteroscopy) • Biopsy samples are very small and may contain inadequate submucosal tissue or proffer limited architectural information • Biopsy samples are prone to artefact due to oedema and crush • Lesions of lymphangiectasia and lymphoma are easily missed	• Longer recovery time, which may be relevant in debilitated patients • Risk of surgical dehiscence leading to septic peritonitis with an associated high mortality rate • Visualisation of mucosal surface from lumen not possible without enterotomy

The patient is demonstrating evidence of hypovolaemia and circulatory compromise due to severe hypoalbuminaemia, and these features should be corrected/supported as far as possible prior to undertaking investigation other than initial laboratory tests. Symptomatic hypocalcaemia should also be corrected prior to undertaking further investigation.

Outcome
In this patient the following clinical findings were determined:

• Abdominal paracentesis
  ○ Clear colourless fluid
  ○ Nucleated cell count 0.2 x 10^9/l
  ○ Fluid protein <4 g/l

- ◦ A cytospin preparation is hypocellular consisting of small numbers of mixed leukocytes (comprising neutrophils, monocytes, a few lymphocytes and rare macrophages). Neutrophils are non-degenerative
  - ◦ Analysis consistent with pure transudate
- Urinalysis demonstrated pale straw-coloured urine with pH 6.5, specific gravity 1.028 and urine protein:creatinine ratio of 0.4. The urine sediment was inactive
- Pre- and post-prandial bile acids were 2 and 5.5 μmol/l (<15) respectively
- Serum free calcium was **0.70** mmol/l (1.18–1.40)
- Canine pancreatic lipase was 142 μg/l (<200)
- Plasma parathyroid hormone (PTH) was **505** pg/ml (20–65) and 25 hydroxycholecalciferol (vitamin D) was **9** nmol/l (60–215)
- cTLI 16.1 μg/l (5.0–32.0)
- Folate 8.1 ng/ml (6.5–11.5)
- B12 **167.0** pg/ml (> 275)

These findings confirm hypovitaminosis D as a likely cause of the hypocalcaemia and implicate, by exclusion of hepatic dysfunction and protein-losing nephropathy, protein-losing enteropathy as a cause of the severe hypoalbuminaemia and consequent transudative ascites. It was considered that concurrent intestinal inflammation had probably offset any concurrent decrease in serum globulin. Low serum B12 (cobalamin) may be found in distal small intestinal malabsorptive disease or in small intestinal bacterial overgrowth (aka intestinal dysbiosis, antibiotic-responsive diarrhoea) and is discussed further later. Low B12 often frequently accompanies exocrine pancreatic insufficiency, excluded here by the robustly normal cTLI.

A pooled sample of three consecutive faecal samples demonstrated the following results:

Assessment	Result
Appearance	Semi-formed
Faecal parasites	No ova, cysts or parasites seen
Campylobacter **spp.**	Not isolated
Salmonella **spp.**	Not isolated
Cl. difficile toxin/antigen	Negative
Cl. perfringens toxin	Negative
Cryptosporidium **spp.**	Negative
Giardia **spp.** antigen	Negative

A summary of an abdominal ultrasound report is given below (see **Figure 13.2**):

- There is plentiful anechoic peritoneal fluid.
- Liver: mild hepatomegaly. Diffuse homogeneous increased echogenicity of the hepatic parenchyma. Gallbladder: normal.
- Gastrointestinal tract: marked echogenicity of the mucosa of the duodenum and jejunum. The duodenum has a mildly thickened wall and the mucosal echogenicity has faint striations. The jejunal mucosa is speckled/echogenic and also mildly thickened (0.49 cm). Jejunal lymph nodes are normal.
- The remainder of the abdominal examination is normal.

The patient received colloid fluid therapy at a rate of 20 ml/kg/24 hours and via a separate intravenous cannula, a constant rate infusion of 10% calcium borogluconate in normal saline to deliver

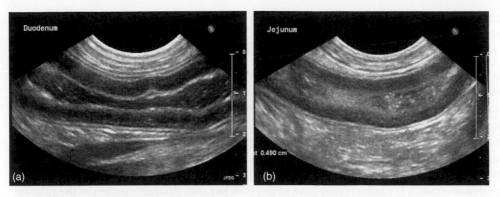

Figure 13.2 (a) Duodenal ultrasound and (b) jejunal ultrasound.

a target of 60 mg/kg/day elemental calcium, but adjusted on the basis of a twice daily assessment of free calcium. 500 mcg of vitamin B12 was also administered parenterally and a fish and potato-based commercial diet was fed.

An upper gastrointestinal endoscopic examination was performed (**Figure 13.3**) and endoscopic biopsies obtained from the stomach and duodenum.

The following histological diagnosis was made:

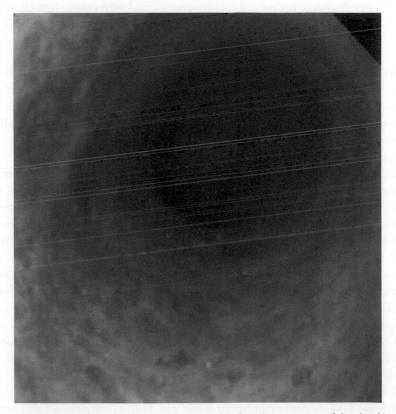

Figure 13.3 Endoscopic view of the duodenum. The normal 'velvety' appearance of the duodenal mucosa is absent and a rather mucoid, pitted appearance is present.

A. Gastritis, lymphocytic-plasmacytic, subacute to chronic, multifocal, mild, stomach.
B. Enteritis, lymphocytic-plasmacytic to neutrophilic, subacute to chronic, multifocal, moderate with villous atrophy, mild to moderate, and some crypt microabscessation, duodenum.

A diagnosis of **protein-losing enteropathy (PLE) due to intestinal inflammation and micro-abscessation** was made with **secondary hypovitaminosis D**

The patient was treated with prednisolone at an initial dose of 2 mg/kg/day and chlorambucil 2 mg once daily for 14 days and then 2 mg every other day, oxytetracycline 250 mg orally every 8 hours and vitamin B12 250 mcg by subcutaneous injection weekly. A diet based on fish and potato (Eukanuba Dermatosis response FP) was fed exclusively. Calcium borogluconate was infused at a dose of 90 mg/kg/day elemental calcium for 3 days whilst oral therapy was undertaken; it was considered that oral vitamin D products may have to be given but after discontinuation of the calcium borogluconate infusion serum calcium levels remained higher than on presentation and the dog was discharged without oral vitamin D products.

Initially the dog brightened and at re-examination one week after discharge stool quality was reportedly improved to produce solid consistency and normal coloured faeces and all signs of coarse tremor and seizure had stopped. On physical examination ascites had resolved. Serum biochemistry a week after discharge demonstrated calcium to have risen to 1.9 mmol/l (2.1–2.8), albumin to 18 g/l (25–40) and globulin to 26 g/l (23–45).

At 7 weeks after discharge clinical improvement continued and serum albumin had risen to 22 g/l (25–40), globulin 34 g/l (23–45) and calcium was 2 mmol/l (2.1–2.8).

At 10 weeks after discharge the patient rapidly deteriorated with concurrent clinical signs suggestive of acute pancreatitis. The owners elected for euthanasia to be performed at this time.

Discussion

The term 'protein-losing enteropathy' (PLE) describes a heterogenous group of intestinal pathologies that result in loss of serum proteins into the GI tract, principally because of either lymphatic obstruction/rupture, widespread ulceration/erosion or mucosal infiltrates (inflammatory or neoplastic). The most commonly reported conditions underlying PLE in dogs are idiopathic inflammatory bowel disease, lymphangiectasia and a diffuse form of intestinal lymphoma, though occasionally infectious and parasitic agents (Parvoviral enteritis, Histoplasmosis, *Ancylostoma* spp.) and diffuse mechanical disruption (such as intussusception) have been reported causes. Crypt abscessation or 'mucoid cryptal ectasia' has also been a commonly reported histopathological finding in dogs with PLE, especially Yorkshire Terriers, and has been reported in the presence of minimal inflammatory change within the lamina propria. Determination of the underlying pathological process requires intestinal biopsy, which may be undertaken by endoscopy or by surgical full-thickness biopsy, and both have advantages and disadvantages. Endoscopic biopsies have advantages of the endoscopist being able to target visually identified abnormalities for biopsies and are generally very safely performed since dehiscence of a surgical wound to the intestinal wall is not a feature. However, gross changes to the wall of the intestine are generally not specific for a particular pathology and endoscopic biopsy collection is limited in the small intestine to the proximal and very terminal small intestine only. Furthermore, pathology whose lesions may be predominantly within deeper layers of the gut wall may be missed and lesions that may be somewhat patchy in distribution or which are easily disrupted/only partly accessed by such small biopsies (namely lymphangiectasia and lymphoma) may be missed. Additionally, endoscopic biopsies may be rendered of poor quality by both crush artefact and because in severely hypoproteinaemic animals mucosal oedema of the intestine may substantially alter the morphology of such small biopsies. Surgical biopsies have the advantage of diagnostic yield and access to areas of the intestine inaccessible to routine endoscopy and allow corrective surgery to be performed should a surgically correctable lesion exist. However, disadvantages include a risk of potentially disastrous surgical dehiscence and a period of convalescence/recuperation in already often debilitated patients.

The diagnosis of lymphangiectasia and intestinal lymphoma are based on characteristic histological findings of lacteal dilatation, rupture and lipogranulomata and lamina proprial infiltration with clonal lymphocyte populations. The diagnosis of idiopathic inflammatory bowel disease is problematic since stereotypical lymphoplasmacytic inflammation of the lamina propria accompanies most major disorders of the intestines and the demonstration of inflammatory infiltrates alone does not vindicate a diagnosis of inflammatory bowel disease. The presence of architectural disruption such as villus blunting, fusion and stunting may lend corroborative evidence to such a presumptive diagnosis but ultimately a diagnosis of IBD should be made only after systematic elimination of other potential causes of intestinal pathology, including evaluation for parasitic and infectious diseases, meticulous exclusion of anatomical and structural/obstructive pathologies and performance of treatment trials for dietary intolerances and intestinal dysbiosis (see below), as well as documenting intestinal inflammation.

The consequences of PLE may include development of ascites and tissue oedema due to reduction of colloid oncotic pressure because of hypoalbuminaemia and of thromboembolic complications due to the generation of a hypercoagulable state in these patients. Malabsorption of vitamin D and magnesium have been reported occasionally in dogs with PLEs and symptomatic hypocalcaemia, as in this case, may result.

Intestinal 'dysbiosis' (also known as small intestinal bacteria overgrowth, SIBO) is a poorly understood syndrome of small intestinal diarrhoea and failure to thrive, which usually occurs secondary to other intestinal pathology, though a primary form (often referred to as antibiotic-responsive diarrhoea, ARD) may be seen in young large breed dogs, especially German Shepherds. The terms bacterial overgrowth is largely one of supposition since laboratory methods to quantify small intestinal bacterial numbers provide massive underestimation due to the inability to culture many commensal intestinal organisms. Although the finding of either/both or reduced vitamin B12 (cobalamin) and increased levels of folate (based on the observation that many bacteria synthesise folate and others bind cobalamin) may offer supportive evidence, such findings are neither sensitive nor specific for a diagnosis of dysbiosis and reduced cobalamin may simply reflect distal small intestinal malabsorption (see **Case 15**).

The principle treatment of PLE comprises two main components in the stable patient, namely dietary modification and modulation of intestinal inflammation. However, many patients present in a severely debilitated state and may require treatment to ameliorate the reduction in colloid oncotic pressure due to hypoalbuminaemia and intensive nutritional supportive efforts. Correction of hypoalbuminaemia is problematic; use of high molecular weight colloids may help temporarily to increase intravascular colloid oncotic pressure and reduce fluid extravasation but do not alter albumin levels. Administration of plasma to provide plasma proteins including albumin is an extremely inefficient way to correct hypoalbiminaemia and transfusate from many animals is needed to make the smallest impact on serum albumin levels. Infusion of human albumin solutions were at one time popular and are undoubtedly associated with the most efficient means of acutely increasing serum albumin, but are associated with major risks including that of fatal vasculopathies. When acute nutritional supportive measures are taken these may involve a combination of both enteral and parenteral nutrition; careful planning is essential and nutritional plans should take into account both the extraordinary protein loss that some such individuals experience and the fact that the absorptive gut is effectively 'crippled' until such a time that medical treatment responses are seen. Dogs with lymphangiectasia are usually treated with an ultra-low fat diet to try and limit further lymphatic dilatation and rupture. In dogs with putative IBD the use of hydrolysed diets or novel protein-source diets is often recommended.

Modulation of intestinal inflammation is usually undertaken with corticosteroid therapy and prednisolone at an initial dose of 2–4 mg/kg/day is usually used, followed by gradual dose tapering based on clinical and clinicopathological response. Additional immunomodulatory agents are also often employed and include azathioprine, chlorambucil and ciclosporin. There are several studies published to support the use of these agents and also other corticosteroid formulations such as budesonide but to date no consensus exists as to the best form of treatment of inflammation associated with PLE.

The prognosis in PLE has been described as guarded and reported variously as 66% mortality rate within 5 months, 32% mortality within 2 years or 58% risk of death and median survival times of 90 days and 701 days have been reported.

Further reading

Allenspach, K., Wieland, B., Grone, A. et al. (2007) Chronic enteropathies in dogs: evaluation of risk factors for negative outcome. *J Vet Intern Med* **21** (4), 700–708

Craven, M., Simpson, J.W., Ridyard, A.E. et al. (2004) Canine inflammatory bowel disease: retrospective analysis of diagnosis and outcome in 80 cases (1995–2002). *J Small Anim Pract* **45** (7), 336–342

Dandrieux, J.R., Noble, P.J., Scase, T.J. et al. (2013) Comparison of a chlorambucil–prednisolone combination with an azathioprine–prednisolone combination for the treatment of canine chronic enteropathies with concurrent protein-losing enteropathy: 27 cases (2007–2010). *J Am Vet Med Assoc* **242** (12), 1705–1714

Dossin. O & Lavoue, R. (2011) Protein-losing enteropathies. *Vet Clin North Am Small Anim Pract* **41** (2), 399–418

Gow, A.G., Else, R., Evans, H. et al. (2011) Hypovitaminosis D in dogs with inflammatory bowel disease and hypoalbuminaemia. *J Small Anim Pract* **52** (8), 411–418

Kimmel, S.E., Waddell, L.S. & Michel, K.E. (2000) Hypomagnesemia and hypocalcemia associated with protein-losing enteropathy in Yorkshire terriers: five cases (1992–1998). *J Am Vet Med Assoc* **217** (5), 703–706

Simpson, K.W. & Jergens, A. (2011) Pitfalls and progress in the diagnosis and management of canine inflammatory bowel disease. *Vet Clin North Am Small Anim Pract* **41** (2), 381–398

Stroda, K., Wakamatsu, N., Gaschen, L. et al. (2012) Histopathological, clinical, endoscopic, and ultrasound features of dogs with chronic enteropathies and small intestinal crypt lesions. Paper presented at the ACVIM Forum 2012, New Orleans.

Willard, M.D., Helman, G., Fradkin, J.M. et al. (2000) Intestinal crypt lesions associated with protein-losing enteropathy in the dog. *J Vet Intern Med* **14**, 298–307

Clinical presentation

An 8 year-old male-neutered Elkhound weighing 28 kg is presented with a 24-hour history of acute onset inappetence, vomiting and depression. The dog has vomited a total of eight times, initially vomiting partially digested food 3 hours after eating and subsequently has vomited bile-stained liquid in large amounts. Abdominal effort is seen to accompany vomiting and no diarrhoea is reported by the owner. The dog has continued to drink water without vomiting.

The dog has an unremarkable previous medical history, is vaccinated annually against distemper, infectious canine hepatitis, parvovirus, parainfluenzavirus and leptospirosis (*L. icterohaemorrhagiae* and *L. canicola*) and is wormed twice yearly with fenbendazole. It has not travelled outside the United Kingdom and receives no regular medication or over-the-counter supplements. No recent history of scavenging or other dietary indiscretion is reported by the owners.

Physical examination demonstrates an overweight dog (body condition score 4/5) that is very subdued and reluctant to walk. Sclerae, conjunctival and oral mucous membranes are icteric and the latter are tacky to the touch. Capillary refill is difficult to ascertain due to icterus but eyes seem slightly sunken. Heart rate is 100/min and peripheral pulse quality is poor. Respiratory rate is 32/min and auscultation of the heart and respiratory tract is normal. The dog's rectal temperature is 39.4 °C. Palpation of the abdomen demonstrates diffuse mid-abdominal discomfort, which is reproducible but poorly localisable. No dermatological changes or lymphadenomegaly are detected.

Questions (there are three questions, two *before* and one *after* the case findings)

1. What is the problem list and differential diagnosis list for this dog?
2. One cause of acute onset vomiting, abdominal discomfort and icterus commonly seen in the dog is acute pancreatitis. What diagnostic tests are available to confirm a diagnostic suspicion of pancreatitis and what other differential diagnoses should be considered for this combination of clinical problems?

    (Answer this before reading onwards.)

Answers

1. What is the problem list and differential diagnosis list for this dog?

The problem list may be described as

- Vomiting
- Abdominal pain
- Jaundice (icterus)
- Lethargy
- Inappetence
- Pyrexia
- Interstitial and intravascular volume depletion without compensatory tachycardia

See Case 12 and Table 12.1 previously for discussion of approach to jaundice. Differential diagnoses for vomiting and abdominal pain are listed in **Tables 14.1** and **14.2**. However, relatively

Canine Internal Medicine: What's Your Diagnosis? First Edition. Jon Wray.
© 2018 John Wiley & Sons Ltd. Published 2018 by John Wiley & Sons Ltd.

Table 14.1 Differential diagnosis of acute vomiting

Differential diagnosis for canine vomiting	
Systemic disorders that may present primarily with vomiting	*M (Metabolic)* • Hypoadrenocorticism • Liver disease (especially leptospirosis) • Kidney disease • Diabetic ketoacidosis • Encephalopathy, vestibular disease *N (Neoplastic, Nutritional)* • Systemic mastocytosis *I (Infectious, Inflammatory, Immune-mediated)* • Sepsis *T (Traumatic, Toxic)* • Drug administration, intoxication
Local disorders that may cause GI signs of vomiting as an 'innocent bystander' effect	*A (Anomalous, Anatomical)* • Diaphragmatic hernia • Torsions/entrapment involving the GI tract *N (Neoplastic, Nutritional)* • Diffuse neoplasia *I (Infectious, Inflammatory, Immune-mediated)* • Pancreatitis • Pansteatitis • Focal peritonitis, abscess or adhesions • Inflammatory hepatobiliary disease

Primary gastric disease
[those in square brackets uncommon]
	A (Anomalous, Anatomical)
	• Foreign body
	• Pyloric stenosis / antral hypertrophy
	• Gastric volvulus
	• Motility disorders
	N (Neoplastic, Nutritional)
	• Gastric neoplasia (focal or diffuse)
	• Dietary intolerance
	• Dietary indiscretion
	• [Gastrinoma]
	I (Infectious, Inflammatory, Immune-Mediated)
	• [Infectious]
	   ◦ Bacterial (eg *Helicobacter*-like infection)
	   ◦ Viral
	   ◦ Protozoal
	   ◦ Fungal
	   ◦ Algal
	   ◦ Parasitic

Differential diagnosis for canine vomiting

	• Polyps
	• Gastric ulceration
	• Chronic gastritis / Inflammatory Bowel Disease
	T (Traumatic, Toxic)
	• Drug side effects, toxins
Vomiting accompanying primarily intestinal disease	*A (Anomalous, Anatomical)*
	• Foreign body
	• Intussusception
	• Motility disorders
	N (Neoplastic, Nutritional)
	• Intestinal neoplasia (focal or diffuse)
	• Dietary intolerance
	• Dietary indiscretion
	I (Infectious, Inflammatory, Immune-Mediated)
	• Infectious (bacterial, viral, protozoal, fungal,
	• algal, parasitic)
	• Inflammatory bowel disease
	• Vomiting associated with colitis
	• *T (Traumatic, Toxic)*
	• Drug and toxin-induced

Table 14.2 Differential diagnosis of abdominal pain

Differential diagnoses of abdominal pain

D (Degenerative)
- Spinal pain due to intervertebral disc disease mimicking abdominal pain

A (Anomalous, Anatomical)
- Gastrointestinal foreign body, intussusception
- Obstructive cholelithiasis
- Torsion of
  ° Liver lobes
  ° Spleen
  ° Mesentery
  ° Colon
- Gastrointestinal ileus (structural or functional)
- Upper and lower urinary tract obstruction especially due to urolithiasis

M (Metabolic)
- Hypoadrenocorticism

N (Neoplastic, Nutritional)
- Intra-abdominal neoplasia especially carcinomatosis, mast cell tumour
- Dietary indiscretion, dietary intolerance

(Continued)

Differential diagnoses of abdominal pain

I (Infectious, Inflammatory, Immune-mediated)

- Pancreatitis
- Pansteatitis
- Cholecystitis
- Gall bladder mucocoele
- Gastritis
- Enteritis
- Colitis
- Necrosis, ulceration, rupture or perforation of the gastrointestinal tract
- Peritonitis
- Abscessation of the liver, pancreas, spleen, mesentery or kidneys

T (Traumatic, Toxic)

- Gastrointestinal irritant toxin ingestion

V (Vascular)

Thrombosis of

- Mesenteric vessels
- Portal vein
- Hepatic vessels

---

few of these would be likely to be associated with icterus and thus icterus may be considered a 'pivotal' problem in this problem list. The differential diagnosis of jaundice was described in **Table 12.1** of **Case 12** and may be defined as 'pre-hepatic', 'hepatic' and 'post-hepatic'.

Of the problems listed the main differential diagnosis list for icterus, vomiting and abdominal pain is

- Pancreatitis
- Acute icteric liver disease with abdominal discomfort
  - Entrapment of liver in diaphragmatic hernia (congenital or acquired)
  - Leptospirosis
  - Hepatic thrombosis
  - Hepatic abscess
  - Hepatic lobar torsion
- Acute disease of the gall bladder and common bile duct
  - Mucocoele
  - Obstructive cholelithiasis
  - Acute cholecystitis

2. **One cause of acute onset vomiting, abdominal discomfort and icterus commonly seen in the dog is acute pancreatitis. What diagnostic tests are available to confirm a diagnostic suspicion of pancreatitis and what other differential diagnoses should be considered for this combination of clinical problems?**

Diagnostic tests for pancreatitis may be divided into

- Supportive/concurrent clinical pathology abnormalities

- Specific clinical pathology abnormalities
- Diagnostic imaging tests

Supportive clinical pathology abnormalities
- Haematology
  - Commonly a neutrophilia +/– left shift consistent with an inflammatory response is seen.
  - Evidence of haemoconcentration or conversely mild anaemia may be detected.
  - Platelet count may be initially elevated due to inflammatory response but in some cases may be low and particularly in severe acute pancreatitis more significant lowering of platelet count may be present due to developing DIC.
- Biochemistry
  - Mild to moderate raises in ALKP and ALT are commonly, though not invariably, seen and may lead to erroneous assumption of primary hepatopathy. A combination of cholestasis and secondary/reactive local hepatopathy is probably responsible.
  - Hyperbilirubinaemia due to extrahepatic partial obstruction of bile flow is very common.
  - Azotaemia is frequently present and very often the relative magnitude of a rise in urea is greater than that in creatinine. Azotaemia may be multifactorial and may represent, alternatively or in combination, dehydration/hypovolaemia, gastrointestinal haemorrhage or development of renal failure as part of a multi-organ dysfunction syndrome seen in some dogs with severe pancreatitis.
  - Electrolyte abnormalities are often seen and may relate to vomiting, acidosis, a decreased glomerular filtration rate and third-space loss in abdominal effusions. Hypochloridaemia, hyponatraemia and either hyper- or hypokalaemia are most frequently seen.

Specific clinical pathology abnormalities
- Serum amylase and lipase
  - Traditionally alterations in amylase and lipase were examined for evidence of pancreatitis but have disappointing sensitivity and specificity.
  - Both amylase and lipase will become elevated in a variety of non-pancreatic conditions and especially where the glomerular filtration rate is reduced.
  - Values exceeding 3–4 times the upper reference interval are commonly reported as indicating greater specificity for pancreatic pathology, although some animals with non-pancreatic pathology will have levels that exceed these limits.
  - The sensitivity for amylase in diagnosing canine pancreatitis has been variably reported as between 14% and 69% and specificity 50–100%, and for lipase sensitivity of 14–71% and specificity of 43–81%. This wide variation reflects differences in sample methodology, study populations and comparison 'gold standard' used.
  - In summary, amylase and lipase, when high and where other reasons for elevation are not present, may offer strong corroborative evidence for pancreatitis but normal values should not be used to exclude it. The author would caution against dismissal of these tests as being of 'historical' value only since clinically there are many patients whose diagnosis is strongly supported by their use.
  - A recent development is that of lipase activity using the substrate 1,2-o-dilauryl-rac-glycero glutaric acid-(6'methylresorufin)-ester (shortened to DGGR lipase) which seems to correlate well with the Spec cPL assay in dogs.
- Canine pancreas-specific lipase immunoreactivity (PLI)
  - Detect pancreatic lipase purely of pancreatic origin and measures in either a semi-quantitative fashion (cassette ELISA cPLI 'SNAP' method) or a laboratory-based quantitative measurement. There appears to be good agreement between the two methods. The original

PLI assay has been replaced by a more widely available immunoassay (Spec cPL).

- ○ A 'grey area' exists for canine Spec cPL between 201 and 399 µg/l, with values >400 µg/l strongly suggestive for pancreatitis.
- ○ The sensitivity of cPLI in diagnosis of clinical pancreatitis in dogs is 72–78% in one study, and in another evaluating dogs with a variety of severities of histological pancreatitis determined at necropsy sensitivity varied between 21% for mild to 71% for moderate-to-severe pancreatitis. Overall a wide range of sensitivities from 21% to 94% has been reported. Specificity is somewhat more consistent with reports between 81% and 100%.
- ○ The performance of cPLI is superior to other diagnostic tests and convincingly abnormal values have high positive predictive value for the presence of pancreatitis. Nonetheless, the variable sensitivity should mandate that, should beware of false-negative results, which are clinically not uncommon. The author's opinion is that cPLI assays improve upon and complement existing diagnostic tests in a way that has improved our diagnostic capabilities, rather than wholesale replacement of them.

- Other diagnostic tests
  - ○ Serum canine trypsin-like immunoreactivity (cTLI) measures trypsinogen and trypsin and may be elevated in acute pancreatitis but has a short serum half-life and has been shown to decrease rapidly after experimental induction of pancreatitis. Sensitivity is low (36–47%) in diagnosis of spontaneous pancreatitis with specificity reported between 75% and 100%.
  - ○ Other tests that have been examined but are either limited by poor test performance or limited by the nature of evaluation include
    - Trypsin-alpha1-antitrypsin complexes.
    - Plasma and urine trypsinogenic activation peptide (TAP).
    - Alpha-2-macroglobulin.
    - Faecal elastase.
    - Phospholipase A2.

Diagnostic imaging

- Radiography
  - ○ Classical radiographic findings in pancreatitis include loss of serosal detail within the cranial right abdomen, displacement of the duodenum and stomach, increased soft tissue opacity within the right cranial abdominal quadrant and gas distension/corrugation of bowel loops adjacent to the pancreas.
  - ○ Sensitivity of radiography is, however, only reported to be 24% and these findings are not specific for pancreatitis.

- Ultrasound
  - ○ The sensitivity of ultrasound for diagnosis of acute pancreatitis is not entirely known since most studies evaluating this are now relatively old and the pace of advances in ultrasound machine quality and familiarity with evaluating the pancreas is rapid. Typical findings are of areas of heterogeneity or hypoechoic foci within the pancreas and surrounding hyperechoic mesenteric fat. Irregularity of the pancreas and obstruction to the common bile duct may also be seen along with foci of fluid accumulation either within the pancreas or surrounding it.
  - ○ Previous sensitivity has been reported as 68% in dogs with severe acute pancreatitis, though we would feel presently in our clinic this would be a marked underestimation.

- Other techniques
  - ○ Contrast-enhanced computed tomography is a well-established diagnostic imaging technique for acute pancreatitis in humans but has not been well-evaluated in veterinary species.
  - ○ Similarly MRI has not been thoroughly evaluated.
  - ○ Endoscopic retrograde cholangiopancreatography (ERCP), a technique whereby a radiographic contrast agent is installed via the major duodenal papilla after endoscopic cannulation has been reported in dogs, but studies evaluating its diagnostic utility are not currently available and a risk of induction of pancreatitis exists with this technique.
  - ○ Ultrasound-guided fine needle aspiration cytology can be performed with a low but not insignificant risk of complication of 7%. A recent study documented the cytological yield to be adequate or good in 74% of cases and correlated well with histological findings, though these were available only for a very small number of cases. Furthermore, this population was biased towards patients with a high index of suspicion of pancreatic neoplasia rather than pancreatitis.

In this patient the following initial diagnostic tests were performed:
- Haematology
- Serum biochemistry, which included serum amylase and lipase
- cPLI
- Abdominal radiographs (see **Figure 14.1**)
- Abdominal ultrasound examination (see **Figures 14.2 and 14.3**)

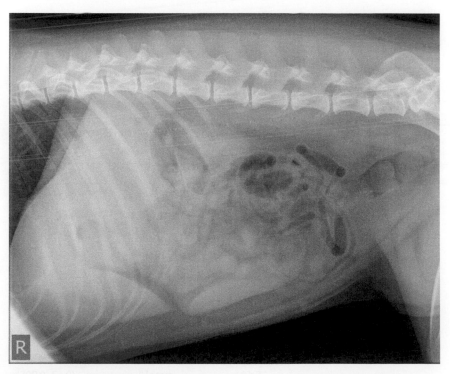

Figure 14.1 Right lateral abdominal radiograph (VD orthogonal view not shown).

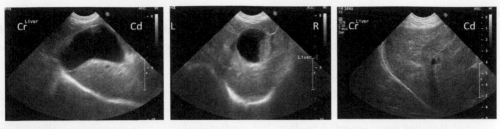

Figure 14.2 (from left to right) Sagittal view of right liver including gall bladder, transverse view showing gall bladder, sagittal view of left liver. Note that patient is in right lateral recumbency for all imaging planes.

Haematology

Parameter	Value	Units	Range
RBC	**5.02**	$\times 10^{12}$/l	(5.5–8.5)
Haemoglobin	**11.5**	g/dl	(12.0–18.0)
Haematocrit	**0.34**	l/l	(0.37–0.55)
Mean cell volume	68.7	fl	(60–77)
Mean cell haemoglobin oncentration	33.4	g/dl	(30.0–38.0)
Mean cell haemoglobin	22.9	pg	(19.5–25.5)
Total white cell count	11.46	$\times 10^9$/l	(6.0–15.0)
Neutrophils	9.21	$\times 10^9$/l	(3.0–11.5)
Lymphocytes	1.74	$\times 10^9$/l	(1.0–4.8)
Monocytes	0.38	$\times 10^9$/l	(0.2–1.4)
Eosinophils	0.12	$\times 10^9$/l	(0.1–1.2)
Basophils	0.02	$\times 10^9$/l	(0.0–0.1)
Platelets	**513**	$\times 10^9$/l	(200–500)
Film comment:	No abnormal findings		

Biochemistry

Parameter	Value	Units	Range
Total protein	64	g/l	(54–77)
Albumin	33	g/l	(25–40)
Globulin	31	g/l	(23–45)
Urea	**8.7**	mmol/l	(2.5–7.4)
Creatinine	71	µmol/l	(40–145)
Potassium	3.4	mmol/l	(3.4–5.6)
Sodium	140	mmol/l	(139–154)
Chloride	108	mmol/l	(105–122)
Calcium	2.6	mmol/l	(2.1–2.8)
Magnesium	0.68	mmol/l	(0.62–0.90)
Inorganic phosphate	1.4	mmol/l	(0.60–1.40)

Parameter	Value	Units	Range
Glucose	5.5	mmol/l	(3.3–5.8)
ALT	**135**	IU/l	(13–88)
AST	**74**	IU/l	(13–60)
ALKP	**419**	IU/l	(14–105)
GGT	**14**	IU/l	(0–10)
Bilirubin	**96**	µmol/l	(0–16)
Cholesterol	5.8	mmol/l	(3.8–7.0)
Triglyceride	**2.1**	mmol/l	(0.56–1.14)
Creatine kinase	167	IU/l	(0–190)
Amylase	**7571**	IU/l	(100–900)
Lipase	**3281**	IU/l	(0–250)
cPLI	**>1000**	µg/l	(<200)

Abdominal radiography demonstrated mild ventral hepatomegaly and some loss of serosal detail in the mid-abdomen with adjacent 'bunching' of the small intestine. A ventrodorsal radiograph did not demonstrate any additional findings.

Abdominal ultrasound demonstrated mild hepatomegaly with a slightly hyperechoic parenchyma but no discrete mass lesions or evidence of heterogeneity. The gall bladder was seen to be large with a small amount of dependent biliary 'sludge'; no evidence of intra- or extrahepatic biliary obstruction was seen. The pancreas appeared relatively hypoechoic (best seen on the image of the right lateral limb in **Figure 14.3**) and surrounded by hyperechoic peritoneum. A small, 6.6 mm diameter hypoechoic nodule was seen in the left limb of the pancreas. A mild cranial mesenteric lymphadenomegaly was identified and a small amount of free abdominal fluid was identified in the cranial mid-abdomen but was too scant to sample.

These findings were felt to be consistent with **acute pancreatitis**, with likely secondary/reactive hepatopathy.

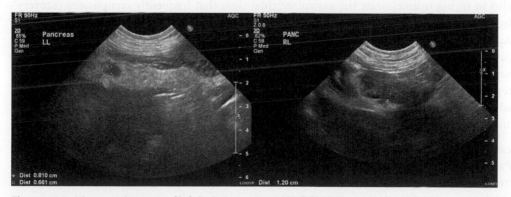

Figure 14.3 Ultrasound images of left limb (LL) and right limb (RL) of pancreas.

Questions (continued)

3. How would you manage this patient?

Answer

The clinical effects of acute pancreatitis may be described as

- Local (pain, inflammation, vomiting, fluid loss)
- Systemic (multi-organ damage, such as acute lung injury, cardiac arrhythmias and acute renal injury, or disseminated intravascular coagulation)
- Consequential (malnutrition due to anorexia, gastrointestinal ulceration, gastrointestinal ileus)

The 'gamut of severity' of acute pancreatitis

Acute pancreatitis varies enormously in severity and in the time-course both for spontaneous resolution and the development of systemic consequences, and management of it must be taken on a case-by-case basis. More than most other acute medical problems, acute pancreatitis runs a gamut of severity from acute–self-limiting–benign to fulminant-multi-organ failure and death, and it is important to have an 'iterative' (repetitively reviewing) approach of repetitive re-evaluation and re-appraisal of this changeable situation.

Fluid therapy
- Many animals with acute pancreatitis have total body water deficit due to the combined effects of anorexia, vomiting and voluminous local secretions from exudative inflamed pancreas. Fluid therapy to replace this and anticipated ongoing losses should be instituted and. Furthermore, may blunt microcirculatory underperfusion of the pancreas, which may in part perpetuate pancreatic injury.
- Crystalloid fluid therapy is undertaken initially though the addition of colloids may be beneficial in some patients. Theoretically the administration of alakalinising fluids such as Hartmann's solution may reduce the activation of trypsin within pancreatic acinar cells though objective evidence is lacking.
- Addition of potassium chloride may be indicated, both in those patients with documented hypokalaemia and hypochloridaemia, which frequently result from prolonged vomiting, but also in trying to ameliorate the gastrointestinal ileus that frequently complicates recovery from acute pancreatitis episodes.
- Administration of fresh frozen plasma has been traditionally popular in acute pancreatitis cases in veterinary medicine though there is no proven benefit. Proponents of its use cite the supply of alpha macroglobulins, which may help 'quench' activated pancreatic zymogens, and replacement of coagulation factors consumed in DIC. It should be remembered though that administration of plasma also supplies blood constituents that actively promote coagulation and it is naïve to suggest that administration of plasma in DIC is solely beneficial.

Analgesia
- Pain is a significant clinical finding in a large number of dogs with acute pancreatitis though overall it is reported to be detected in only approximately 40% of cases. Nonetheless analgesia remains an important part of management
- Opioids such as the full μ-agonists (morphine, methadone, fentanyl, hydromorphone, meperidine) or partial μ-agonist buprenorphine are most commonly used, full agonists being preferred as more effective in the setting of severe pain. Increasing biliary sphincter pressure is a theoretical disadvantage and is more potently caused by morphine and methadone,

though in experimental models of pancreatitis, the local effects of pancreatitis on this may far outweigh any opioid-induced effects. Of probably greater concern and impact on recovery is the effect of opioids on delaying gastric emptying and intestinal propulsive contractions, and this may compound the ileus, which often accompanies pancreatitis.

- The NMDA antagonist ketamine may be particularly useful in both reducing central initiations and sensitisation of pain due to visceral inflammation but also in having some opioid-sparing effect. It is used as a constant rate infusion either alone or in combination with lidocaine, also as a constant rate infusion.
- Non-steroidal anti-inflammatory drugs (NSAIDs) are generally best avoided in the setting of acute pancreatitis as these patients are frequently hypovolaemic.

Antiemetics

- Maropitant is an effective NK-1 receptor antagonist antiemetic with both central and peripheral effects and is effective in controlling mild to moderate nausea in patients with pancreatitis.
- Ondansetron, a serotoninergic antagonist, may be given additionally in uncontrolled nausea.
- The use of metoclopramide, a D2 receptor antagonist, is popular, though in a rodent model of pancreatitis, dopamine infusion actually improved the response to acute pancreatitis, leading to theoretical recommendations that metoclopramide be avoided. However, use of metoclopramide as a constant-rate infusion may also help ameliorate ileus, which frequently develops in pancreatitis patients.

Ileus in pancreatitis

It is the author's opinion that many cases of acute pancreatitis in dogs have their recovery prolonged by development of ileus. Ileus may develop due to local effects of pancreatic inflammation, but is also compounded by electrolyte disturbances (especially hypokalaemia), use of opioid analgesics and the additive effects of anorexia.

Correction of ileus by fluid therapy, early enteral nutrition, potassium supplementation in fluids as appropriate and considered use of gastrointestinal prokinetic agents may reduce this.

Antibiotics

- There is little evidence to support the use of antibiotic administration in cases of canine acute pancreatitis.

Nutrition

- Previous recommendations to fast patients with pancreatitis are based on the belief that pancreatic secretions would provoke further pancreatic inflammation, but in acute pancreatitis this has been shown to decrease anyway.
- Enteral nutrition should be introduced early and absolutely by day 5 of anorexia (including the pre-hospitalisation period).
- Major impediments to provision of enteral nutrition include intractable vomiting and ileus and attention to these should precede enteral feeding.
- Even if total calorie needs are not met by enteral nutrition, provision of local (especially amino acid) substrate to enterocytes prevents enterocyte apoptosis and gastrointestinal inflammation.

- Parenteral nutrition as the sole route of feeding has been shown to confer a poorer prognosis and higher rate of complications, but supplementation of enteral nutrition with partial parenteral nutrition may be useful in selective patients.
- Veterinary studies have shown that in most pancreatitis cases gastric or oesophageal feeding is as well tolerated as jejunal feeding. Nonetheless, a variety of non-surgical means of placement of jejunal feeding tubes are available for veterinary patients.
- Feeding of diets that are low in fat is recommended due to the high prevalence of hyperlipidaemias in patients with pancreatitis and some liquid enteral veterinary diets may be too high in fat content to be ideal for this purpose.

Surgery in canine pancreatitis

Surgical intervention should be assiduously avoided in the setting of acute pancreatitis and there are few indications to perform it.

Limited indications might be

- For diagnostic (biopsy) purposes where there exists significant diagnostic doubt that pancreatitis versus pancreatic neoplasia exists.
- Where surgical placement of a feeding tube is required.
- Where an identifiable local focus of pancreatic inflammation is identified that is not resolving on serial diagnostic imaging tests such as ultrasound and necrosectomy is to be performed.
- Where a pancreatic abscess is identified.

Outcome

The initial concern with this patient was a combination of interstitial and intravascular dehydration without a good compensatory response (see **Case 3** and **Table 3.1**), vomiting and mild-to-moderate abdominal pain. Note that anorexia had not been present for long in this patient.

Treatment was instituted with crystalloid fluid therapy (Hartmann's solution) at an initial rate of 550 ml/h for 4 hours, then 120 ml/h thereafter for the first 24 hours. In addition to the interstitial and intravascular dehydration some further vomiting was anticipated. After the first 4 hours and given the low-normal serum potassium, it was anticipated that whole-body potassium would be likely to decrease further (through the combined effects of anorexia, vomiting and administration of large amounts of crystalloid fluid with only 4 mmol/l potassium content) and potassium chloride was supplemented in fluids at a rate of 20 mmol potassium chloride/litre of crystalloid.

Analgesia was administered initially in the form of methadone 0.2 mg/kg i.v. q4 hours and serial pain-scoring assessments were performed q4 hours. After 24 hours analgesia was changed to buprenorphine 0.02 mg/kg i.v. q6 h, and then 8 hourly, based on sustained improvement in the patient's pain score.

Maropitant citrate was administered at a dose of 1 mg/kg s.c. q24 h and metoclopramide was administered as a constant rate infusion at a dose of 0.5 mg/kg/24 h. Two further episodes of emesis occurred 1 and 6 hours after admission but not thereafter.

No food was offered for the first afternoon, evening and night of admission but starting the following morning a combination of baby rice and a dextrose/glutamine/electrolyte solution was syringe fed per os in small amounts q4–6 hours. This was well tolerated and did not induce emesis. After a further 24 hours a small amount of fresh cooked chicken was given and consumed without emesis and 48 hours after admission small amounts of a low fat tinned commercial dog food were eaten. Intravenous fluid therapy was reduced and subsequently discontinued 4 days after admission and the patient was discharged 5 days after admission as he was eating, emesis had ceased and no clinical evidence of abdominal discomfort or hypovolaemia recurred after discontinuation of fluid therapy and parenteral analgesia. Serum urea, creatinine and electrolytes were performed 2 days after admission (see the table below) and bilirubin and markers of hepatocellular injury were re-performed after 5 days. The dog was maintained at home with a low-fat complete commercial tinned diet and was re-examined as an outpatient 5 days after discharge. Resolution of clinical and biochemical icterus was noted and physical examination at this time was normal. A repeat ultrasound examination of the pancreas (**Figure 14.4**) showed resolving alterations in echogenicity of the pancreas and the surrounding mesentery.

Parameter	Initial value	After 2 days	After 5 days	After 10 days	Units	Range
Urea	**8.7**	7.3	7.0	7.3	mmol/l	(2.5–7.4)
Creatinine	71	78	75	75	µmol/l	(40–145)
Potassium	3.4	4.2	4.2	4	mmol/l	(3.4–5.6)
Sodium	140	148	143	144	mmol/l	(139–154)
Chloride	108	110	111	107	mmol/l	(105–122)
ALT	**135**	–	**108**	67	IU/l	(13–88)
AST	**74**	–	56	43	IU/l	(13–60)
ALKP	**419**	–	**281**	100	IU/l	(14–105)
GGT	**14**	–	**11**	9	IU/l	(0–10)
Bilirubin	**96**	–	**45**	8	µmol/l	(0–16)

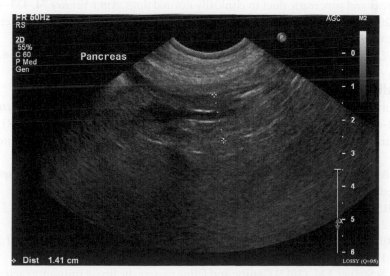

Figure 14.4 Follow-up ultrasound appearance of the right limb of the pancreas. The pancreatic duct can be clearly seen in the centre of the pancreas.

Discussion

Management of pancreatitis is supportive and symptomatic rather than specific and in the majority of cases spontaneous resolution occurs. Occasional sequelae such as development of exocrine pancreatic insufficiency or endocrine pancreatic insufficiency (i.e. diabetes mellitus) may subsequently be seen and weight loss after apparent recovery from acute pancreatitis should prompt evaluation for these.

The exact cause of acute pancreatitis in dogs is not known though proposed risk factors include breed, being overweight, having concurrent hyperlipidaemia or endocrinopathy with dogs of terrier breeds and Miniature Schnauzers being at increased risk. Some attention has been focussed on evaluation of the genes encoding for inhibitors of trypsin activation, particularly serine protein inhibitor Kazal type 1 (SPINK1, previously known as pancreatic secretory trypsin inhibitor), since a subgroup of human patients with predisposition to pancreatitis have mutations in this gene and thus lack the protective properties of the protein product it encodes. However, whilst studies have found variability in gen coding SPINK1, mutations have been documented in individuals both with and without pancreatitis. Abnormal pancreatic ductal anatomy, ductal blockage, reflux and alteration in ductal pH by biliary contents and ischaemia are all proposed to be contributory mechanisms for acute pancreatitis in dogs but none have been systematically evaluated in this species. Dietary indiscretion is frequently cited as a provocative cause of acute pancreatitis in dogs, though in our clinic we identify very few patients in which a dietary history is compatible with this.

A combination of clinical history, clinical pathology testing and ultrasound evaluation of the pancreas currently appears the best means of diagnosing pancreatitis and these diagnostic methods have been recently reviewed (see Dossin 2011; Steiner 2014; Xenoulis 2015; Penninck et al. 2013).

Novel therapeutic strategies may include administration of pancreatic enzyme supplements and the use of corticosteroids, but a positive benefit of these is yet to be demonstrated in canine patients.

References

Dossin, O. (2011) Laboratory tests for diagnosis of gastrointestinal and pancreatic diseases. *Top Companion Anim Med* **26**, 86–97

Penninck, D.G., Zeyen, U., Taeymans, O.N. & Webster, C. R. (2013) Ultrasonographic measurement of the pancreas and pancreatic duct in clinically normal dogs. *Am J Vet Res* **74**, 433–437

Steiner, J.M. (2014) Review of commonly used clinical pathology parameters for general gastrointestinal disease with emphasis on small animals. *Toxicol Pathol* **42**, 189–194

Xenoulis, P.G. (2015) Diagnosis of pancreatitis in dogs and cats. *J Small Anim Pract* **56**, 13–26

Further reading

Kook, P.H., Kohler, N., Hartnack, S., Riond, B. & Reusch, C.E. (2014) Agreement of serum Spec cPL with the 1,2-o-dilauryl-rac-glycero glutaric acid-(6'-methylresorufin) ester (DGGR) lipase assay and with pancreatic ultrasonography in dogs with suspected pancreatitis. *J Vet Intern Med* **28**, 863–870

Mansfield, C. & Beths, T. (2015) Management of acute pancreatitis in dogs: a critical appraisal with focus on feeding and analgesia. *J Small Anim Pract* **56**, 27–39

Watson, P. (2015) Canine and feline pancreatitis: a challenging and enigmatic disease. *J Small Anim Pract* **56**, 1–2

Watson, P. (2015) Pancreatitis in dogs and cats: definitions and pathophysiology. *J Small Anim Pract* **56**, 3–12

Xenoulis, P.G. & Steiner, J.M. (2012) Canine and feline pancreatic lipase immunoreactivity. *Vet Clin Pathol* **41**, 312–324

Clinical presentation

A 1 year 1 month-old female-neutered Standard Poodle (**Figure 15.1**) is presented with a history of weight loss and diarrhoea. The dog has been healthy up until three weeks ago, has received primary vaccinations and is regularly wormed every 5–6 months with febantel/praziquantel/pyrantel. The dog has no history of travel outside the United Kingdom and lives with one other (unrelated) adult Poodle who is clinically well. The dog eats a commercial complete canned adult maintenance dog food.

The dog has recently developed diarrhoea, which is described by the owners as pale yellow and voluminous, occasionally becoming watery. No faecal incontinence, tenesmus or haematochezia has been reported and accidental soiling within the house has been noted on one occasion only. The dog's appetite has remained very good and vomiting has not been reported; water intake and urinating behaviour is normal. The dog's weight has decreased from 26 kg to 22.3 kg during this time.

Initially the owners repeated worming and fed the dog some plain chicken and boiled rice for one week, neither of which appeared to improve the diarrhoea.

Physical examination reveals a very bright dog in thin body condition (body condition score 2/5). The dog appears normovolaemic, well-hydrated and heart rate and respiratory rate, rectal temperature and abdominal palpation are normal.

Questions

1. Is this dog's diarrhoea small-intestinal or large-intestinal in nature or mixed? Why?
2. What are the principle differential diagnoses for this dog's clinical signs?
3. What investigation would you perform?

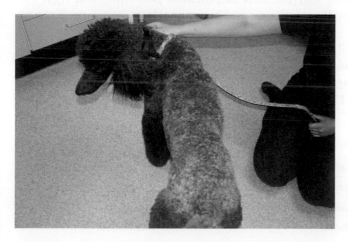

Figure 15.1 The patient at presentation.

Canine Internal Medicine: What's Your Diagnosis? First Edition. Jon Wray.
© 2018 John Wiley & Sons Ltd. Published 2018 by John Wiley & Sons Ltd.

Answers

1. Is this dog's diarrhoea small-intestinal or large-intestinal in nature or mixed? Why?

Features that may distinguish small and large intestinal diarrhoea are listed in **Table 15.1**.

In this patient the absence of haematochezia, dyschezia or faecal mucous, lack of urgency and presence of large amounts of faeces accompanied by weight loss are all characteristic of small intestinal diarrhoea.

2. What are the principle differential diagnoses for this dog's clinical signs?

Diarrhoea, along with vomiting, which is absent in this case, is one of the cardinal clinical signs of gastrointestinal pathology.

The 'mantra of three' (causes of gastrointestinal signs)

However, before homing-in on the gastrointestinal tract as the sole origin of clinical signs such as diarrhoea, it behoves clinicians to consider that just because the symptomology is of gastrointestinal signs it does not exclude the possibility of extraintestinal disease. A useful mantra is to always consider that vomiting/diarrhoea may be due to

- Systemic diseases that may manifest as primarily gastrointestinal signs.
- Diseases and disorders that occur local to the GI tract and that might 'affect' it as an 'innocent bystander'.
- Primary gastrointestinal disorders including those of the pancreas.

By considering these *in this order* (i.e. considering GI disease last) errors of omission caused by lack of consideration are avoided.

Examples of systemic diseases that may manifest as primarily gastrointestinal signs include endocrinopathies such as hypoadrenocorticism and hypothyroidism, and gastropathy of uraemia.

Examples of diseases local to the GI tract include pancreatitis, mesenteric abscessation, pansteatitis and portal hypertension due to obstructive liver disease.

When considering differential diagnoses related to the GI tract, it is helpful to consider these mechanistically/aetiologically (**Table 15.2**).

Table 15.1 Characteristics of small and large intestinal diarrhoea

Characteristic	Small intestinal diarrhoea	Large intestinal diarrhoea
Frequency	Normal to increased	Usually very increased
Volume	Usually increased	Usually normal to decreased
Nature of blood if present	Melaena	Fresh blood
Presence of mucus	Absent	Often present
Presence of urgency	Normal to mild increase in urgency	Usually increase in urgency
Presence of tenesmus	Absent	Often present
Presence of weight loss	Often	Usually not

Table 15.2 Differential diagnosis for small intestinal diarrhoea

Systemic disorders that may present with primary signs of small intestinal diarrhoea		*M (Metabolic)* • Hypoadrenocorticism • Hypothyroidism • Liver disease • Kidney disease • Thyrotoxicosis (rare in dogs) *I (Infecious, Inflammatory, Immune-mediated)* • Endotoxaemia • Polysystemic infections, e.g. leptospirosis, infectious canine hepatitis, distemper
Local disorders that may cause small intestinal signs as an innocent bystander effect		*N (Neoplastic, Nutritional)* • Abdominal carcinomatosis *I (Infectious, Inflammatory, Immune-mediated)* • Pancreatitis • Pansteatitis • Hepatic disease • Adhesions • Mesenteric abscessation • Peritonitis *V (Vascular)* • Portosystemic shunt • Portal hypertension
Exocrine pancreatic insufficiency (EPI)		
Primary gastrointestinal disease	*A (Anamalous, Anatomical)*	• Chronic or intermittent intussusception • Motility disorders • 'Irritable bowel syndrome'
	N (Neoplastic, Nutritional)	Focal neoplasia, especially: • Adenocarcinoma • Leiomyoma • Leiomyosarcoma • Gastrointestinal stromal tumour (GIST) • Mast cell tumour Diffuse neoplasia, especially: • Lymphoma • Diffuse mast cell tumour Dietary • Dietary change • Overeating/dietary indiscretion • Dietary intolerance

(Continued)

I (Infectious, Inflammatory, Immune-mediated)	
Infectious	• Parasitic (e.g. hookworms *Uncinaria steno-cephala*, *Ancylostoma caninum*, roundworms *Toxocara canis*, *Toxascaris leonina* and tapeworms *Dipylidium caninum*, *Taenia* spp, *Echinococcus multilocularis** and *granulosa*)
	• Protozoal (e.g. *Giardia* spp., *Cryptosporidium* spp., *Isospora* spp., others)
	• Bacterial (e.g. *Salmonella*, *Campylobacter* spp., *Clostridium perfringens*, *Clostridium difficile*, *E.coli*)**
	• Viral (e.g. parvovirus, enteric coronavirus)
	• Fungal (e.g. *Histoplasma capsulatum**), Oomycetes (e.g. *Pythium insidiosum**)
	• Algal (e.g. *Prototheca* spp.)
	• Rickettsial (e.g. *Neorickettsia helminthoeca**)
Infectious/inflammatory disorders of uncertain aetiology	• Small intestinal bacterial overgrowth (SIBO)/ intestinal dysbiosis/antibiotic-responsive diarrhoea (ARD)
	• Haemorrhagic gastroenteritis (HGE)
Inflammatory/ immune-mediated	• Idiopathic inflammatory bowel disease (iIBD)
	• Lymphangiectasia
T (traumatic, Toxic)	• Drug-induced
	• Non-steroidal anti-inflammatory drugs
	• Cytotoxic chemotherapy agents
	• Digoxin
	• D-penicillamine
	• Antibiotics

*Not endemic to the United Kingdom.
**May be isolated from faeces of healthy dogs.

As well as considering the lengthy differential diagnosis one must apply clinical 'common sense' based on the history and presenting signs. For example, drug-induced diarrhoea can be quickly eliminated based on taking a history and diffuse neoplastic infiltration or serious systemic infection are extremely unlikely in a patient whose appetite is excellent.

3. What investigation would you perform?

Application of clinical common-sense to diarrhoea: reason rather than over-reaction

Many cases of diarrhoea are acute/self-limiting and investigation may be unwarranted, associated with poor diagnostic yield and be both costly to owners and risk exposure of patients to unnecessarily intrusive investigation. A decision to investigate is based on

- Persistence of the condition or repetitive episodes.
- Association with 'constitutional' signs of illness such as prolonged inappetence, depression, loss of condition, weakness, ascites.
- Identification of immediately life-threatening consequences such as massive gastrointestinal haemorrhage, evidence of hypovolaemic shock identified on physical examination, likelihood of life-threatening systemic illness.
- Assessment of whether diarrhoea is a prominent/predominant problem or whether it is a minor clinical problem associated with a more prominent disease.

It is commonsensical to evaluate the possibility of and treat obvious causes of diarrhoea such as dietary change, dietary indiscretion and heavy parasite burden before undertaking extensive diagnostic evaluation.

Rational investigation also exhausts, prior to performing further tests, those diagnostic tests that are cost-effective and involve minimal intrusion/risk of morbidity to the patient.

Investigation might reasonably initially be (**Figure 15.2**)
- A complete blood count usually proffers non-specific information in small intestinal diarrhoea and changes usually reflect consequences of (e.g. haemoconcentration with large amounts of fluid loss, anaemia with chronic GI blood loss, neutrophilia in response to inflammation) diarrhoea rather than leading to differentiation between causes.
- Demonstration of hypoalbuminaemia, usually (but not exclusively) with hypoglobulinaemia suggests protein-losing enteropathy (PLE) and given the likely severity of the underlying disease process and guarded prognosis this entails, further investigation is always indicated. Hypoalbuminaemia may also be due to hepatic functional disease and protein-losing nephropathy and whilst neither would be expected to cause hypoglobulinaemia, in isolated hypoalbuminaemia testing for both is recommended.

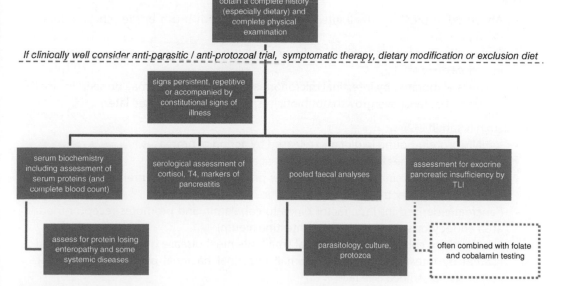

Figure 15.2 Rational investigation of persistent diarrhoea: Step 1.

- Biochemistry may also be used to evaluate for the possibility of renal and hepatic disease (remembering that azotaemia may be pre-renal in animals with substantial fluid loss and that modest raises in hepatobiliary enzymes are frequently due to 'reactive' hepatopathy) and normal basal cortisol and total T4 should exclude hypoadrenocorticism and hypothyroidism respectively.
- Pancreatitis may be suspected clinically with an unequivocally elevated level of serum pancreatic lipase immunoreactivity (cPLI) but bear in mind that whilst this test offers significant advantages over other serum tests in sensitivity of detection of pancreatitis, false negative results are still relatively common. Amylase and lipase should not, in this author's opinion, be relegated as diagnostic tests. Whilst it is true that sensitivity is generally lower than cPLI, they are not without use in identifying some cases of pancreatitis.
- Faecal analyses for parasitic ova and protozoa, especially *Giardia* spp. is cost effective but identification of *Giardia* spp. can be difficult and trial therapy, for example with 5–7 day course of fenbendazole, is rational.
- Faecal culture results may be very difficult to interpret since many organisms that may be associated with infectious diarrhoea (*Salmonella*, *Campylobacter* spp., *Clostridia* spp., *E.coli*) may also be isolated very frequently from healthy dogs and a cause/effect relationship when positive culture is identified cannot be assured. Many laboratories do not 'speciate' such positive cultures and may furthermore report, as significant, organisms that would be normally expected to be identified in faeces. Greater 'weight' can be placed on positive cultures if accompanied by signs of febrile illness, bloody diarrhoea, or neutrophilic histology or cytology of bowel wall preparations, in young animals or in environments where multiple dogs are affected. Faecal culture cannot be used to diagnose small intestinal bacterial overgrowth.
- The diagnostic test of choice for exocrine pancreatic insufficiency is the TLI test, which is both sensitive and specific, and not faecal proteolytic activity. It is often combined with assessment of folate and cobalamin (see the box below).

Folate and cobalamin

Folate

- Absorbed in proximal small intestine by reaction with brush border enzyme folate deconjugase.
- Dietary insufficiency is unlikely and low levels usually reflect severe proximal small intestinal disease.
- Folate is elaborated by intestinal microflora and elevated levels may be seen in small intestinal bacterial overgrowth/antibiotic-responsive diarrhoea (see later).

Cobalamin (vitamin B12)

- Initially protein-bound in diet and released by action of proteases.
- In stomach becomes bound to R-proteins at an acid pH.
- R-protein–cobalamin complex undergoes proteolysis in the neutral pH of the small intestine and under the action of pancreatic-derived proteases.
- Pancreatic-derived intrinsic factor binds to cobalamin and promotes receptor-mediated endocytosis in the distal small intestine (ileum).
- Low levels of cobalamin reflect distal small intestinal disease or competition for utilisation by intestinal microflora in small intestinal bacterial overgrowth/antibiotic-responsive diarrhoea (see later).

Should investigation thus far have not demonstrated a convincing cause of the diarrhoea, the principle groups of primary gastrointestinal disease that remain as differential diagnoses include
- Dietary intolerance.
- Inflammatory or diffusely infiltrative gastrointestinal disease.
- Focal mass lesions.
- Mechanical and functional diseases.
- Small intestinal bacterial overgrowth/antibiotic-responsive diarrhoea/intestinal dysbiosis.

Further investigation (assuming clinical signs persist) at this stage might include the steps in **Figure 15.3**.

Diagnostic imaging

- Diagnostic imaging should be considered by both radiography and by ultrasound. Both of these types of imaging study have a role to play in investigation of chronic small intestinal signs and can be viewed as offering 'complementary information' to each other.
- Principle clinical 'questions' that diagnostic imaging can help to answer are
  ◦ Is there a condition for which surgical correction is the most appropriate form of treatment (e.g. chronic intussusception)?
  ◦ Is there focal disease for which surgical exploration and biopsy/excision is the most appropriate course of action (e.g. focal mass lesion)?

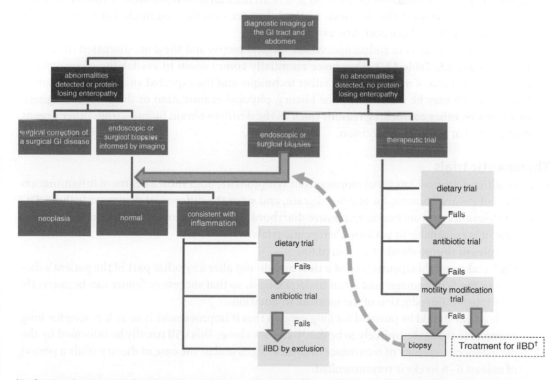

†Performing therapeutic trials with immunomodulatory agents should generally be avoided and should certainly be considered only if adequate, logical and interpretable attempts to exclude other pathologies, including if necessary by a therapeutic trial response, has preceded this.

Figure 15.3 Rational initial investigation of persistent diarrhoea: Step 2.

- ○ If the equipment and skill for endoscopic evaluation and biopsy is available
  - Is there evidence of non-surgically correctable pathology within diagnostic 'range' of endoscopic evaluation?
  - Is there evidence of non-surgically correctable pathology that is clearly outside the 'range' of endoscopic evaluation?

Histopathology from intestinal biopsies

- Histopathology is invaluable to determine the presence of disease and with some diffuse infiltrative conditions (e.g. GI lymphoma) may provide a definitive diagnosis. However, one must be cognisant of the fact that the intestinal mucosa displays a relatively limited 'repertoire' of responses to a variety of luminally derived and mucosal insults and that it is seldom the case that a pathognomonic lesion is identified on histopathology that allows for a definitive aetiological diagnosis. In particular, the clinician should be wary of confident pronouncements that a particular histological appearance is consistent with 'dietary intolerance' or 'inflammatory bowel disease', since inflammation may occur with a wide variety of disorders and the presence of widespread inflammation is seen in idiopathic inflammatory bowel disease, in dietary intolerances with a resultant inflammatory component and in dogs with antibiotic responsive diarrhoea.
- Thus confidence in a diagnosis of idiopathic inflammatory bowel disease is not so much based on histopathological finding of inflammatory infiltrates within the lamina propria (though this is a *sine qua non* for diagnosis of iIBD and severe architectural changes such as villous blunting and fusion may support the diagnosis further), but rests on the exactitude with which other differential diagnoses have been first excluded.
- There are pros and cons to endoscopic versus surgical biopsy and these are discussed in further detail in **Case 13, Table 13.3**. The choice essentially comes down to availability of equipment and expertise, risks of morbidity with either technique and the expected anatomical location of disease (which may be informed by the history, physical examination or diagnostic imaging). There may be other compelling reasons (such as the desire to obtain biopsies from other organs at surgery) that inform this decision.

Therapeutic trials

- Since ultimately most intestinal biopsies from symptomatic dogs show a degree of inflammation that is not pathognomonic for any one disease, and since the differential diagnoses include dietary intolerance and antibiotic-responsive diarrhoea, as well as idiopathic inflammatory bowel disease, it is reasonable to perform therapeutic trials.
- A few rules of thumb should be adhered to:
  - ○ Undertake one therapeutic trial at a time and do not alter any other part of the patient's dietary or medical management when undertaking it, so that success or failure can be correctly attributed to introduction of the measure in question.
  - ○ Such a trial should be pursued for long enough that if improvement is seen, it is seen for long enough for this to be unlikely to be due to chance alone. This will usually be informed by the persistence/frequency of recurrence of clinical signs and in the case of dietary trials a period of at least 6–8 weeks is recommended.
  - ○ Interpretation of a trial is only as good as compliance with it. In particular, it is essential to impress on owners the reasoning behind dietary trials and that failure of compliance may result in a 'false-failure' diagnosis, which could, in the worst case scenario, lead to an erroneous diagnosis of disorders that prompt unnecessary lifelong medical therapy.

- Dietary trials are usually undertaken with either a single protein-source diet, which is not something routinely encountered by the patient before or after a diet (usually chicken or soya based), in which the protein has been chemically processed to produce low molecular weight protein derivatives, which should be less immunogenic.

- Blood tests purporting to demonstrate dietary intolerances do not distinguish between primary dietary immunogenic intolerances and elaboration of antibodies to foodstuffs occurring as a consequence of loss of the mucosal barrier function. Such tests are not currently recommended by most medical specialists including the author.

- SIBO/antibiotic-responsive diarrhoea may be suspected based on low cobalamin and/or elevated folate levels, but such findings are both insensitive and, in the case of cobalamin, non-specific in diagnosing this disorder. Therapeutic trials are usually undertaken with one of:
  - Oxytetracycline 10–20 mg/kg p/o TID for 4 weeks or
  - Tylosin 10–15 mg/kg p/o BID for 4 weeks or
  - Metronidazole 10 mg/kg p/o BID for 4 weeks.

Caution needs to be undertaken with metronidazole since development of adverse neurological signs of central vestibular disease can be seen in some dogs, albeit usually at higher doses, and the agent's immunomodulatory effects may confound the supposition that a positive response is generated by an antimicrobial effect (though to some degree the same problem can be levelled at oxytetracycline and tylosin).

'Small intestinal bacterial overgrowth (SIBO)'/'antibiotic-responsive diarrhoea'/ 'intestinal dysbiosis'

These are differing names signifying effect, diagnosis by therapeutic response and proposed aetiology (respectively) of the same condition. SIBO is predominantly used here, due to more widespread familiarity of the term. A condition of altered intestinal floral homeostasis ('dysbiosis'), resulting in proliferation of some bacterial species within more proximal areas of the gut, is suspected to occur in dogs. However, objective measures (such as quantitative duodenal juice cultures) to document this disorder are difficult and rarely performed, and previous diagnostic criteria based on them have been questioned. Proponents of the term 'antibiotic-responsive diarrhoea' defend this term as perhaps more intellectually 'honest' since the condition is often suspected due to positive response to therapy (see above) rather than being based on diagnostic tests of folate and cobalamin, which have been shown to have low sensitivity and specificity for this condition. Whilst SIBO may occur as a primary condition in some dogs, most notably in German Shepherds, in many the condition appears to occur secondary to other digestive derangements caused by a variety of gastrointestinal pathologies.

- Finally, whilst diagnostically undesirable, there are some circumstances whereby it may be appropriate to undertake trial treatment with immunomodulatory agents for idiopathic inflammatory bowel disease. Such circumstances might include
  - The preclusion of any further diagnostic evaluation by the owner on cost or concern grounds.
  - Failure of other rational treatment trials has been complete.
  - Severe patient morbidity due to, for example, severe protein-losing enteropathy where the risks of anaesthesia for surgical or endoscopic biopsies are considered high.

If pursuing such a therapeutic trial strategy it should be remembered and communicated with owners that

- ○ Such a trial represents a diagnostic point of no-return in that subsequent reversal of this decision in favour of further diagnostics may render such tests uninterpretable.
- ○ Not all cases of idiopathic inflammatory bowel disease respond to treatment and failure of response is not necessarily an indication that iIBD is not the cause. Overall complete remission from signs of iIBD is experienced in about a quarter of patients, improvement but not resolution of clinical signs is seen in about half and in the remainder little or no response is seen. In the author's experience, veterinary surgeons oftentimes overestimate the efficacy of medical management for iIBD.

Diagnosis and outcome

In this case initial laboratory findings were as shown in the following tables.

Haematology

Parameter	Value	Units	Range
RBC	6.57	$\times 10^{12}$/l	(5.5–8.5)
Haemoglobin	15.6	g/dl	(12.0–18.0)
Haematocrit	0.46	l/l	(0.37–0.55)
Mean cell volume	70.6	fl	(60–77)
Mean cell haemoglobin concentration	33.6	g/dl	(30.0–38.0)
Mean cell haemoglobin	23.7	pg	(19.5–25.5)
Total white cell count	7.06	$\times 10^9$/l	(6.0–15.0)
Neutrophils	3.58	$\times 10^9$/l	(3.0–11.5)
Lymphocytes	2.48	$\times 10^9$/l	(1.0–4.8)
Monocytes	0.65	$\times 10^9$/l	(0.2–1.4)
Eosinophils	0.28	$\times 10^9$/l	(0.1–1.2)
Basophils	0.06	$\times 10^9$/l	(0.0–0.1)
Platelets	203	$\times 10^9$/l	(200–500)
Film comment:	Unremarkable morphology		

Biochemistry

Parameter	Value	Units	Range
Total protein	53	g/l	(54–77)
Albumin	30	g/l	(25–40)
Globulin	23	g/l	(23–45)
Urea	2.5	mmol/l	(2.5–7.4)
Creatinine	88	µmol/l	(40–145)
Potassium	4.6	mmol/l	(3.4–5.6)
Sodium	146	mmol/l	(139–154)
Chloride	109	mmol/l	(105–122)

Parameter	Value	Units	Range
Calcium	2.7	mmol/l	(2.1–2.8)
Magnesium	–	mmol/l	(0.62–0.90)
Inorganic phosphate	1.4	mmol/l	(0.60–1.40)
Glucose	5.6	mmol/l	(3.3–5.8)
ALT	**343**	IU/l	(13–88)
AST	53	IU/l	(13–60)
ALKP	**135**	IU/l	(14–105)
GGT	3	IU/l	(0–10)
Bilirubin	4	µmol/l	(0–16)
Cholesterol	**3.1**	mmol/l	(3.8–7.0)
Triglyceride	0.7	mmol/l	(0.56–1.14)
Creatine kinase	98	IU/l	(0–190)
Fasting bile acid	1.4	µmol/l	(0–10)
Post-prandial bile acid	3.2	µmol/l	(0–15)

Endocrine tests

Basal cortisol	75	nmol/l	(27.5–125)
Total T4	22	nmol/l	(15–50)

Faecal analysis/culture

Appearance	Semi-formed, pale
Faecal parasites	No ova, cysts or parasites seen.
Campylobacter spp.	Not isolated
Salmonella	Not isolated
Clostridium spp.	Not isolated
C. difficile toxinantigen	Negative
C. perfringens toxin	Negative
Giardia antigen	Negative
Cryptosporidium	Negative

TLI	<1	µg/L	(6.1–35)
Folate	**19.9**	ng/ml	(8.2–13.5)
B12	**266**	pg/ml	(>275)

The serum biochemical findings were of a very marginally raised ALKP, which, being only just outside the normal reference interval, was not on its own considered significant. However, the ALT was raised above 3 times the reference interval and whilst only modestly raised was considered potentially more significant. Bile acid stimulation was normal. Mild hypocholesterolaemia may indicate hepatic dysfunction, hypoadrenocorticism or gastrointestinal disorders, resulting in a lack of lipoprotein production or excessive lipid loss by enterocytes. Basal cortisol was sufficient to exclude hypoadrenocorticism.

Trypsin-like immunoreactivity (TLI) was very low and is diagnostic of exocrine pancreatic insufficiency (EPI). A subnormal serum cobalamin (vitamin B12) is consistent, either with distal small intestinal disease or with competition for this vitamin by intestinal bacterial overgrowth. Elevation in folate is a relatively uncommon finding in dogs and is most consistent with elaboration by intestinal bacteria.

Abdominal imaging was undertaken in the light of the clinical signs and modest elevation in ALT and ALKP. Orthogonal abdominal radiographs demonstrated no specific abnormalities. Abdominal ultrasound demonstrated a normal appearance to the liver and the gastrointestinal tract. Whilst the left limb of the pancreas could not be clearly identified, the right limb appeared structurally normal.

A final diagnosis of **exocrine pancreatic insufficiency (EPI) with secondary small intestinal bacterial overgrowth (SIBO)** was made.

The patient was treated with the addition of 2 teaspoons/meal of a powdered porcine pancreatic enzyme supplement (Pancrex V powder, Penn Pharmaceuticals) comprising pancreatin powder of 1400 units/g free protease, 25 000 units/g lipase and 30 000 units/g amylase. The dog was fed its previous canned adult maintenance diet with no specific dietary modifications made, in 3 meals/day and with the pancreatin powder mixed thoroughly into each meal before feeding.

Cobalamin was supplemented by subcutaneous injection of 250 µg given weekly for four occasions and then monthly thereafter and oxytetracycline was administered at an approprimate dose of 20 mg/kg p/o TID for an initial period of 8 weeks.

Over this time the dog's diarrhoea resolved and a weight gain of 2 kg was seen. After 8 weeks of treatment, trial discontinuation of oxytetracycline was undertaken, which resulted in some worsening of stool quality. This resolved with reintroduction of oxytetracycline.

Discussion

EPI results when >90% of the secretory capacity of the exocrine pancreas is lost, most commonly as a result of pancreatic acinar atrophy (PAA) but also occasionally due to chronic pancreatitis or pancreatic neoplasia. Breed predispositions for EPI include the German Shepherd dog, Rough Collie, Chow Chow and Cavalier King Charles Spaniel with a genetic predisposition (likely an autosomal recessive trait) reported in the first two of these and the Eurasian dog. The pathogenesis of PAA in dogs is not well understood, though autoimmune pathology is thought to play a role and in some dogs subclinical EPI may be identified by serial assessment of trypsin-like immunoreactivity. Clinical signs usually develop in dogs between 1 and 4 years of age and typically involve increased faecal volume, pale faeces, diarrhoea, weight loss and flatulence, with weight loss being the most consistent of these. Some patients may also demonstrate polydipsia, the aetiology of which is uncertain. Diagnosis is reliably made by severely subnormal serum levels of trypsin-like immunoreactivity (TLI, <2.5 µg/l), though dogs with values that fall between this and the lower limit of the reference interval may be suspected to have 'subclinical' EPI. TLI assays are species-specific and measure a combination of trypsinogen, which 'overspills' from the pancreas into blood, and small amounts of trypsin, both free and bound to protease inhibitors. Faecal pancreatic elastase has been evaluated for diagnosis of exocrine pancreatic insufficiency but lacks the sensitivity and specificity of TLI. Faecal proteolytic activity is not recommended as a diagnostic test. Whilst development of a ravenous appetite is very common in malabsorptive disorders such as EPI, a lack of ravenous appetite, as in this case, should not be used to exclude it.

The mainstay of therapy in EPI is replacement therapy with pancreatic enzyme supplements. These may be pharmaceutical replacements or employ use of chopped porcine or bovine pancreas, but whilst the latter are useful, effective and cheap, availability in many countries has become scarce. Pancreatic enzyme supplements offer a routinely available and consistent replacement but products may vary both in their content, their formulation (powder, granules, capsules) and in the addition of enteric coatings. Whilst some pancreatic enzymes (such as trypsin) may pass through the acid pH of the stomach with minimal degradation, others (most notably lipases) are severely and rapidly degraded by acid pH, resulting in a marked reduction in the amount of functional enzyme delivered to the small intestine after administration. Some products therefore have an enteric coating designed to limit acid digestion within the stomach and one study has shown a greater degree of weight gain in animals treated with the enteric coated product versus the same medication with no coating. Other studies have suggested that powdered products may result in more consistent improvement and some differences in activity may also be due to the rate of emptying from the stomach of powdered versus granular products. Given the somewhat conflicting nature of studies to date, it may be reasonable to suspect that different individuals may respond better to different products and that failure of response might prompt trial treatment with another product. Whilst sometimes advocated, there is currently little evidence to support routine administration of antacid medications in an attempt to reduce gastric digestion of pancreatic enzyme supplements.

Although both dietary fat restriction (to limit delivery of malassimilated lipid to the small intestinal lumen) and, conversely, dietary fat supplementation (to compensate for fat maldigestion) have been recommended, studies assessing the impact of dietary formulations on success of treatment for EPI have not established clear therapeutic benefits of any one dietary modification.

Hypocobalaminaemia is detected in >80% of dogs with EPI and may be due to both lack of pancreatic intrinsic factor and due to lack of bacteriostatic activity of pancreatic secretions allowing 'small intestinal bacterial overgrowth'. In some dogs administration of pancreatic enzyme supplements may reverse hypocobalaminaemia but in the majority this is ineffective and parenteral administration is advisable. Whilst it is commonplace to suspect secondary SIBO (see how above) concurrently in dogs with EPI, objective evidence for this and evaluation of effectiveness of antimicrobial treatment for this is lacking.

Therapeutic failure occurs in a substantial minority of dogs with EPI and it is worthwhile discussing with owners at the outset that studies have shown an approximate 60% rate of good control of clinical signs, approximately 20% partial response and approximately 20% of dogs showing a poor response. Co-morbid conditions may sometimes contribute to poor responsiveness and may include concurrent inflammatory bowel disease in some dogs.

Endoscopic examination and biopsy was not undertaken in this dog since a laboratory diagnosis of EPI was made. Failure of therapeutic response, were it seen, would prompt further investigation including endoscopy and biopsy.

Further reading

Batchelor, D.J., Noble, P.J., Cripps, P.J., Taylor, R.H., McLean, L., Leibl, M.A. & German, A.J. (2007) Breed associations for canine exocrine pancreatic insufficiency. *J Vet Intern Med* **21**, 207–214

Batchelor, D.J., Noble, P.J., Taylor, R.H., Cripps, P.J. & German, A.J. (2007) Prognostic factors in canine exocrine pancreatic insufficiency: prolonged survival is likely if clinical remission is achieved. *J Vet Intern Med* **21**, 54–60

Dossin, O. (2011) Laboratory tests for diagnosis of gastrointestinal and pancreatic diseases. *Top Companion Anim Med* **26**, 86–97

German, A.J. (2012) Exocrine pancreatic insufficiency in the dog: breed associations, nutritional considerations, and long-term outcome. *Top Companion Anim Med* **27**, 104–108

Mas, A., Noble, P.J., Cripps, P.J., Batchelor, D.J., Graham, P. & German, A.J. (2012) A blinded randomised controlled trial to determine the effect of enteric coating on enzyme treatment for canine exocrine pancreatic efficiency. *BMC Vet Res* **8**, 127

Watson, P.J. (2003) Exocrine pancreatic insufficiency as an end stage of pancreatitis in four dogs. *J Small Anim Pract* **44**, 306–312

Westermarck, E. & Wiberg, M. (2003) Exocrine pancreatic insufficiency in dogs. *Vet Clin North Am Small Anim Pract* **33**, 1165–1179, viii–ix

Westermarck, E. & Wiberg, M.E. (2006) Effects of diet on clinical signs of exocrine pancreatic insufficiency in dogs. *J Am Vet Med Assoc* **228**, 225–229

Westermarck, E. & Wiberg, M. (2012) Exocrine pancreatic insufficiency in the dog: historical background, diagnosis, and treatment. *Top Companion Anim Med* **27**, 96–103

Clinical presentation

A 10 year 1 month-old male-neutered Golden Retriever (**Figure 16.1**) is presented with a one-week history of daily regurgitation of both food and saliva. The dog has had intermittent regurgitation for approximately 1 month but in the last week has developed more frequent clinical signs, coughing and increased respiratory effort. On examination the dog is quiet and has an increased respiratory rate of 36/min and a slightly choppy/restrictive respiratory pattern. Cardiac auscultation is normal and peripheral pulse rate and quality is normal. Rectal temperature is 38.9 °C. Auscultation of the thorax demonstrated increased bronchovesicular sounds on the right side of the thorax.

The radiographs (**Figure 16.2**) (taken under light sedation) and a complete blood count are performed soon after admission.

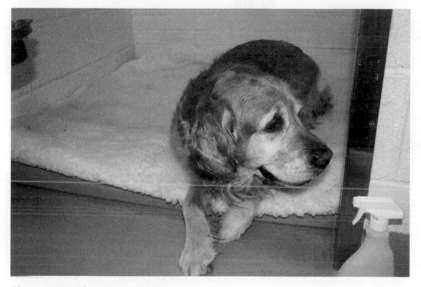

Figure 16.1 The patient at presentation.

Canine Internal Medicine: What's Your Diagnosis? First Edition. Jon Wray.
© 2018 John Wiley & Sons Ltd. Published 2018 by John Wiley & Sons Ltd.

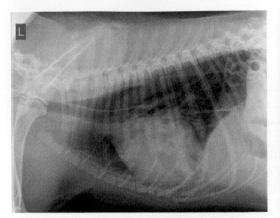

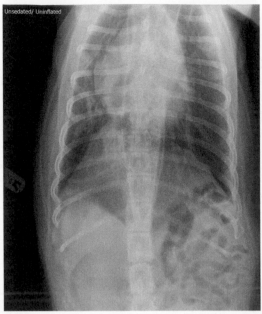

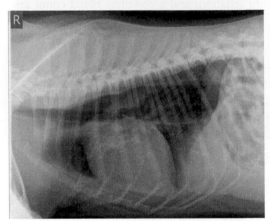

Figure 16.2 Left lateral, right lateral and dorsoventral thoracic radiographs at presentation.

Haematology

Parameter	Value	Units	Range
RBC	**5.14**	× 10^{12}/l	(5.5–8.5)
Haemoglobin	12.0	g/dl	(12.0–18.0)
Haematocrit	**0.35**	l/l	(0.37–0.55)
Mean cell volume	67.2	fl	(60–77)
Mean cell haemoglobin concentration	34.6	g/dl	(30.0–38.0)
Mean cell haemoglobin	23.2	pg	(19.5–25.5)
Total white cell count	**27.37**	× 10^9/l	(6.0–15.0)
Neutrophils	**23.1**	× 10^9/l	(3.0–11.5)
Lymphocytes	2.52	× 10^9/l	(1.0–4.8)
Monocytes	**1.59**	× 10^9/l	(0.2–1.4)
Eosinophils	0.12	× 10^9/l	(0.1–1.2)
Basophils	0.03	× 10^9/l	(0.0 0.1)

Parameter	Value	Units	Range
Platelets	464	$\times 10^9/l$	(200–500)
Film comment:	Red cell morphology unremarkable		
	White cell morphology shows moderate numbers of mildly toxic neutrophils with Dohle bodies and foamy cytoplasm		
	Platelet morphology unremarkable		

Questions

1. How may regurgitation be differentiated from vomiting in the dog?
2. What are the two main radiographic findings discernible from the thoracic radiographs supplied?
3. Interpret the results of the complete blood count.
4. What differential diagnoses should be considered for the underlying cause of the dog's regurgitation? What further investigation should be considered?
5. How should this dog be managed in the interim?

Answers

1. How may regurgitation be differentiated from vomiting in the dog?

Differentiating regurgitation from vomiting

Distinguishing between these is a vital first step with any patient that is orally expelling food or liquid since the differential diagnosis, investigation and consequences of the two differ.

Regurgitation is typified by a passive production of undigested food, fluid, saliva or a mixture, whereas vomiting is typified by abdominal effort ('heaving') prior to vomiting; owners generally report little to no effort when dogs are regurgitating. Often regurgitated food will be produced 'like a sausage' and regurgitation of saliva, which has pooled within the oesophagus (and which has lost much of its aqueous content) will appear like 'egg white'. Note that timing from feeding can be rather unreliable, since many dogs with oesophageal disorders will accumulate food and saliva for many hours before regurgitation. Similarly, measurement of the pH of produced fluid/food may be misleading since gastro-oesophageal reflux of acidic gastric contents occurs episodically normally.

2. What are the two main radiographic findings discernible from the thoracic radiographs supplied?

The most obvious finding is of generalised oesophageal dilatation with air (megaoesophagus). This is seen best on the left lateral view and is typified by the 'dorsal tracheal stripe sign', the dorsal border of the trachea being highlighted by air within the oesophagus between the thoracic inlet and the sixth ribs on this view. The dorsal and ventral oesophageal walls can be seen to continue roughly parallel to each other until they reach the diaphragm. These parallel, thin, soft tissue lines can be seen clearly crossing the left crus of the diaphragm on the left lateral film and the right crus of the diaphragm on the right lateral film.

Radiography to identify megaoesophagus

Take care when assessing oesophageal gas distension by radiography since images taken under general anaesthesia, and if excessive aerophagia has occurred, may demonstrate moderate amounts of oesophageal air *normally* and should not be overinterpreted as evidence of megaoesophagus.

It is seldom necessary, and increases the chances of aspiration, to perform barium oesophagrams and these should be avoided. Occasional subtle oesophageal dysmotility may require barium swallows to be performed with fluoroscopic examination, but static barium radiographs offer very poor diagnostic benefit versus risk.

The other finding is of a patchy/ill-defined increase in pulmonary opacity consistent with an alveolar infiltrate seen in the region of the right middle lung lobe. This is seen most clearly on the dorsoventral radiograph and overlying the heart base on the left lateral recumbency radiograph. In conjunction with the clinical signs and the presence of megaoesophagus, aspiration pneumonitis is the primary consideration.

3. **Interpret the results of the complete blood count.**

There is a very mild normocytic, normochromic anaemia of haematocrit 0.35 l/l (0.37–0.55). There is a moderate, mature neutrophilia (which may be consistent with inflammation, including infection) of 23.01 × 10^9/l (3.0–11.5) and a mild monocytosis of 1.59 × 10^9/l (0.2–1.4), which together with the neutrophilia suggests an established inflammatory response. Some of the neutrophils show mild toxic changes, which may be consistent with marked inflammation or infection. The anaemia is very mild but should be interpreted in the light of the dog's hydration status. Commonly normocytic, normochromic anaemias of this level are seen as an anaemia of chronic illness, but early blood loss, haemolysis, bone marrow abnormalities or endocrinopathy (especially hypothyroidism) could not be excluded.

4. **What differential diagnoses should be considered for the underlying cause of the dog's regurgitation? What further investigation should be considered?**

A diagnosis of megaoesophagus can be confidently made from the radiographs. Megaoesophagus may be acquired and is also seen as a congenital idiopathic disorder in the Wire-Haired Fox Terrier and Miniature Schnauzer as well as in some breeds due to congenital myasthenia gravis.

Differential diagnoses for megaoesophagus are shown in **Table 16.1**, but note that idiopathic megaoesophagus is the most common diagnosis. The role of hypothyroidism in causing megaoesophagus is controversial and a cause-and-effect link has not been demonstrated.

Initial further investigation should be subsequent to
- A thorough medical, dietary, vaccination, travel, worming and environmental history.
- A thorough general physical examination, which should include a proactive assessment for evidence of dysautonomia (findings of which might include mydriasis, bradycardia, enlarged atonic bladder, constipation).
- A specific and thoroughly performed neurological examination, which should include observation for gait disturbances/fatigue with exercise/exertion (see Case 2).

Table 16.1 Differential diagnosis of megaoesophagus

Primary	Idiopathic megaoesophagus
Secondary	To neurological/neuromuscular disease

- Myasthenia gravis
  - Focal pharyngeal/oesophageal involvement
  - As part of generalised myasthenia gravis
  - As part of a paraneoplastic syndrome of myasthenia gravis and megaoesophagus with thymoma
- Immune-mediated (polymyositis, systemic lupus erythematosus, dermatomyositis)
- Toxic (tetanus, snake envenomation, acrylamide)
- Dysautonomia

Endocrinopathy-related

- Hypoadrenocorticism
- Hypothyroidism

Obstructive*

*This latter is rare – usually focal oesophageal dilatation cranial to the point of obstruction is seen, but very rarely generalised dilatation may be seen due to obstructive disease at the lower oesophageal sphincter (including lesions of Spirocerca lupi in countries where it is endemic) or as persisting gaseous distension after hiatal herniation.

Importance of concurrent neuromuscular signs

Because of the association between megaoesophagus and more generalised neurological/neuromuscular disorders, it is very important to pay very close attention to gait and neurological examination. Having identified megaoesophagus in a patient it is a sensible practice to further review this in the light of the discovery.

Further rational evaluation would include
- Assessment of serum biochemistry, which might proffer information with regard to parameters such as electrolyte disturbances, hypoglycaemia and hypercholesterolaemia, which might be diagnostically helpful in the context of some of the differential diagnoses discussed.
- Performance of an ACTH stimulation test or a basal cortisol level to exclude the possibility of hypoadrenocorticism.
- Performance of diagnostic evaluation for hypothyroidism but bearing in mind that
  - A true cause-and-effect relationship between hypothyroidism and megaeosophagus is controversial.
  - The patient has clinical signs of aspiration pneumonitis and such test results are likely to be affected by the presence of a severe non-thyroidal illness (in particular total T4 is likely to be lowered by the presence of aspiration pneumonitis).
- Performance of diagnostic testing for myasthenia gravis.
  - Assessment of acetylcholine receptor antibody positivity is highly specific (i.e. false positive is unlikely) but a greater proportion of animals with focal myasthenia gravis are thought to be 'sero-negative' than those with generalised myasthenia gravis.

- ◦ Electrophysiological tests such as
  - Repetitive nerve stimulation.
  - Evaluation for 'jitter', though neither of these are specific for myasthenia gravis.

To 'scope or not to 'scope?

A dilemma is often whether oesophagoscopy ought to be considered in patients with megaoeso-phagus. Animals with megaoesophagus are prone to further aspiration when anaesthetised or during recovery and prior to considering diagnostic steps involving anaesthesia for endoscopy, the clinician should carefully consider:

- How diagnostically useful is the procedure likely to be (since obstructive causes of gen-eralised megaoesophagus are extremely unlikely and megaoesophagus is not an endo-scopic diagnosis)?
- What contingency planning should be made (i.e. meticulous suctioning of oesoph-ageal and gastric contents, close supervision during recovery) prior to performing oesophagoscopy?
- What procedures should be planned to be undertaken at the same time to minimise compounding the risk of aspiration by multiple anaesthetics? For instance:
  - ◦ If aspiration pneumonitis is present, should bronchoalveolar lavage samples be taken to culture and better target antimicrobial therapy?
  - ◦ If the animal is unable to tolerate oral feeding and is becoming malnourished should a per-endoscopic gastrostomy (PEG) tube be placed?
  - ◦ Should electrophysiological testing be performed whilst the dog is anaesthetised?

---

5. How should this dog be managed in the interim?

The most important initial step is to institute strict postural feeding and water adminis-tration, that is feeding the patient with the whole head, neck and thorax raised to a height that ensures that the entire oesophagus is positioned as near to vertical as possible. Using a water and food bowl raised on a stand is not sufficient since this does not beneficially al-ter the cervical or thoracic oesophageal orientation other than shifting it to the horizontal plane. Malnourished patients may require provision of a gastrostomy feeding tube until corrected.

The clinical signs of coughing, depression and elevated respiratory rate and effort, the inflammatory leukogram and the radiographic findings are suggestive of aspiration pneumonitis.

Suitable management may include provision of broad-spectrum antibacterial medication, which should be lipophilic, bacteriocidal and attain high concentrations in airway fluid film compared with plasma concentrations. The intravenous route is appropriate in the face of de-hydration or debilitation but is not necessarily advantageous over other routes in well-hydrated animals, though oral medications may not be adequately absorbed if entrapped within a dilated oesophagus. Inhaled antimicrobial administration has become popular but environmental de-livery of antimicrobials has implications for responsible confinement of these agents to target infected tissues. Judicious oxygen administration and provision of regular saline nebulisation and coupage may aid resolution of the aspiration pneumonitis.

Diagnosis

The dog in this case had no findings consistent with neuromuscular causes of the megaoesophagus, hypoadrenocorticism or hypothyroidism and acetylcholine receptor antibody testing was negative. Initial postural feeding resulted in clinical resolution of the episodes of regurgitation. A provisional diagnosis of **idiopathic megaoesophagus** was made.

The patient was initially administered cefuroxime (Zinacef, GlaxoSmithKline) at a dose of 20 mg/kg i.v. q8 hours and received regular nebulisation with saline and thoracic coupage for 10–15 minutes q6 hours. At 3 days after admission, respiratory rate and effort had settled and the dog appeared much brighter. Repeat thoracic radiographs showed the aspiration pneumonitis to be resolving (**Figure 16.3**). The dog was discharged after a further 4 days and was treated with oral antimicrobials for a further 6 weeks in total. The dog has been maintained since with no medical management and postural feeding and drinking only.

Discussion

Regurgitation is a clinical sign of disordered swallowing, which is a form of dysphagia. Dysphagia may be described as oral, pharyngeal or oesophageal, but oral dysphagia results in an inability to prehend or masticate food rather than regurgitation.

Megaoesophagus is probably the commonest cause of oesophageal dysphagia and can often be detected on thoracic radiographs, provided these are of adequate quality. The cardinal finding is the dorsal tracheal stripe sign caused by the air-filled cranial thoracic oesophagus, allowing the dorsal wall of the trachea to be more clearly seen. Megaoesophagus may be generalised or focal. Generalised megaoesophagus precludes oesophageal obstruction by a vascular ring anomaly. Focal megaoesophagus may be genuine or the result of a transient area of more marked oesophageal dilatation being detected on a static imaging technique such as thoracic radiography. Oesophageal dysfunction that does not result in dilatation requires a real-time imaging technique such as fluoroscopy to assess.

Idiopathic megaoesophagus has been well-studied and is caused by dysfunction within the afferent vagal arm of the swallowing reflex, altered oesophageal viscoelastic properties and poor vagal responsiveness to intraluminal oesophageal distension.

Though idiopathic megaoesophagus is the most common differential diagnosis, a thorough evaluation for other causes of megaoesophagus should be undertaken since no effective treatment exists for idiopathic megaoesophagus. Of particular concern is the possibility that cases of focal mysaesthenia gravis may be ruled out prematurely on the basis of a negative acetylcholine receptor antibody test (we do not know the sensitivity of this test in focal myasthenia gravis in dogs, but it is known that false negative results frequently occur in man).

The importance of aspiration pneumonitis

Megaoesophagus, as in this case, is often complicated by aspiration pneumonitis; respiratory effort and a soft/moist cough are typical clinical signs and it is important to remember to ask during the clinical history about any association between eating/drinking and cough or 'splutter' that might be associated with respiratory signs secondary to dysphagia.

The normal rectal temperature does not preclude the possibility of severe, even life-threatening inflammatory disease. Aspiration pneumonitis is not invariably complicated by infection, though it is common to assume that it is synonymous with a bacterial pneumonia. In fact, aspiration is a direct chemical/mechanical injury caused by ingress of saliva particulate matter

(a)

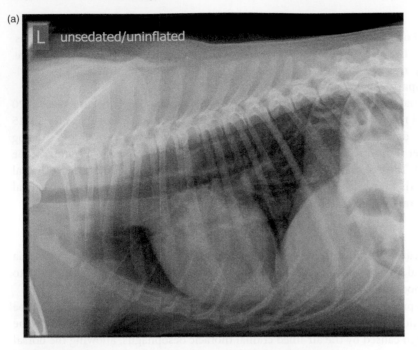

(b)

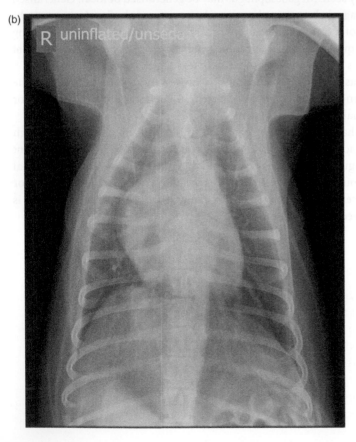

Figure 16.3 (a) Left lateral thoracic radiograph and (b) dorsoventral thoracic radiograph after 3 days of treatment.

and possibly low-pH gastric contents into the respiratory tract. The exact pathological consequences depend on precisely what has been inhaled but three distinct phases may be seen of

- I: immediate (airway neurogenic, increased permeability, oedema and a bronchospasm
  response),
- II: inflammatory (neutrophil accumulation, proteolysis, platelet activation and alveolar
  infiltrate development) and
- III: chronic inflammatory with or without secondary bacterial infection.

Most bacteria isolated during phase III are commensals of the oropharynx. It should be remembered that radiographic signs of aspiration often 'lag' behind clinical findings by 24–48 hours.

It is important to emphasise the role of postural feeding in idiopathic megaoesophagus since this
is the bedrock of management. Too often veterinary surgeons recommend that food bowls and water
bowls are elevated but using stands and similar height devices does not result in elevation of the cervical and thoracic oesophagus, just the head and oropharynx. It is very important to feed such dogs in
an upright position such as on a stepladder, stairs or in an especially manufactured chair (**Figure 16.4**).

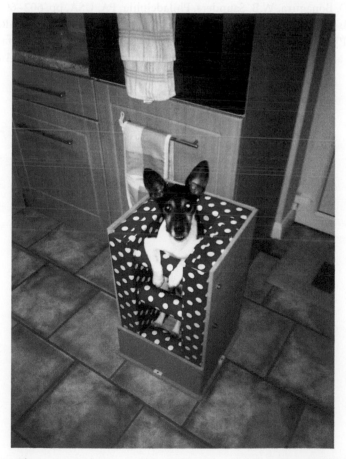

Figure 16.4 Patient with megaoesophagus ready for feeding in a specially constructed 'Bailey' chair.

The prognosis with megaoesophagus is always guarded but is hugely variable. Some patients live for many years with postural feeding alone, whilst other animals succumb (usually to the effects of recurrent aspiration pneumonitis) quickly after diagnosis.

Further reading

Boudrieu, R.J. & Rogers, W.A. (1985) Megaoesophagus in dog: a review of 50 cases. *J Am Anim Hosp Assoc* **21**, 33–40

Dewey, C.W., Bailey, C.S., Shelton, G.D., Kass, P.H. & Cardinet, G.H., III (1997) Clinical forms of acquired myasthenia gravis in dogs: 25 cases (1988–1995). *J Vet Intern Med* **11**, 50–57

Gaynor, A.R., Shofer, F.S. & Washabau, R.J. (1997) Risk factors for acquired megaesophagus in dogs. *J Am Vet Med Assoc* **211**, 1406–1412

Holland, C.T., Satchell, P.M. & Farrow, B.R. (1996) Vagal esophagomotor nerve function and esophageal motor performance in dogs with congenital idiopathic megaesophagus. *Am J Vet Res* **57**, 906–913

McBrearty, A.R., Ramsey, I.K., Courcier, E.A., Mellor, D.J. & Bell, R. (2011) Clinical factors associated with death before discharge and overall survival time in dogs with generalized megaesophagus. *J Am Vet Med Assoc* **238**, 1622–1628

Mears, E.A. & deNovo, R.C. (2000) Canine megaesophagus. In *Kirk's Current Veterinary Therapy*, Vol. XIII, ed. J.D. Bonagura, W.B. Saunders, Philadelphia, PA, USA, pp. 602–607

Ovbey, D.H., Wilson, D.V., Bednarski, R.M., Hauptman, J.G., Stanley, B.J., Radlinsky, M.G., Larenza, M.P., Pypendop, B.H. & Rezende, M.L. (2014) Prevalence and risk factors for canine post-anesthetic aspiration pneumonia (1999–2009): a multicenter study. *Vet Anaesth Analg* **41**, 127–136

Respiratory

Respiratory

Equine Internal Medicine: What's Your Diagnosis? First edition. Ian West.
© 2014 John Wiley & Sons Ltd. Published 2014 by John Wiley & Sons Ltd.

Clinical presentation

An 11 month-old female-entire Shetland Sheepdog (**Figure 17.1**) is presented for a history of progressively worsening cough and tachypnoea. Coughing (which has been described as harsh and 'reaching') and reduced exercise tolerance were first noted 10 days previously and a course of oxytetracycline had been prescribed at this time with a provisional diagnosis of infectious tracheobronchitis. However, clinical signs had progressed and the other dog in the household had shown no coughing in the interim. Physical examination demonstrated a dyspnoeic dog with orthopnoeic posture and shallow, rapid breathing. Respiratory rate is 108/min with equal inspiratory and expiratory phases and there is normal resting heart rate and pulse rate (with no evidence of murmur or arrhythmia). Mucous membranes are cyanosed and there is marked bilateral generalised inspiratory wheezes and crackles. Frequent paroxysms of harsh coughing are noted. Rectal temperature is 38.5 °C and remaining physical examination was normal. The dog has no previous medical history and has not travelled outside the United Kingdom.

Questions

1. What 'type' of dyspnoea is this dog demonstrating?
2. What are the potential causes of cough in this dog?
3. What initial management should be undertaken?
4. After initial stabilisation the thoracic radiographs in Figure 17.2 were taken. Interpret these radiographs and list the likely differential diagnoses.
5. What further investigation should be undertaken in this patient, assuming it is safe to do so?

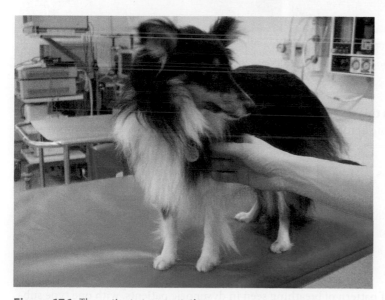

Figure 17.1 The patient at presentation.

Canine Internal Medicine: What's Your Diagnosis? First Edition. Jon Wray.
© 2018 John Wiley & Sons Ltd. Published 2018 by John Wiley & Sons Ltd.

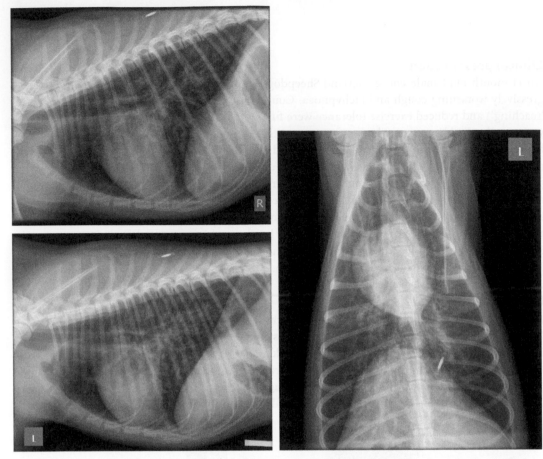

Figure 17.2 (from top to bottom) Right lateral recumbency, left lateral recumbency and ventrodorsal thoracic radiographs. The ventrodorsal radiograph has some rotation.

Answers

1. What 'type' of dyspnoea is this dog demonstrating?

Dyspnoea describes a state of difficulty in breathing.

'Ventilation' is determined by measuring dissolved blood CO_2

Note that the terms 'hyperventilation' and 'hypoventilation' should not be used to describe respiratory effort since ventilation is, by definition, adequacy of removal of carbon dioxide produced through cellular metabolism, which can only be determined by blood gas analysis and not by clinical observations. Instead the terms 'hyperpnoea' and 'hypopnoea' should be used.

There are three 'types' of pattern of breathing seen in dyspnoeic patients, with one type subdivided into two. Most commonly we describe dyspnoeic breathing patterns as either being rapid-and-shallow ('restrictive') or slow-and-forceful ('obstructive'). These patterns and their significance are summarised in **Table 17.1**.

This dog has a rapid and shallow breathing pattern characteristic of a 'restrictive' dyspnoea.

Table 17.1 Types of respiratory pattern

Respiratory pattern	Characteristics	Significance
Restrictive (choppy)	Rapid and shallow/subtle *Inspiratory:expiratory effort/ length usually equal*	Usually seen due to diffuse lung parenchymal, pleural space fluid or air accumulation, fibrosis, pain or loss of thoracic wall/diaphragm integrity
Obstructive (inspiratory)	Slow and forceful *Inspiratory effort/length greater than expiratory effort/length*	Indicates obstructive disease of the upper airways, for example in laryngeal paralysis
Obstructive (expiratory)	Slow and forceful *Expiratory effort/length greater than inspiratory effort/length*	Indicates obstructive disease of the lower airways, for example in small airway bronchospasm
Paradoxical	Rapid and forceful *Caudal thorax collapses inwards during inspiration and abdomen billows outwards*	Paradoxical respiration is not a 'localising' pattern but instead indicates that the patient has been dyspnoeic for sufficient time/severity that intrinsic muscles of respiration are fatigued and abdominal recruitment/abnormal diaphragmatic motion is present. It is often an indication of impending respiratory failure

2. **What are the potential causes of cough in this dog?**

Cough is a clinical sign caused by initiation of a protective mechanism to rid the airways of potentially harmful substances. It is initiated by a cough stimulus (may be mechanical, inflammatory, chemical, etc.) acting upon cough receptors. This latter are most commonly and most densely:

- Myelinated rapidly adapting stretch receptors within the tracheobronchial tree.
- Bronchial C-fibres.

Cough characteristics

Harsh/hacking/loud coughing is most commonly caused by activation of cough receptors within the larger airways. Coughing that is more 'soft', 'wet' or 'moist' is most commonly due to lower airway and lung parenchymal disease. Pleural space disease can also provoke coughing.

The timing of coughing may sometimes be diagnostically helpful but may also be over-interpreted. Coughing that is provoked by eating or drinking, particularly if accompanied by 'spluttering', should raise in the clinician's mind the possibility of aspiration due to dysphagia. A cough that is predictably provoked by excitement is most commonly seen in dynamic airway collapse such as tracheal and/or bronchial collapse.

A cough at night is frequently afforded a significance that the author feels is often over-emphasised. It is likely that some owners are simply more aware of a cough at night compared with one during the day because (i) they are out of the household more during the day themselves, (ii) it is quieter at night in most households so a cough is more noticeable, (iii) a coughing dog is annoying when one is trying to get to sleep!

In this dog, whilst the coughing is harsh and hacking there is also evidence of hypoxaemia (cyanosis), suggesting impaired gas exchange. The respiratory rate and pattern is 'restrictive' and is more commonly associated with parenchymal and interstitial lung disease, pleural space disease, pain and fibrosis. Thus a disorder anatomically distributed at more than one respiratory 'level'/site is anticipated. Common differential diagnoses for a cough are shown in **Table 17.2**.

In this dog cardiac causes of a cough would be unlikely since there has been no history or physical examination findings consistent with the likelihood of congestive heart failure. Infectious tracheobronchitis would be highly unlikely in the presence of another dog in the household who has not started to cough in the time-frame given.

3. **What initial management should be undertaken?**

The dog is dyspnoeic and cyanosed. Cyanosis is recognised when the amount of deoxyhaemoglobin within the blood exceeds 3–5 g/dl (normal oxyhaemoglobin content of blood is 12–18 g/dl in dogs in our laboratory). Detection of cyanosis is dependent on ambient lighting conditions and also whether the patient is anaemic, since detection depends on both the amount and saturation of haemoglobin.

Significance of cyanosis

Cyanosis is always a late finding in progressive hypoxaemia and provision of oxygen support by the best tolerated method is indicated as a matter of urgency.

Anxious, dyspnoeic dogs may also benefit from anxiolysis in the form of opiate-based sedatives and in rapidly deteriorating patients a decision may need to be made to induce anaesthesia, intubate and ventilate the patient on an emergency basis.

4. **After initial stabilisation the thoracic radiographs in Figure 17.2 were taken. Interpret these radiographs and list the likely differential diagnoses.**

The most striking finding is a generalised marked bronchointerstitial infiltrate. Bronchial patterns are characterised by findings of 'donuts', 'signet rings' and 'tramlines' caused by thickening of the bronchus. Clear examples of this can be seen on the right lateral thoracic radiograph overlying the heart base in intercostal spaces 5 and 6 and dorsocaudal to the heart base in intercostal spaces 7–9. On the left lateral radiograph similar 'donuts' can be seen in intercostal space 3 and caudal to the cardiac apex. There is also an unstructured ('hazy') interstitial pattern characterised by increased lung opacity and obscured pulmonary vasculature. This can be seen best on the VD radiograph in the left-central portion of the lungfields.

Of the differential diagnoses listed above, inflammatory, infectious and parasitic airway disease would be most likely. A diffuse infiltrative neoplastic process such as lymphoma or airway/interstitial haemorrhage could not be excluded.

5. **What further investigation should be undertaken in this patient, assuming it is safe to do so?**

Once the patient is stabilised, appropriate investigation would include
- Assessment of a complete blood count
  - May demonstrate polycythaemia associated with appropriate response to prolonged hypoxaemia.

Table 17.2 Differential diagnosis for cough

D (Degenerative)	Tracheal collapse
	Bronchomalacia
A (Anomalous, Anatomical)	Airway foreign body
	Presence of pleural fluid of any aetiology
	Carinal / bronchial compression due to
	– Cardiomegaly
	– Enlarged tracheobronchial lymph nodes
	– Cardiac mass lesions
N (Neoplastic, Nutritional)	Neoplasia
	• Primary
	• Secondary (metastatic)
	• As part of a diffuse infiltration (e.g. lymphoma)
I (Infectious, Inflammatory, Immune-mediated)	Infectious tracheobronchitis
	Infectious bronchopneumonia caused by
	– Bacteria
	– Viruses
	– Fungi
	– Protozoa
	Parasitic respiratory disease caused by
	• *Angiostrongylus vasorum*
	• *Crenosoma vulpis*
	• *Capillaria aerophila*
	• *Oslerus osleri*
	Granulomatous airway disease caused by
	• Infectious (usually fungal or mycobacterial)
	• Parasitic
	• Eosinophilic granuloma
	• Lymphomatoid granulomatosis
	Aspiration pneumonitis
	Canine chronic bronchitis
	Eosinophilic bronchopneumonopathy
	Idiopathic pulmonary fibrosis
T (Traumatic, Toxic)	As sequel to thoracic trauma
	Inhaled irritant toxins
	Paraquat toxicity
V (Vascular)	Pulmonary arterial disease
	– Thromboembolism
	– (*Dirofilaria immitis* – not seen in UK)
	Pulmonary oedema

- ○ May demonstrate anaemia consistent with intrapulmonary blood loss.
- ○ May demonstrate eosinophilia consistent with parasitism or eosinophilic bronchopneumonopathy.
- ○ May demonstrate neutrophilia consistent with an active inflammatory response, which may include (but is not limited to) infection.
- Performance of faecal analysis by the Baermann technique to evaluate for *Angiostrongylus vasorum* and *Crenosoma vulpis* larvae (these may be difficult to distinguish) and eggs of *Capillaria aerophila*. *Oslerus osleri* is most often detected by identification of parasitic tracheobronchial nodules at endoscopy, but larvae are best seen in faeces by zinc sulfate flotation rather than the Baermann technique.
- Performance of *Angiostrongylus vasorum* antigen test.
- Bronchoscopy and bronchoalveolar lavage for
  - ○ Cytology
  - ○ Culture
- Assessment of arterial blood gas and/or co-oximetry results may proffer information regarding the severity of the hypoxaemia but are unlikely to add to the clinical diagnosis since cyanosis is already recognised.
- Similarly, it is unlikely that biochemistry will proffer information that is diagnostically helpful in most cases of coughing in dogs.

Diagnosis

- The patient was initially administered oxygen via an oxygen cage and was given butorphanol at a dose of 0.2 mg/kg i.v. as an anxiolytic. Dyspnoea soon abated allowing further evaluation.
- Haematology demonstrated:

Haematology

Parameter	Value	Units	Range
RBC	6.60	$\times 10^{12}/l$	(5.5–8.5)
Haemoglobin	15.8	g/dl	(12.0–18.0)
Haematocrit	0.47	l/l	(0.37–0.55)
Mean Cell Volume	71.7	fl	(60–77)
Mean Cell Haemoglobin concentration	33.5	g/dl	(30.0–38.0)
Mean cell haemoglobin	24.0	pg	(19.5–25.5)
Total white cell count	**25.05**	$\times 10^9/l$	(6.0–15.0)
Neutrophils	**12.53**	$\times 10^9/l$	(3.0–11.5)
Lymphocytes	3.51	$\times 10^9/l$	(1.0–4.8)
Monocytes	**2.0**	$\times 10^9/l$	(0.2–1.4)
Eosinophils	**7.01**	$\times 10^9/l$	(0.1–1.2)
Basophils	0.00	$\times 10^9/l$	(0.0–0.1)
Platelets	273	$\times 10^9/l$	(200–500)

Parameter	Value	Units	Range
Film comment:	Red cell morphology: normal		
	White cell morphology: no left shift or toxic changes seen		
	Platelet morphology: small numbers of clumps seen		

- The most pertinent finding was a marked peripheral eosinophilia and a mild established inflammatory response.
- Faecal analyses (3 samples) by the Baermann technique demonstrated no parasitic larvae or eggs. This case preceded availability of antigen testing for *Angiostrongylus vasorum*.
- Bronchoscopy and bronchoalveolar lavage were performed. This demonstrated generalised airway erythema and large quantities of mucopus to be present within all major bronchial divisions. A bronchoalveolar lavage sample demonstrated the following:

MICROBIOLOGY

Source of sample — BAL

Culture and sensitivity

Aerobic culture — No bacterial growth

Anaerobic culture — No anaerobes isolated

Fungal culture — Negative to date

CYTOLOGY (BAL)

Appearance — Pale pink, turbid with stringy clots

Cytological findings

On cytospin preparation examination the cellularity is high and the preservation is good. The background is lightly basophilic and contains a small amount of blood. There are high numbers of mixed inflammatory cells. The vast majority of these cells (80%) are eosinophils. There are also moderate numbers of neutrophils and lower numbers of activated macrophages. Low numbers of mast cells are present.

INTERPRETATION

Eosinophilic inflammation

A diagnosis of eosinophilic bronchopneumonopathy (EBP) was made.

Treatment

Due to the severity of the clinical signs, initially dexamethasone sodium phosphate (Dexadreson, MSD Animal Health) was administered at a dose of 0.5 mg/kg intravenously once and terbutaline (Bricanyl, AstraZeneca) at a dose of 0.01 mg/kg intramuscularly once. Thereafter oral prednisolone was administered at a dose of 1 mg/kg p/o BID for 1 week followed by 1 mg/kg p/o SID for 4 weeks, then 0.5 mg/kg p/o SID for 4 weeks and then 0.5 mg/kg p/o every other day for 4 weeks before trial discontinuation.

Clinical signs rapidly improved and dyspnoea rapidly and permanently resolved within the first 24 hours of treatment. The respiratory rate gradually normalised over the subsequent 6 days and thoracic radiographs taken 7 days after admission demonstrated resolving bronchointerstitial

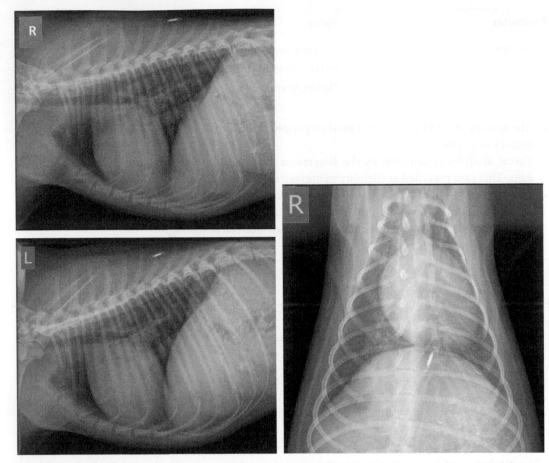

Figure 17.3 (from top to bottom) Right lateral recumbency, left lateral recumbency and dorsoventral thoracic radiographs 1 week after the initiation of therapy.

infiltrates (**Figure 17.3**). A subsequent lateral radiograph taken during the convalescent period and after discontinuation of medication showed no radiographic recurrence and no further clinical signs recurred when the dog was off all medication.

Discussion

Eosinophilic bronchopneumonopathy (EBP) has been also known as pulmonary infiltration with eosinophils (PIE), eosinophilic pneumonia and pulmonary eosinophilic granuloma. It is a poorly reported condition in veterinary medicine despite widespread experience in treating cases (Clercx et al. 2000; Corcoran et al. 1991). A breed predispositions in Siberian Huskies has been reported and this breed represents the majority of cases seen in our practice (predisposition in Malamutes and Rottweilers is also reported). Intractable coughing is the most frequently reported clinical signs and loss of exercise tolerance is commonly seen in working Huskies. EBP is probably not a very common disorder though it represents a large proportion of patients, especially younger dogs, presented to referral centres for evaluation of coughing, perhaps reflecting a low degree of clinical suspicion for it and difficulties in diagnosis. An underlying aetiology has not been determined and although it has been sometimes referred to as 'allergic bronchitis' there is little evidence currently to support

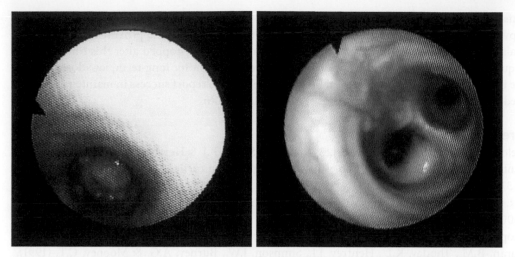

Figure 17.4 Bronchoscopic findings in examples of eosinophilic bronchopneumonopathy.

an allergic aetiology and moreover the stark breed predispositions and the observation that many patients do not show a relapse in the condition when treated with discontinuous therapy would not support this.

The severity of clinical signs is variable and the patient in this case was particularly severely affected. A substantial minority of patients also present with signs attributable to nasal cavity inflammation and finding of eosinophilic rhinitis in patients with EBP undergoing nasal biopsies is not uncommon (Clercx et al. 2000). A bronchointerstitial thoracic infiltrate is the most common radiographic abnormality, though alveolar infiltrates, nodular interstitial infiltrates (which appear to be due to eosinophilic granulomata but may be mistaken for neoplastic lung nodules) and bronchiectasis may also be commonly seen.

The major differential diagnoses are of airway parasitism (see Shaw et al. 1996) and airway eosinophilia as part of a systemic hypereosinophilic syndrome (HES) or due to mast cell tumour or lymphoma. Peripheral eosinophilia is documented in approximately 50–60% of dogs with EBP but its absence must not be used to exclude it and care must be taken in breeds such as the Husky, Rottweiler and German Shepherd dog, where a relative eosinophilia is found in normal dogs (Lilliehook and Tvedten 2003). It is common to see exhuberant amounts of mucopus in the airways (see **Figure 17.4** examples from other patients) and this may be so concreted as to appear almost solid. It is vital to recognise that observation of mucopus does not distinguish between highly cellular but sterile material and an infectious process and assessment by cytology and culture is always necessary.

Corticosteroid responsiveness of EBP

EBP is characterised by rapid and exquisite sensitivity to corticosteroid administration and failure to show a dramatic response should lead to critical reappraisal of the diagnosis and, if not already performed, trial anti-parasitic therapy.

The optimum therapeutic strategy has not been elucidated though it is common practice to treat with an initial brief period of a high anti-inflammatory/low immunosuppressive dose of prednisolone followed by tapering over a 2–3 month period. It is not known precisely how long therapy should be continued though clinical experience suggests that approximately half of the animals treated may successfully have oral corticosteroid therapy stopped after this time without subsequent relapse. The remainder appear to have a requirement for long-term, low-dose prednisolone in order to control their clinical signs and some authors report success in maintenance with inhaled corticosteroids such as fluticasone (Bexfield et al. 2006).

References

Bexfield, N.H., Foale, R.D., Davison, L.J., Watson, P.J., Skelly, B.J. & Herrtage, M.E. (2006) Management of 13 cases of canine respiratory disease using inhaled corticosteroids. *J Small Anim Pract* **47**, 377–382

Clercx, C., Peeters, D., Snaps, F., Hansen, P., McEntee, K., Detilleux, J., Henroteaux, M. & Day, M.J. (2000)

Eosinophilic bronchopneumopathy in dogs. *J Vet Intern Med* **14**, 282–291

Corcoran, B.M., Thoday, K.L., Henfrey, J.I., Simpson, J.W., Burney, A.G. & Mooney, C.T. (1991). Pulmonary infiltration with eosinophils in 14 dogs. *J Small Anim Pract* **32**, 494–502

Shaw, D.H., Conboy, G.A., Hogan, P.M. & Horney, B.S. (1996) Eosinophilic bronchitis caused by *Crenosoma vulpis* infection in dogs. *Can Vet J* **37**, 361–363

Lilliehook, I. & Tvedten, H. (2003) Investigation of hypereosinophilia and potential treatments. *Vet Clin North Am Small Anim Pract* **33**, 1359–1378, viii

Further reading

Clercx, C. & Peeters, D. (2007) Canine eosinophilic bronchopneumopathy. *Vet Clin North Am Small Anim Pract* **37**, 917–935, vi

Clinical presentation

A 10 year-old male-neutered Yorkshire Terrier is presented for further investigation of episodes of respiratory distress. The dog has had a systolic left apical heart murmur noted in its clinical records since 3 years previously and the murmur has become louder over this time from grade II/VI when first noted to grade IV/VI now. The dog has intermittently coughed when excited for the last 2 years but in the last 4–5 months the episodes of coughing have become both more frequent and more severe and now the dog has paroxysms of harsh 'barking' coughing whenever excited or agitated and on three occasions in the last month has presented to out-of-hours emergency clinics in respiratory distress with cyanosis. On each occasion he has been provided with oxygen therapy, anxiolysis in the form of butorphanol injections and has been administered parenteral furosemide and dexamethasone. On each occasion he has recovered uneventfully over several hours. His primary veterinary practice have started treatment with furosemide at a dose of 1 mg/kg p/o BID and an ACE-inhibitor (benazepril). The episodes of cough and less severe episodes of respiratory compromise have continued unchanged until three days ago when he had another severe bout of coughing and respiratory distress, which was treated in the same way as the previous ones. However, he has remained lethargic since this bout and though the coughing has subsided, remains tachypnoeic.

The owner reports that when not coughing the dog's respiratory rate and effort appears normal and his enthusiasm for and ability to exercise is normal, but any excitement predictably provokes paroxysms of coughing. These are not initiated by eating or drinking and they feel that his bark is unchanged. They describe the cough as always having a harsh, 'honking' characteristic.

On physical examination the dog is slightly quiet and in normal body condition. Respiratory rate is 36/min with a rapid and shallow respiratory pattern. Heart rate is 108/minute and rhythm is sinus. Peripheral pulse quality is normal. Auscultation demonstrates a grade IV/VI pansystolic left apical heart murmur and some moist rales (crackles) bilaterally at peak inspiration. Palpation of the trachea at the thoracic inlet provokes paroxysms of harsh coughing terminated by a non-productive retch. Rectal temperature is 39.3 °C. Remaining examination is normal.

Questions

1. What is the problem list for this dog?
2. What are the principle differential diagnoses for the cause of the cough and can the history and physical examination findings help marshal these into an order of likelihood?
3. How would you investigate this patient further?

Canine Internal Medicine: What's Your Diagnosis? First Edition. Jon Wray.
© 2018 John Wiley & Sons Ltd. Published 2018 by John Wiley & Sons Ltd.

Answers

1. What is the problem list for this dog?

A suitable problem list would be:

- Cough, paroxysmal, harsh in nature, provoked by excitement
- Episodes of respiratory embarrassment provoked by cough
- Grade IV/VI pansystolic left apical heart murmur
- Tachypnoea with rapid, shallow respiratory pattern and accompanied by moist rales
- Pyrexia and depression currently

2. What are the principle differential diagnoses for the cause of the cough and can the history and physical examination findings help marshal these into an order of likelihood?

A cough has a long list of differential diagnoses in dogs (see **Table 17.2** in the previous case for an expanded list), but these may include:

- Obstructive conditions of the airways due to degenerative disease
  - Tracheal collapse
  - Bronchial collapse
- Anatomical causes including
  - Airway foreign bodies
  - Presence of pleural fluid of any aetiology
  - Carinal/bronchial compression due to external masses
- Neoplasia, which may be primary, secondary or diffuse
- Infectious, inflammatory, immune-mediated, allergic and irritation disorders of the airways
  - Infectious tracheobronchitis and bronchopneumonia
  - Respiratory parasites
  - Granulomatous airway disease
  - Aspiration pneumonitis
  - Canine chronic bronchitis
  - Eosinophilic bronchopneumonopathy
  - Idiopathic pulmonary fibrosis
- As sequel to thoracic trauma
- After inhaled irritants or consumption of toxins with primarily respiratory toxicity such as paraquat
- Vascular disorders including those caused by *Dirofilaria immitis* in endemic countries
- Pulmonary oedema*

Cough in congestive heart failure and cardiomegaly

*Some debate surrounds the relevance of a cough as a feature of pulmonary oedema due to congestive heart failure. Pulmonary cough receptors are likely to be a very weak inducer of cough and are sparsely populated in the canine lung. Furthermore, studies show little association between the presence of a cough and the presence of pulmonary oedema in dogs, though experience would suggest that those patients presenting with fulminant pulmonary oedema whose airways are flooded with oedema fluid often cough due to excitation of bronchial C-fibre receptors and rapidly adapting stretch receptors of larger airways. However, in the majority of dogs with congestive heart failure it is polypnoea rather than a cough that is the principle feature. Veterinary dogma also suggests that marked left atrial enlargement 'compresses' the left mainstem bronchus caudal to the carina and that this causes the cough. However, dogs with marked cardiomegaly of the left side for other reasons, for example patent ductus arteriosus, tend not to cough despite often having enormous degrees of dorsal deviation of the airways. It is perhaps more likely, and certainly the author's experience, that a cough in dogs with left atrial enlargement is usually due to concurrent airway pathology, which may permit compression/irritation in a way that normal healthy airways would resist.

In this patient, the cough is described as being loud and harsh. This is a feature most commonly of a cough originating from the upper or larger airways rather than pulmonary parenchymal disease, which commonly results in a softer 'wet' cough. The cough is also described as being predictably initiated by excitement. This is a cardinal feature of large airway disease with a dynamic component. This is also suggested by the provocation of coughing by palpation of the trachea at the thoracic inlet, which suggests tracheal collapse specifically. Although the dog has a grade IV/VI pansystolic left apical murmur, which, given its age, breed and progression, is most likely due to myxomatous mitral valve disease, there are features that suggest that the dog has not previously been in congestive heart failure (that the dog has been exercising with undiminished capacity and that respiratory rate and effort between bouts of coughing has been normal). Furthermore, the clinical signs have not been improved by administration of furosemide. However, currently and on physical examination there are not features present, such as the presence of a sinus arrhythmia, which could be helpful in eliminating congestive heart failure as a potential cause and the dog is currently tachypnoeic with some moist rales (crackles) being present (see below). Thus it could be considered that it is possible that congestive heart failure may be currently developing.

Lung 'sounds'

The term lung 'sounds' is a misnomer since the respiratory sounds heard with auscultation are vibrations caused by rapid, turbulent airflow in larger airways; by the time inspired air has reached smaller bronchi (from the third division onwards) airflow becomes slowed, laminar, smooth and, importantly, silent. Thus the sounds that are heard with the stethoscope on application of it to the thoracic wall are bronchial sounds (sometimes described as bronchovesicular) that are transmitted as 'pseudosounds' through lung parenchyma to the thoracic wall. They do not originate in lung tissue at all.

Adventitial or abnormal lung sounds are relatively infrequently heard and are limited to wheezes (high-pitched, medium intensity, 'whistling' sounds caused by airway narrowing), rhonchi (low-pitched, higher intensity, 'sighing' sounds most often heard in airway disease) and crackles/rales (high-pitched, brief, rustling sounds made by small airspaces snapping open). Whilst crackles are often taken to be a cardinal sign of pulmonary oedema it is vital to remember that crackles are detected in many primary respiratory disorders and that most patients with congestive heart failure will not have audible crackles present unless the oedema is extremely severe.

3. How would you investigate this patient further?

In this patient, although the history and clinical examination are more suggestive of a dynamic airway collapse, specifically tracheal collapse (nature of the cough, provocation with palpation of the trachea at the thoracic inlet), developing congestive heart failure should be excluded prior to airway evaluation, which always requires general anaesthesia. Should congestive heart failure be developing then satisfactory resolution of this prior to general anaesthesia should be undertaken for patient safety. The use of cardiac biomarkers such as NT-ProBNP may be helpful in determining the likelihood that a patient is in congestive heart failure but utility is limited in those situations in which both significant cardiac and concurrent respiratory disease might be present and also by the time taken to receive results. Thoracic radiography either conscious or under light sedation represents good diagnostic value in both evaluation of changes consistent with cardiogenic pulmonary oedema and some evaluation of the airways, though the dynamic nature of changes in these needs to be borne in mind.

In this case rational investigation might include

- Assessment of a haemogram to determine the presence of eosinophilia, which may be seen in the setting of eosinophilic bronchopneumonopathy, parasitism and neoplasia.
- Assessment of a faecal sample for evidence of larvae or eggs of respiratory parasites. A blood test for *Angiostrongylus vasorum* antigen is now available and has impressive (but not perfect) sensitivity in detection of infection.
- Thoracic radiography.
- Echocardiography.
- Evaluation of the airways:
  - Dynamic** structural assessment by
    - Radiography of the extra- and intrathoracic airways during both inspiration and expiration and/or
    - Fluoroscopy and/or
    - Tracheobronchoscopy.
  - By direct visualisation of
    - Laryngeal function under a light plane of anaesthesia.
    - Evaluation of the trachea, carina and segmental bronchi by tracheobronchoscopy.
  - By collection of material for cytological and microbiological (culture) evaluation by bronchoalveolar lavage.
  - By specific evaluation of airway samples for organisms that may be detected by non-routine methods:
    - PCR for *Bordetella bronchiseptica*
    - Mycoplasma culture

Problems with 'static' imaging methods for 'dynamic' airway disorders

**Dynamic airway collapse can be difficult to determine using static imaging methods such as conventional radiography and both fluoroscopy and endoscopic examination have advantages over conventional radiography in which false-negative diagnoses are common. However, fluoroscopy is not widely available outside specialist centres and endoscopic airway examination is significantly dependent on the experience and familiarity of the operator with normal anatomy and variation. It is important to remember that the intrathoracic trachea and bronchi will have a tendency to collapse during *expi*ration, whilst the extrathoracic trachea collapses most during *inspi*ration. To maximise the chances of detecting airway collapse with conventional static radiography it is therefore imperative to pay great attention to radiographic positioning, to temporarily extubate the patient provided it is safe to do so and to make sure careful veterinary supervision of the airway is continuously present, as well as timing exposures during both inspiratory and expiratory phases.

Diagnosis

In this patient haematology was normal and faecal analysis was negative for parasitic larvae. This patient's investigation pre-dated the *A. vasorum* antigen blood test.

Thoracic radiographs (**Figure 18.1**) taken under sedation demonstrated predominantly left-sided cardiomegaly with a left atrial 'tent' seen on the right lateral radiograph and mild tracheal elevation. Although assessment is slightly hampered by the films being slightly expiratory and the patient's overweight body condition probably contributing to a mild generalised increase in the interstitial component of the lungfields, no overt evidence of pulmonary venous congestion or infiltrates consistent with pulmonary oedema were seen. The trachea can be seen to reduce in diameter from the thoracic inlet to the intrathoracic portion and further abruptly narrow dorsoventrally at the level of the carina. In this instance, the expiratory nature of this film probably actually increased the degree to which intrathoracic airway collapse could be seen.

An echocardiographic assessment (**Figure 18.2**) demonstrated myxomatous mitral valve disease and marked prolapse of the anterior mitral valve leaflet associated with a large volume mitral regurgitant jet directed posterolaterally. Echocardiographically only relatively mild left atrial enlargement was seen and this was most appreciated on a right parasternal long axis rather than the short axis dimension. No evidence of systolic dysfunction was seen.

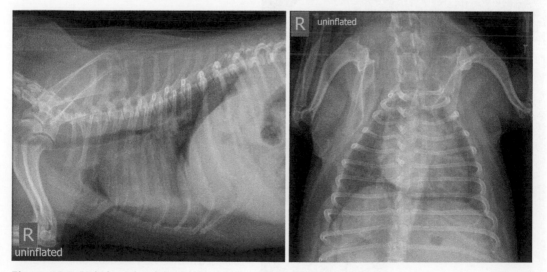

Figure 18.1 Right lateral and dorsoventral radiographs taken under light sedation.

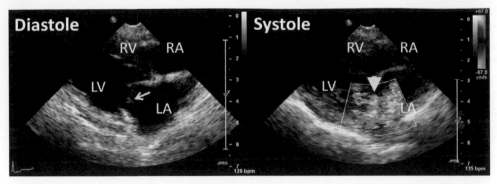

Figure 18.2 Right parasternal long axis 4 chamber echocardiographic views at the end diastole without colour-flow Doppler (left) and during systole with colour-flow Doppler (right). The anterior mitral valve leaflet can be seen to be prolapsing behind the posterior leaflet (arrow, left image) and a substantial volume of mitral regurgitation is seen during systole (arrowhead, right image).

Endoscopic examination (**Figure 18.3**) and fluoroscopy (**Figure 18.4**) demonstrated severe, grade IV/IV, tracheal collapse throughout most of the length of the trachea. Mild bronchial collapse concurrently was also seen though this was very much less marked. Some increase in the amount of intraluminal mucus and some mucopus was seen within the airways and bronchoalveolar lavage samples yielded turbid fluid, cytological assessment of which was consistent with marked inflammatory change comprising predominantly degenerate neutrophils. Many intracellular and extracellular rod-shaped bacteria could be seen but aerobic and anaerobic cultures failed to yield any growth from these samples.

A diagnosis of severe (grade IV/IV) tracheal collapse with secondary bacterial bronchopneumonia was made. Though the dog had myxomatous mitral valve disease (ACVIM classification B2 – structural remodelling without evidence of congestive heart failure), this was not felt to be contributory to the dog's clinical signs.

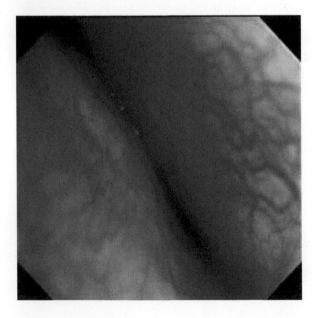

Figure 18.3 Endoscopic view of severely collapsed mid-cervical trachea. Complete obliteration of the lumen is seen.

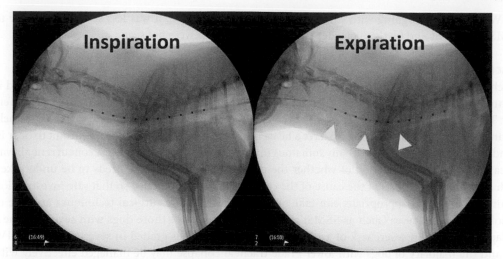

Figure 18.4 Lateral fluoroscopic images during inspiration and expiration showing marked generalised tracheal collapse (arrowheads). A marker catheter with 1 cm spaced radio-opaque markings is present within the oesophagus for procedural planning.

Treatment and outcome

Due to the severity of the collapse and the frequent episodes of dyspnoea requiring emergency treatment, a self-expanding metallic stent (SEMS) made of NiTiNOL (nickel-titanium) was placed after careful fluoroscopic measurements and planning for 'foreshortening' (these stents will reduce in length from their on-the-catheter size during deployment) (**Figure 18.5**). Concurrently the bacterial bronchopneumonitis was treated with a combination of enrofloxacin and metronidazole for a period of 4 weeks.

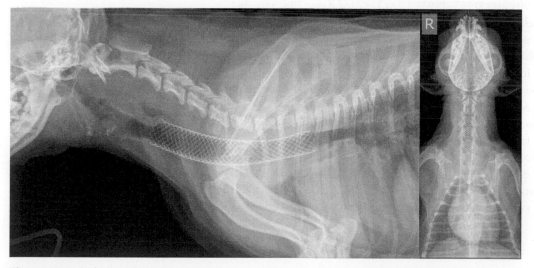

Figure 18.5 Right lateral and DV cervical/thoracic radiographs showing deployed SEMS in place. This radiograph was taken 1 week after placement and a degree of foreshortening of the stent has occurred from the original expanded length.

Whilst some coughing with excitement continued to be seen, it was less severe than prior to SEMS placement and further episodes of respiratory distress were not seen.

Discussion

Tracheal and bronchial collapse occurs due to malacia of the airway cartillagenous support and is common in some small breeds of dog such as the Yorkshire Terrier, Pomeranian and Maltese Terrier. These breeds also have a high prevalence of myxomatous mitral valve disease so it is extremely common for these coughing dogs to have a heart murmur at presentation. It is important to bear in mind that coughing in dogs with myxomatous mitral valve disease may suggest concurrent airway disease and critical evaluation of whether the patient is in heart failure needs to be undertaken both so that misdiagnosis of the cause of the cough is not made but also so that safe investigation of airway disease, if appropriate, can take place. Both traditional surgical techniques and use of endoluminal prostheses (such as SEMS) are valid treatments for those dogs with severe tracheal collapse resulting in severe risk of asphyxia. Tracheal collapse is graded in severity from I to IV/ IV, and the majority of dogs with lower grade tracheal collapse may be managed effectively with medical treatment such as judicious combinations of antitussive agents and anti-inflammatory doses of corticosteroids along with weight loss. These dogs are not, in the author's opinion, suitable for endoluminal prostheses and this treatment is reserved for those patients with life-threatening degrees of collapse where asphyxiation is a serious risk or where complete failure of concerted medical treatment has occurred. Surgical or endoluminal stenting will not resolve coughing and all such procedures are associated with some risk of complications, including some that may be catastrophic for the patient, and assessment should preferably be undertaken by an individual experienced in these methods of management.

Further reading

Beal, M.W. (2013) Tracheal stent placement for the emergency management of tracheal collapse in dogs. *Top Companion Anim Med* **28**, 106–111

Buback, J.L., Boothe, H.W. & Hobson, H.P. (1996) Surgical treatment of tracheal collapse in dogs: 90 cases (1983–1993). *J Am Vet Med Assoc* **208**, 380–384

Gellasch, K.L., Da Costa Gomez, T., McAnulty, J.F. & Bjorling, D.E. (2002) Use of intraluminal nitinol stents in the treatment of tracheal collapse in a dog. *J Am Vet Med Assoc* **221**, 1719–1723, 1714

Johnson, L.R. & Fales, W.H. (2001) Clinical and microbiologic findings in dogs with bronchoscopically diagnosed tracheal collapse: 37 cases (1990–1995). *J Am Vet Med Assoc* **219**, 1247–1250

Johnson, L.R. & McKiernan, B.C. (1995) Diagnosis and medical management of tracheal collapse. *Semin Vet Med Surg (Small Anim)* **10**, 101–108

Macready, D.M., Johnson, L.R. & Pollard, R.E. (2007) Fluoroscopic and radiographic evaluation of tracheal collapse in dogs: 62 cases (2001–2006). *J Am Vet Med Assoc* **230**, 1870–1876

Moritz, A., Schneider, M. & Bauer, N. (2004) Management of advanced tracheal collapse in dogs using intraluminal self-expanding biliary wallstents. *J Vet Intern Med* **18**, 31–42

Sura, P.A. & Krahwinkel, D.J. (2008) Self-expanding nitinol stents for the treatment of tracheal collapse in dogs: 12 cases (2001–2004). *J Am Vet Med Assoc* **232**, 228–236

Clinical presentation

A 9 year-old male-neutered Cocker Spaniel weighing 18 kg is presented with a 2 week history of malaise, gradually reducing appetite, weight loss and increased respiratory rate. The dog is fully vaccinated, is fed a commercial complete dog food and has never travelled outside the United Kingdom. It is treated for ecto-/endoparasites every 4 months with imidacloprid/moxidectin and has no previous medical problems or known exposure to toxins.

Physical examination demonstrates a quiet and anxious dog in slim body condition. Respiratory rate is 44/min with a rapid restrictive (choppy) respiratory pattern and an orthopnoeic stance. Heart rate is 124/min and peripheral pulse quality is normal. Mucous membrane colour, hydration and rectal temperature are normal and abdominal palpation is unremarkable. On auscultation of the thorax the heart sounds are muffled bilaterally and no normal bronchovesicular sounds can be heard in the ventral third of the thorax, though are heard normally dorsal to this. Thoracic percussion is noticeably dull over the ventral third of the thorax.

Thoracic radiographs were taken, as shown in **Figure 19.1**.

Questions

1. Describe the radiographic findings (Figure 19.1). What are the differential diagnoses for this?
2. How should this patient be initially managed and what should be done to differentiate between these differential diagnoses?
3. A photomicrograph of some of the pleural space content is shown in Figure 19.2. Describe the findings and state which of the differential diagnoses this supports.
4. How should this patient be definitively managed?

Answers

1. **Describe the radiographic findings. What are the differential diagnoses for this?**

On both lateral radiographs the dorsocaudal aerated lung tissue is retracted from the dorsal costophrenic angle whilst retaining a triangular shape. A soft tissue/fluid radio-opacity is seen dorsal and caudal to the retracted lung lobes. Similar retraction of the cranioventral portions of aerated lung tissue are seen with a rounded appearance (sometimes referred to as 'scalloping') of the lung seen cranially on the right lateral view and overlying the cardiac silhouette on the left lateral view; a widened interlobar fissure line is also seen dorsal to the heart base on the left lateral view. The apex of the cardiac silhouette is effaced by a similar soft tissue/fluid opacity and this extends over the ventral one-third or so of the thorax, obscuring the line of the diaphragm ventrally.

On the dorsoventral view, all lung lobes are seen to be retracted from normal contact with the thoracic wall and a soft tissue/fluid opacity is seen to occupy this widened pleural space and between lung lobes, particularly the right cranial and right middle lobe, and right caudal and right middle lobe. The cardiac silhouette and diaphragmatic line cannot be clearly determined on the DV view.

These findings are consistent with a pleural effusion.

Canine Internal Medicine: What's Your Diagnosis? First Edition. Jon Wray.
© 2018 John Wiley & Sons Ltd. Published 2018 by John Wiley & Sons Ltd.

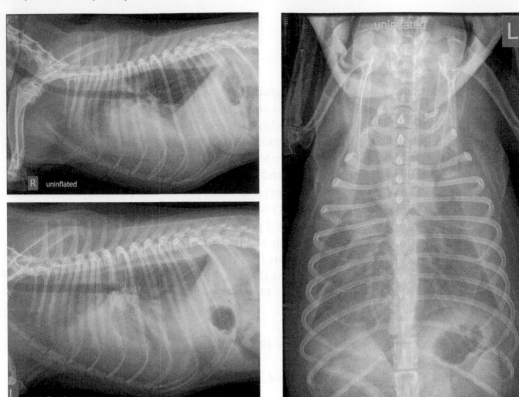

Figure 19.1 Right and left laterally recumbent and dorsoventral views of the thorax of the patient upon admission.

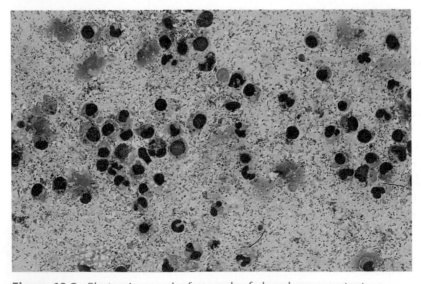

Figure 19.2 Photomicrograph of a sample of pleural space content (Wright-Giemsa ×50).

Causes of pleural effusion may include:

- Blood
- Chyle
- Pure transudate
- Modified transudate
- Exudate
  - Non-septic
  - Septic

Pleural effusion may also be neoplastic (either due to diffuse infiltrative disease or secondary to focal/massive or nodular neoplasia) and occur secondary to diaphragmatic rupture; the nature of the fluid in both of these may be alternatively a modified transudate or non-septic exudate dependent on duration and cellular/protein content.

2. How should this patient be initially managed and what should be done to differentiate between these differential diagnoses?

The patient is dyspnoeic and provision of oxygen therapy and relief of the pleural effusion with subsequent re-expansion of collapsed lobar tissue is indicated. A variety of methods of oxygen supplementation are available including administration of 'flow-by' oxygen, use of nasal oxygen prongs or a nasal cannula, an oxygen cage and modification of 'buster collars' to achieve an oxygen-rich environment local to the patient's face. All have pros and cons, but the most commonsense approach is to use the method that is best tolerated by the individual patient (which will usually depend on the degree of dyspnoea) and the necessity for veterinary access for any physical interventions. In severely dyspnoeic animals it may be safer and more expedient to induce anaesthesia as rapidly and safely as possible and to intubate and ventilate the patient.

Thoracocentesis may be performed with goals of diagnosis (only a small amount of pleural fluid required), performing therapeutic evacuation of as much pleural fluid as possible, or both; in the setting of dyspnoea caused by pleural fluid, therapeutic evacuation is required.

Whilst needle drainage (with, for example, a butterfly cannula and extension tube) may be sufficient for this in cats and very small dogs, this is unacceptably time-consuming in a middle-sized dyspnoeic dog. Placement of thoracostomy tubes and drainage is more appropriate and whilst smaller-bore tubes may be placed for rapid evacuation of large amounts of pleural fluid (either standard tubes with an internal trocar or 'Seldinger method' over-the-wire tubes) it is advantageous to place large-bore thoracostomy tubes in purulent effusions. Not only will this allow rapid evacuation of fluid that may be rather viscous and tenacious (in the case of pyothorax versus, for instance, chylous effusion) but they are more secure to be left secured *in situ* for ongoing drainage and possibly pleural lavage. Proponents of smaller (e.g. Seldinger-type) tubes cite potential reduction in trauma during placement but no clinical studies evaluating the optimal tube type have been performed in veterinary medicine.

Placement of thoracostomy tubes may be unilateral or bilateral depending on the distribution of fluid present. The author prefers to perform this under general anaesthesia both for optimal provision of oxygen and for patient comfort, but it may also be performed in sedated patients using an intercostal nerve block.

Placement of thoracostomy tubes

The sites for thoracostomy tube placement are shown in **Figures 19.3** and **19.4**. The level of placement within the intercostal space depends on whether fluid (ventral placement position) or air (dorsal placement position) is present. The operator should aim to penetrate the intercostal space cranial to a rib to avoid the caudal neurovascular bundle and to ensure that a subcutaneous 'tunnel' of approximately 2 intercostal spaces in length is achieved between the skin exit of the tube and the point of pleural space penetration to act as a protection against air ingress (**Figure 19.5**).

To achieve this a tunnel may be 'dissected' by either a rapid forward subcutaneous 'drilling' motion of a thoracostomy tube with a sharp trocar in place, cranial to the site of skin incision to the point where intercostal penetration is planned, or alternatively to perform the same action with curved haemostats, then to grasp the tube tip (without the trocar in place) with the same curved haemostats and use them to push through the intercostal tissues. The author feels that both these methods are unnecessarily time-consuming and feels a better alternative is for an assistant to firmly grasp a dorsal-to-ventral fold of skin and subcutis of the thoracic wall just caudal to the scapular and to maintain strong cranial traction on this whilst a tube is placed; utilising the normal elasticity of these tissues, upon release after placement of the tube, provided that firm traction has been applied, the tissues will slide caudally to create a lengthy subcutaneous tunnel without the need for time-consuming and locally traumatic dissection.

When placing a thoracostomy tube with a trocar in place, it is important to place this through the intercostal tissues with a controlled thrust, maintaining a good grip with one hand a short distance from the sharp tip to avoid overpenetration. The practice of striking the outer 'pommel' of a trocar with the heel of one's hand in order to penetrate the intercostal space is strongly discouraged as it leaves little control over accidental overpenetration. The author has seen several catastrophic injuries caused by such placement behaviour and considers this practice below the standard of care. The tube is clamped and a connector allowing drainage and, if desired, infusion of sterile lavage solution is applied and the tube connected to the thoracic wall via a 'finger trap'/'Roman sandal' suture. Fluid is evacuated

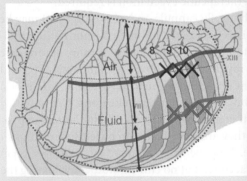 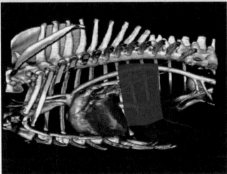

Figure 19.3 (left) Correct sites for thoracostomy tube placement depending on whether air or fluid is present in the pleural space. The solid blue and green lines represent the tube. (right) 3D computed tomography rendering showing cutaway thoracic wall and placement site (pink block) in relation to the diaphragm and cardiovascular structures.

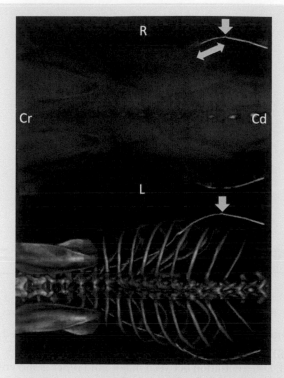

Figure 19.4 Volume-rendered CT images of a dog with bilateral thoracostomy tubes. The upper image shows the costal and intercostal musculature, the lower shows thoracic skeletal structures only. The site of skin entry can be seen as a slight 'wrinkle' in the tube (yellow arrow) and the length of the subcutaneous tunnel before the tube penetrates intercostally is shown by the double-headed green arrow.

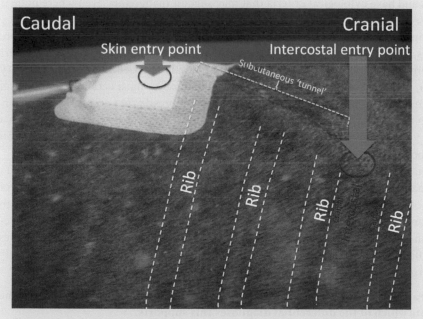

Figure 19.5 Correct entry point just cranial to a rib, and demonstration of the subcutaneous 'tunnel' of adequate length.

from the pleural space as soon as the tube is secured. The tube(s) is/are bandaged securely in place (**Figure 19.6**).

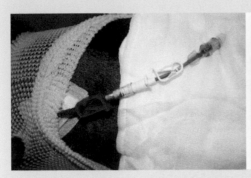 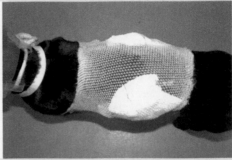

Figure 19.6 (left) Thoracostomy tube (head towards left) secured in place with a finger-trap suture, red C-clamp in place and a 'moduflo' connecter. (right) Bilateral tubes secured to the thorax in a dog.

Fluid analysis helps differentiate the major differential diagnoses. Fluid should be analysed for protein content, cell content and cytology and should be cultured for aerobic and anaerobic bacteria where a septic exudate is diagnosed. Differentiation between major fluid types is shown in **Table 19.1**. It should be noted that reactive mesothelial cells are commonly determined in pleural effusions and have cytological criteria that may suggest malignancy even where none is present.

Additional clinicopathological findings may suggest one pleural fluid aetiology to be more likely than others, for instance the presence of evidence of heart disease involving the right heart or serum biochemical evaluation demonstrating severe hypoalbuminaemia. An inflammatory leukogram, fever, malaise, coughing and dyspnoea are common to most aetiologies of pleural effusion and do not particularly help in differentiation. Some breed types and historical information may help marshal differential diagnoses. For example, hunting/sporting breeds with a preceding history of cough may be more likely to have pyothorax secondary to migrating an inhaled foreign body.

Diagnostic imaging with radiography, thoracic ultrasound or by computed tomography (CT) is useful in evaluating both the extent and distribution of fluid, the presence of obvious foci of potential origin of infection (such as a lung lobar abscess, lobar bronchopneumonia or foreign body) and by monitoring sequelae such as lung cortication. CT is particularly useful in this respect though it should be borne in mind that identification of migrating inhaled foreign bodies is notoriously difficult and objective evidence for these may be lacking, even when subsequently found during surgical exploration.

3. **A photomicrograph of some of the pleural space content is shown (Figure 19.2). Describe the findings and state which of the differential diagnoses this supports.**

The predominant cell type is neutrophils and these demonstrate both hypersegmentation and hyposegmentation, karyolysis, foamy basophilia and nuclear vacuolation. Plentiful macrophages are also seen. There are very many bacteria seen in the background and within cells and these are a mixture of both longer and shorter rod-morphology organisms, suggesting a mixed infection.

Table 19.1 Differentiation between common fluid aetiologies

	Pure transudate	Modified transudate	Exudate	Other
Pathogenesis	Extravasation of low-protein fluid due to decreased vascular colloid oncotic pressure (usually in hypoalbuminaemic states). Occasionally pure transudates may occur in early stages of right-sided congestive heart failure, though modified transudate is more common *Note: it is rare for this to occur in the pleural space in isolation without ascites also being present*	Extravasation of fluid principally from increased hydrostatic pressure in vessels due to right-sided congestive heart failure or tamponade However, modified transudates may also be neoplastic in origin or represent local fluid production from lung lobe torsion or diaphragmatic rupture	The most common cause is inflammation which may be septic or non-septic. The most common cause of septic effusion is pyothorax Non-septic exudates may also be neoplastic in origin, or represent local fluid production from lung lobe torsion or diaphragmatic rupture	Other considerations are: • Chyle • Blood Specific analysis of fluid including cytology, triglyceride content compared with serum (chyle) Chyle is typically rich in small lymphocytes and has a triglyceride content greater than that of plasma; over time chylous effusion becomes steadily more neutrophil-rich. Chylous effusions may be classified as modified transudates or exudates depending on cellularity
Fluid protein	<20 g/l	20–50 g/l	>30g/l	
Fluid nucleated cell count	<1500/ml	<5000/ml	>5000/ml	
Nucleated cell type	Variable but low in number	Mostly neutrophils, macrophages and reactive mesothelial cells	Neutrophils and macrophages. Degenerative neutrophils and possible intracellular bacteria are hallmarks of septic exudates	
Common aetiologies	Severe hypoalbuminaemia	Commonly right-sided congestive heart failure and cardiac tamponade	Pyothorax	

These findings are supportive of a diagnosis of **pyothorax** (also known as empyema).

4. **How should this patient be definitively managed?**

   Considering the frequency with which pyothorax is diagnosed in dogs, there is surprisingly little consensus on the optimum way to manage it and a lack of good evidence-base upon which to rest treatment recommendations. The author would recommend caution and intellectual flexibility in assessing any firm dogmatic pronouncements as to the 'best' way to treat pyothorax.

   Most animals may be successfully managed by a combination of
   • Systemic antibacterial therapy.
   • Draining voluminous septic effusions.

- Consideration of surgical exploration for extirpation of foci of originating infection *which should be kept 'under review'.*
- Additional supportive therapy on a case-by-case basis.

Systemic antimicrobial therapy

A wide variety of bacterial isolates have been reported from naturally occurring cases of canine pyothorax with high prevalence of polymicrobial infections and anaerobic isolates. It is not infrequent for no organisms to be cultured despite cytological evidence of bacterial infection. Organisms commonly originate from the oral cavity and upper GI tract and the upper respiratory tract. Common aerobic isolates include *E.coli, Streptococcus* spp., *Staphylococcus* spp., *Pasteurella* spp., *Actinomyces* spp. *and Nocardia* spp. and anaerobic isolates *Bacteroides* spp., *Peptostreptococcus* spp., *Fusobacterium* spp., and *Prevotella* app.

Empirical antimicrobial choices

Empirical antimicrobial therapy in dogs should include medications with activity against gram positive aerobes, gram negative aerobes of enteric origin and obligate anaerobes. A combination of a beta-lactamase resistant aminopenicillin and a fluoroquinolone may satisfy these requirements, but choice should also be modified as culture and sensitivity results become available. There is often a tendency to adopt an excessive 'polypharmacy' approach to antibiotic therapy in pyothorax, which is both unnecessary and usually borne from misunderstanding of antimicrobial pharmacology.

The optimum route of administration is unclear with many clinicians favouring the intravenous route, at least initially, though this may not be clearly advantageous over the oral route except in patients that are dehydrated or vomiting. Intravenous administration of antimicrobials may be continued until objective improvements in sepsis are seen, patients are well hydrated and eating and reduction in fluid removed from thoracostomy tubes is seen. Administration of antimicrobials into the pleural space is not recommended.

The optimum duration of antimicrobial therapy is unknown with various recommendations of 4–6 weeks and for 2 weeks beyond resolution of radiographic evidence of pleural effusion.

Drainage of pleural effusions

Whilst it is generally accepted that voluminous septic pleural effusions should be evacuated, both to relieve dyspnoea and lung collapse and to reduce the local bacterial load, the necessity of ongoing drainage is unknown. Indeed, there is a report of one case series of 15 canine patients with pyothorax with successful outcome and prolonged follow-up in which a single drainage episode was performed (Johnson and Martin 2007). However, it is perhaps more common clinical practice to perform drainage via indwelling thoracostomy tubes until the volume and cellularity of septic pleural exudation reduces.

The frequency of drainage of effusion depends somewhat on the rate of accumulation of pleural space contents and the volume previously drained. It should be remembered that pleural irritation from the presence of tubes will, in itself, produce approximately 2 ml/kg/24 h of fluid. We will usually perform drainage in our hospital every 4 hours initially, then with reducing frequency as dictated by the amount of fluid being produced and the animal's respiratory rate and effort.

The authors of some studies recommend pleural lavage, usually with sterile warm physiologic saline at a dose of 10–20 ml/kg divided between each tube per lavage, as an adjunct to drainage, and some recommend the addition of anticoagulants such as heparin or fibrinolytics such as tissue plasminogen activator (TPA). Again the optimal fluid type and the usefulness of any additives has not been evaluated in veterinary medicine and it should be considered that introduction of fluid into the pleural space is not entirely benign, and the attendant reduction in aerated lung volume, degree of pleural contact and possible risk of bacterial introduction may all be counterproductive. The author's approach is to consider lavage on a case-by-case basis, performing it when pleural exudate is particularly tenacious, where 'pocketing' of fluid is occurring and where adequate drainage does not appear to be achieved despite optimal tube position, but not performing it when fluid is evacuated with ease. Generally thoracostomy tubes are removed when they are no longer productive (through lack of fluid or because of mechanical dysfunction of the tube) or where fluid removal is <2 ml/kg/24 h (i.e. indistinguishable from fluid provoked by the presence of tubes within the pleural space). It may be reasonable to leave tubes in situ for 24 hours without drainage and monitor by radiography, ultrasound or subsequent fluid drainage to discover whether ongoing mechanical drainage is necessary.

When to consider surgery in pyothorax

The veterinary literature contains both recommendations for both routine surgical intervention and for good success rates with medical therapy alone, and such recommendations are probably heavily influenced by the bias of report authors (surgical versus medical specialists). Indications for surgery include removal of intrathoracic foreign bodies, resection of non-foreign body septic foci (such as pulmonary abscesses), to perform surgical drainage and removal of locally infected tissues where tube drainage has been ineffective and to perform decortication of fibrous plaques of material that may limit lung expansion.

A decision to perform surgery may be informed by diagnostic imaging findings, particularly the presence of an obviously abnormal focus such as a pulmonary abscess, based on a high degree of suspicion of a migrating foreign body (based on, for instance, prior history of coughing in a hunting/sporting breed, development of flank swellings consistent with a migrating foreign body abscess or diagnostic imaging findings, particularly with computed tomography) or where medical therapy combined with tube drainage is not eliciting adequate improvement after 3–7 days. It has often been cited that isolation of *Actinomyces* spp. is associated with the presence of a migrating foreign body, though this oropharyngeal commensal has been isolated from cases where no foreign body is found, where medical treatment alone has been successful and a critical review of the veterinary literature suggests that other organisms, particularly *Staphylococcus* spp., are just as likely to be associated with migrating foreign bodies, but do not receive such dogmatic recommendations.

Surgery is associated with increased expense, risk of patient morbidity, lengthened hospitalisation and wound complications.

It is encouraged not to consider pyothorax a 'surgical' or a 'medical' condition, but to consider the need for surgical intervention in each case based on its own merits and always to consider (and repeatedly discuss with owners) the need for surgery to be kept constantly 'under review' during the initial phases of treatment.

Additional supportive care

- Both the presence of pleural space infection and of indwelling thoracostomy tubes are painful and systemic analgesia, usually with parenteral opioid analgesia, is recommended. Delivery of intrapleural analgesia via bupivacaine administered via thoracostomy tubes may be performed, but absorption and local effects in the presence of pleural fluid may be variable.
- Careful attention to maintaining sterility, security and lack of patient interference with thoracostomy tubes is essential and at least twice daily inspection of entry sites is recommended.
- Patients with pyothorax may be hypo- or anorexic and may exude prodigious amounts of protein-rich fluid. A pre-emptive nutritional support plan is often needed and naso-oesophageal, oesophageal and gastric feeding tubes often aid in nutritional support of such patients.
- Dehydration and systemic electrolyte disturbances, particularly hypokalaemia, may develop due to a combination of anorexia and repetitive fluid drainage and should be corrected.

Outcome

In this patient, despite the convincing cytological evidence of pyothorax, no bacterial growth was obtained on cultures of pleural fluid by aerobic and anaerobic culture. Bilateral thoracostomy tubes were placed and drained initially every 4 hours, decreasing to every 8 hours after 72 hours. Empirical antibiotic therapy in the form of clavulanate-amoxycillin at a dose of 20 mg/kg p/o BID and enrofloxacin 5 mg/kg p/o SID. Drainage appeared to result in adequate removal of purulent fluid bilaterally and pleural lavage was not performed in this patient. The volume of fluid produced declined rapidly over a six-day period and at this time radiographs were repeated and demonstrated no regions of fluid accumulation and that normal bilateral lung aeration was present. The tubes were left in situ, clamped and without drainage for 24 hours and radiographs repeated. Since no fluid was seen to be r-accumulating the thoracostomy tubes were then removed.

Antimicrobial therapy was continued for 8 weeks in total. Interim thoracic radiographs were repeated 1 week after removal of the thoracostomy tubes and again 3 weeks after discontinuation of antimicrobial therapy. No reaccumulation of pleural fluid was noted in either set of radiographs.

Discussion

The aetiology of pyothorax in dogs is often unknown and a specific route of pleural infection or underlying cause is reported in only 2–33% of dogs. Foreign body (usually grass awn) migration, parapneumonic spread from infected foci within lung tissue (such as ruptured pulmonary abscess, extension of lobar bronchopneumonia), haematogenous spread, oesophageal perforation and introduction during surgical or thoracocentesis procedures are all reported as routes of pleural infection. Despite the frequency with which foreign body migration is suspected, it is surprisingly uncommon that foreign material is positively identified upon surgical exploration of persistent pyothorax. This may be due to foreign material not being present or that degradation of plant material has occurred prior to surgery.

Increasingly computed tomography is utilised in veterinary practice to evaluate dogs with pyothorax with the advantage over radiography that small amounts of fluid can be detected with greater sensitivity and that cross-sectional imaging allows evaluation of all thoracic structures, without the effects of radiographic superimposition. Our experience with CT is that it allows a greater sensitivity for detection of focal lesions such as abscessation and extending lobar pneumonia and in determining 'patterns' of tracking foreign bodies. However, there are some foreign bodies that are identified at surgery where CT has not been diagnostic of them and it is suspected that CT, when performed early in the course of pyothorax, yields results that bias towards surgical exploration.

Prognosis appears to be generally good. An overall survival rate in dogs has been reported as 83% (range 29–100%), with a recurrence rate of 0–14%. It has been suggested that the prognosis for dogs with recurrent disease is poor.

Such variable treatment recommendations, approaches to thoracic drainage and reported influences on survival have been reported in the veterinary literature that unifying treatment recommendations supported by a good evidence base do not exist. Many differing means of treatment are successful and it is important to maintain the clinical flexibility to keep all treatment options under review on a case-by-case basis.

Reference

Johnson, M.S. & Martin, M.W. (2007) Successful medical treatment of 15 dogs with pyothorax. *J Small Anim Pract* **48**, 12–16

Further reading

Demetriou, J.L., Foale, R.D., Ladlow, J. et al. (2002) Canine and feline pyothorax: a retrospective study of 50 cases in the UK and Ireland. *J Small* Anim *Pract* **43**, 388–394

Boothe, H.W., Howe, L.M., Boothe, D.M. et al. (2010) Evaluation of outcomes in dogs treated for pyothorax: 46 cases (1983–2001). *J Am Vet Med Assoc* **236**, 657–663

Lee, K.C. (2014) Surgical or medical management of pyothorax in dogs? *Vet Record* **174**, 605–606

MacPhail, C.M. (2007) Medical and surgical management of pyothorax. *Vet Clin North Am Small Anim Pract* **37**, 975–988, vii

Rooney, M.B. & Monnet, E. (2002) Medical and surgical treatment of pyothorax in dogs: 26 cases (1991–2001). *J Am Vet Med Assoc* **221**, 86–92

Stillion, J.R. & Letendre, J.A. (2015) A clinical review of the pathophysiology, diagnosis, and treatment of pyothorax in dogs and cats. *J Vet Emergency Crit Care* **25**, 113–129

Walker, A.L., Jang, S.S. & Hirsh, D.C. (2000) Bacteria associated with pyothorax of dogs and cats: 98 cases (1989–1998). Journal of the American Veterinary Medical Association **216**, 359–363

Ear, Nose and Throat

Clinical Informatics... What's Your Diagnosis? First Edition. Jon Wee...

© 2018 John Wiley & Sons Ltd. Published 2018 by John Wiley & Sons Ltd.

Clinical presentation

A 10 year-old male-neutered Labrador Retriever (**Figure 20.1**) is referred for investigation of suspected congestive heart failure. The owner presented the dog to her primary veterinary surgeon due to a complaint of progressive exercise intolerance during the period from May to July (United Kingdom early summer), and continued panting with exertion and on hot days but not when the dog is in the house. An occasional 'reaching' cough has also been reported. The primary veterinary surgeon has auscultated a heart murmur, which is described as grade II/VI systolic and left apical in nature, but has been noted previously for 2 years. The heart rate on this examination is recorded as 116/minute and the rhythm as a sinus arrhythmia. On clinical examination the primary veterinary surgeon felt that the dog's oral mucus membranes were slightly cyanosed. Oral furosemide was prescribed at a dose of 1 mg/kg p/o BID but the owners have noticed no improvement in the panting or exercise tolerance.

The owner reports that the previous summer, she had also been concerned about the dog's exercise tolerance and felt that he panted excessively then, but that signs had resolved in the autumn.

When examined, in addition to similar findings to the primary veterinary surgeons, prolonged panting and some stridor is noted. When the dog is not panting the respiratory rate is 16/min and an exaggerated inspiratory phase to respiration is seen with a deep-and-slow respiratory pattern.

Questions

1. From the history and both sets of physical examination findings is heart failure likely to be present in this dog?
2. What is cyanosis and what is its significance?
3. What additional questions would it be helpful to ask the owner of this dog?
4. How should this patient be evaluated?

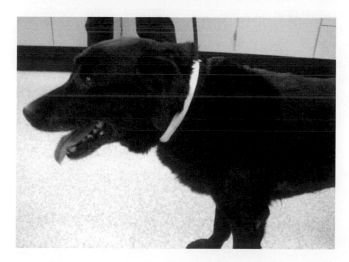

Figure 20.1 The patient at presentation.

Canine Internal Medicine: What's Your Diagnosis? First Edition. Jon Wray.
© 2018 John Wiley & Sons Ltd. Published 2018 by John Wiley & Sons Ltd.

Answers

1. **From the history and both sets of physical examination findings is heart failure likely to be present in this dog?**

   The primary presenting sign of exercise intolerance may have many aetiologies, though cardiac and respiratory causes tend to predominate. The presence of exercise intolerance, cough and heart murmur often provokes the assumption that congestive heart failure is present, and in many situations this might be true, but in this case there are three diagnostic clues that suggest that the dog may have a respiratory cause of the clinical signs rather than cardiac. It should be remembered that heart murmurs, especially those left apical systolic murmurs due to mitral insufficiency, are very common in dogs, and that the majority of patients with valvular heart disease will not develop congestive heart failure during their lifetime.

   The owner reports that panting occurs with exertion and on warm days but not during normal household activity. Congestive heart failure, once developed, does not tend to come and go with exertion and exercise-induced change in respiratory pattern tends to be a feature of primary respiratory tract disorders. The owner reports that similar changes were seen in the summer months the previous year, then abated during the cooler part of the year. Again, heat intolerance and a slowly progressive respiratory compromise is a typical finding in obstructive forms of airway disease rather than cardiac disease.

Sinus arrhythmia

The physical examination finding of sinus arrhythmia is a big diagnostic clue. Sinus arrhythmia describes a 'regularly irregular' rhythm in which the heart rate will accelerate during inspiration and decelerate during expiration. Only by (i) listening for a sufficient length of time and (ii) by getting into the habit of always watching the patient's respiratory pattern during auscultation will clinicians appreciate the regular cycle of the change in frequency of the heart rate and appreciate this to be linked to respiration. A sinus arrhythmia is mediated by alteration in vagal tone, increase in vagal tone occurring in expiration and causing slowing of the sinus rate and a decrease in vagal tone with associated speeding up of the sinus rate during inspiration. In congestive heart failure, sympathetic stimulation and downregulation of parasympathetic stimulation occurs and sinus arrhythmia is lost. Furthermore, vagal tone is increased in many respiratory disorders, especially those which are obstructive in nature so the presence of a sinus arrhythmia is a hugely important diagnostic clue that this patient is not in heart failure.

Cyanosis is also more commonly detected in respiratory disease than cardiac disease (see below).

Respiratory pattern and noise

The respiratory patterns are described in **Case 17** (**Table 17.2**); in this patient the slow-and-forceful breathing pattern with exaggerated inspiratory phase characterises obstructive (inspiratory) dyspnoea.

'Stridor' describes a spontaneously audible noise with a fixed, high-pitched timbre (from Latin: *stridere*, to screech) and is generally caused by fixed obstruction to airflow within the upper respiratory tract. 'Stertor' is a lower pitched, snoring or sonorous sound (from Latin: *stertere*, to snore) with an oscillating element to it. Typically it arises from more mobile obstructions within the respiratory tract especially arising from the nasopharynx and soft palate and fluid accumulations. Note that these terms describe sounds and are not synonymous with an anatomical location.

This dog has both signs of stridor and an inspiratory obstructive breathing pattern, suggesting a somewhat fixed obstructive lesion of the upper airways. The history of heat and exercise intolerance and preservation of sinus arrhythmia would also support this.

2. What is cyanosis and what is its significance?

Cyanosis is a blueish discolouration of the mucous membranes caused by an increase in the proportion of deoxyhaemoglobin in erythrocytes. Normal haemoglobin content of canine blood is 12–18 g/dl, of which the majority is oxyhaemoglobin. Once levels of deoxyhaemoglobin exceed 3-5 g/dl, cyanosis is detected.

Cyanosis is indicative of hypoxia and may be described as shown in **Table 20.1**.

Cyanosis is more commonly caused by respiratory than cardiac disease

Cyanosis is always indicative of severe hypoxia. As a rule of thumb respiratory causes are very much more common than cardiac causes with the exceptions of patients presenting in respiratory distress due to fulminant and effusive pulmonary oedema. Intracardiac right-to-left shunting defects (usually Tetralogy of Fallot, reversed PDA or Eisenmenger's physiology) are relatively rare.

Principle causes of respiratory hypoxia are:

- Decreased inspired oxygen content
- Alveolar hypoventilation
- Ventilation-perfusion mismatch
- Diffusion impairment
- Respiratory shunt, usually due to pulmonary thromboembolism

Table 20.1 Types of cyanosis

'Peripheral' or 'regional' cyanosis	Affects just one area, for instance due to local vascular compromise, causing regional lack of arterial perfusion
'Central' cyanosis	Where generalised hypoxia exists; this may be due to
	• Respiratory disorders and disorders of gas exchange (which are common)
	• Right to left intracardiac shunting defects (which are rare)
	• Haemoglobinopathies (which are very rare)
'Differential' cyanosis	Where cyanosis exists only in those caudal tissues supplied by branches of the descending aorta but not cranial structures
	• Caused by reversed PDA (since the PDA joins the aorta distal to the brachicephalic trunk and left subclavian artery)

3. **What additional questions would it be useful to ask the owners of this dog?**

The history and physical examination findings suggest upper airway obstruction and the most common cause of this in an older medium-sized breed would be laryngeal paralysis. It is helpful to ask whether dysphonia has been noted by assessing the quality of the patient's bark. Patients with laryngeal paralysis are at risk of developing aspiration pneumonitis due to a failure of ability to guard the *rima glottidis* during swallowing and owners should be questioned about coughing/spluttering occurring during eating or drinking, episodes of dyspnoea, unexplained febrile illnesses and previous 'chest infections' (though strictly speaking aspiration pneumonitis is not an infection but a chemical/mechanical pneumonia, which may or may not become secondarily complicated by bacterial pneumonia; see **Case 16**). Laryngeal paralysis may also develop as part of a polyneuropathy or polymyopathy and as a neuropathy secondary to hypothyroidism. A 'verbal neurological assessment' should always be part of clinical history taking and a history of unexplained weight gain and lethargy despite normal appetite and dermatological changes consistent with hypothyroidism should also be discussed.

4. **How should this dog be investigated?**

Although routine laboratory testing is seldom of much help in the majority of patients with primary respiratory disease, the presence of polycythaemia as an appropriate response to prolonged hypoxia and the presence of leukocytosis consistent with an inflammatory response due to aspiration pneumonitis may be helpful in assessing the severity of the primary problem and potential secondary complications. Other than in determining the presence of hyperlipidaemia in many hypothyroid dogs, serum biochemistry is usually unhelpful. Arterial blood gas analysis could be undertaken to quantify the severity of arterial hypoxaemia, though since the patient has been visibly cyanosed and has evidence of respiratory compromise, it is redundant to differentiate between peripheral and central cyanosis and only the degree of hypoxaemia, not its presence or absence, would be answered by arterial blood gas analysis. The patient has a heart murmur that is most likely due to mitral valvular insufficiency, but history and physical examination findings have already precluded heart failure being present. Echocardiography could be undertaken but is not necessary either to determine the diagnosis (since this is respiratory in nature) or manage this patient. Were physical examination findings such as poor peripheral pulse quality or frequent premature contractions to be detected, an argument could be made that the heart murmur may represent mitral insufficiency secondary to dilated cardiomyopathy, but in this patient the murmur has been present unchanged for two years and it is unlikely that clinical dilated cardiomyopathy has been present for this long.

The most helpful forms of investigation in this patient would be:

- Radiography of the thorax and the upper respiratory tract to
  - Evaluate cardiac size.
  - Evaluate for presence of concurrent neurological disease such as megaoesophagus.
  - Evaluate for presence of evidence of aspiration pneumonitis.
  - Evaluate for presence of intrathoracic pathology, especially neoplastic lesions, which might compress/invade the recurrent laryngeal nerve (see **Figure 20.2**).
  - Evaluate the gas lucencies of the nasopharynx, oropharynx, larynx and trachea. Note that strict attention to positioning and performance of this with the patient extubated but carefully monitored is essential for correct interpretation.

(For the principle clinical suspicion in this patient of laryngeal paralysis, no pathognomonic radiographic signs are usually seen.)

- Serological assessment of thyroid function (see **Case 5**).

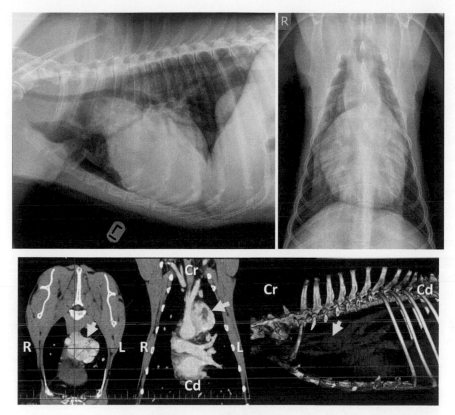

Figure 20.2 Left lateral and DV thoracic radiographs of a (different) 11 year old dog with bilateral laryngeal paralysis (top). Note that there are diffuse alveolar-interstitial infiltrates affecting portions of all of the lung lobes on the right side with a ventral distribution suggestive of aspiration pneumonitis. Additionally on the DV view the cranial mediastinum is focally widened cranial to the cardiac silhouette and this corresponds on the lateral view with an area of increased radio-opacity at the cranial heart base, causing focal elevation of the trachea adjacent to intercostal spaces 2–4. A CT scan (bottom, from left to right: transverse, dorsal and 3D volume rendered images) subsequently confirmed the presence of a large lobulated mediastinal mass (yellow arrowheads) which was impinging on the recurrent laryngeal nerves. Thoracic radiography should not be omitted in the evaluation of laryngeal paralysis in dogs.

- Examination of the upper airways, beginning with an assessment of laryngeal function by direct visualisation under a light plane of anaesthesia or by ultrasound.

Evaluation for laryngeal paralysis

Laryngeal paralysis is best evaluated by inducing a very light plane of anaesthesia (light enough that swallowing can still occur) and directly visualising laryngeal motion. Note that these patients are often hypoxic and some patients with laryngeal paralysis present in respiratory distress (**Figures 20.3** and **20.4**). It is a very good idea to plan ongoing patient management before performing evaluation and in particular to consider whether the expertise exists to surgically manage laryngeal paralysis should it be detected under the same anaesthetic. There are some important rules of thumb when evaluating laryngeal function if misdiagnosis is not to be risked:

- Always be patient in achieving a light plane of anaesthesia in order to evaluate the larynx – loss of ability to swallow indicates too deep a plane of anaesthesia to assess laryngeal function and a false positive diagnosis of laryngeal paralysis becomes likely.
- Patients should always be evaluated in sternal recumbency, *never* in lateral recumbency, since differences in symmetry of movement are being examined for and gravitational effects severely compromise this in laterally recumbent patients.
- Always have a good light source and ability to depress the caudal tongue such as a broad-bladed laryngoscope.
- Always evaluate laryngeal motion in the context of the respiratory phase and it is necessary to have an assistant say out loud what the respiratory phase is. Frequently patients with bilateral laryngeal paralysis show paradoxical movement of the larynx whereby during inspiration the arytenoids are drawn medially by the Venturi effect (sic) and blown laterally during expiration. If the larynx is simply examined without context of the respiratory phase, bilateral motion will be diagnosed and laryngeal paralysis falsely excluded. This is a very common reason for misdiagnosis, in the author's experience.

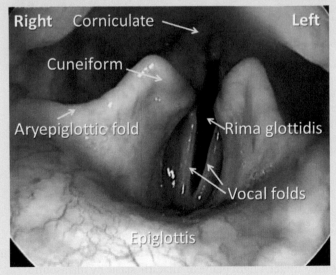

Figure 20.3 Magnified endoscopic view of the larynx of a dog with bilateral laryngeal paralysis showing the relevant anatomical structures. This image is taken during inspiration when the rima glottides should be wide open and the arytenoids abducted. Note the erythema and oedema along the medial margin of the corniculate processes of the arytenoids, which is a common finding. Although endoscopy allows for magnification it is unnecessary to use it to evaluate the larynx and a simple laryngoscope with a good light source is sufficient; endoscopy is merely reproduced here to demonstrate anatomy. In experienced hands the laryngeal function can also be assessed by diagnostic ultrasound in the conscious or sedated animal. Movement of a hyperechoic structure representing the interface of the cuneiform process of the arytenoid cartilage should be seen bilaterally during inspiration. In laryngeal paralysis one or both of these structures is not seen to be moving.

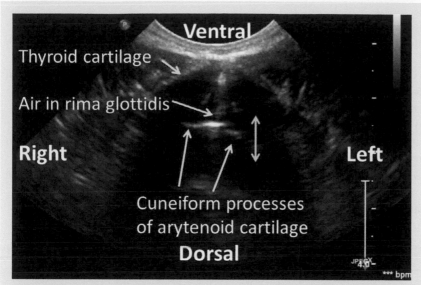

Figure 20.4 Transverse ultrasound image of the larynx of a dog with unilateral (right-sided) laryngeal paralysis. Note the image orientation – the dog is in dorsal recumbency and the ventral surface of the neck is at the top of the image. To either side of the central gas-reverberation artefact caused by air in the rima glottidis is a hyperechoic structure representing the cuneiform cartilage. This has an up-and-down motion on ultrasound in normal animals but is static when laryngeal paralysis is present. Here the left-sided hyperechoic structure was seen to move and the right-sided one was static.

Diagnosis

In this dog haematological assessment was normal and total T4 was also normal excluding hypothyroidism. Thoracic radiography demonstrated no evidence of enlargement of the cardiac silhouette and no evidence of prior aspiration pneumonitis or space occupying lesions. Radiographs of the upper airways were unremarkable. Evaluation of the larynx under a light plane of anaesthesia demonstrated bilateral laryngeal paralysis.

A final diagnosis of **idiopathic bilateral laryngeal paralysis** was made.

The dog underwent unilateral arytenoid lateralisation surgery and made an excellent recovery. Exercise tolerance and heat intolerance both improved dramatically and excessive panting ceased. Occasional throat-clearing coughs continued to be heard – this is a feature of intermittent low-grade aspiration of saliva in laryngeal paralysis and is not helped by surgery.

Discussion

In the author's experience, laryngeal paralysis is one of the most common causes of reduced exercise tolerance and tachypnoea/panting in older dogs, particularly middle-sized breeds. It is commonly mistaken for congestive heart failure but the two can almost always be differentiated by careful history taking and a good physical examination. It is important to always evaluate the larynx under the correct conditions to make this diagnosis and to recognise that the long anatomical pathways of the laryngeal nerves predispose them to injury from thoracic pathology and also that laryngeal neuropathy may be a manifestation of other systemic and secondary polyneuropathies.

Further reading

MacPhail, C.M. & Monnet, E. (2001) Outcome of and postoperative complications in dogs undergoing surgical treatment of laryngeal paralysis: 140 cases (1985–1998). *J Am Vet Med Assoc* **218**, 1949–1956

Panciera, D.L. (2001) Conditions associated with canine hypothyroidism. *Vet Clin North Am Small Anim Pract* **31**, 935–950

Rudorf, H., Barr, F.J. & Lane, J.G. (2001) The role of ultrasound in the assessment of laryngeal paralysis in the dog. *Vet Radiol Ultrasound* **42**, 338–343

Snelling, S.R. & Edwards, G.A. (2003) A retrospective study of unilateral arytenoid lateralisation in the treatment of laryngeal paralysis in 100 dogs (1992–2000). *Aust Vet J* **81**, 464–468

Venker-van Haagen, A.J. (1998) Laryngeal paralysis: an emergency management. *Vet Q* **20** (Suppl 1), S3–4

White, R.A. (1998) Laryngeal paralysis: an introduction. *Vet Q* **20** (Suppl 1), S2–3

Clinical presentation

A 5 year-old male-neutered Labrador is presented with a 6 week history of sneezing and nasal discharge. The discharge has been consistently worse on the right side than the left and, whilst initially serous, has become progressively more purulent. For the last 48 hours epistaxis has been noted intermittently from the right nares. The owner reports that the dog seems to be uncomfortable and resents handling around the nose, and the nasal planum has become crusted and sore, especially under the right nares where it has also become depigmented (**Figure 21.1**). There has been no alteration in the shape or symmetry of the dog's nose or face and no ocular discharge has been seen. The dog has not travelled outside the United Kingdom and there is no history of trauma.

Questions

1. **What are the pertinent features of this dog's history and appearance? What other relevant information may be gained from history and physical examination in a dog presenting with haemorrhagic nasal discharge?**
2. **What are the principle differential diagnoses for epistaxis in the dog? From the information available, which of these would be most likely?**
3. **What investigation would you recommend?**

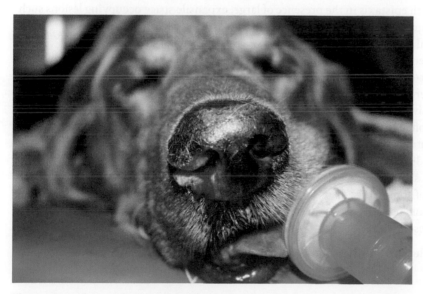

Figure 21.1 The patient at presentation.

Answers

1. Pertinent features of history and appearance

- The discharge is haemorrhagic
  - This suggests that a destructive process is occurring or that a haemorrhagic tendency might exist.
  - Since the clinical signs have been persistently asymmetrical (worse on the right side than the left) and the epistaxis is also occurring on this side, it is more likely that localised asymmetrical destructive disease is occurring rather than there being a systemic bleeding tendency.
  - Epistaxis preceded by purulent discharge, rather than frank haemorrhage initially, suggests a local disease process rather than a systemic bleeding tendency. It would be unwise to completely dismiss the possibility of this latter, but more commonly bilaterally symmetrical signs would be expected.
- Lack of travel outside the UK (where leishmaniasis and monocytic ehrlichiosis are not currently endemic)
  - Helpful in making some differential diagnoses for epistaxis, particularly some infectious ones, unlikely.
- Lack of history of trauma
  - Suggests that the epistaxis is less likely due to nasal injury (though the possibility of unwitnessed trauma or intranasal trauma caused by foreign body cannot be excluded).
- Lack of alteration in facial shape or symmetry
  - Does not particularly help narrow the differential diagnosis though alteration in these, and the presence of ipsilateral ocular discharge, exophthalmos or ptosis are most commonly seen with epistaxis in the presence of large, expansile space occupying lesions such as tumours, and occasionally with very extensive/destructive mycotic infections.
- The dog is painful
  - Although potentially any disease process affecting the nose might be uncomfortable, the process most commonly associated with marked discomfort is destructive rhinitis due to sinonasal aspergillosis.
  - Counterintuitively, many dogs with nasal tumours do not appear uncomfortable or unwell and this often leads to delayed recognition of this particular pathology.
- Crusting and ventral nasal depigmentation is observed, particularly ventral to the right nares
  - Important finding as it is seen most commonly with fungal rhinitis.
  - Some caution should be exercised though since nasal depigmentation will also occur in the presence of some other disorders, including but not limited to, discoid lupus erythematosus and mucocutaneous pyoderma (though asymmetrical and ventral distribution is unusual in these).

What other relevant information may be gained from the history and physical examination?

- History
  - Speed of onset of clinical signs may sometimes be helpful as occasionally epistaxis may be seen associated with foreign body inhalation, and in such instances, though epistaxis may only develop gradually, clinical signs of sneezing may appear abruptly.
  - Evidence of constitutional signs of illness or history of blood loss, petechiation or bruising of other anatomical locations may raise the suspicion that epistaxis may be a manifestation of a more systemic disease state or bleeding diathesis.

- ○ Travel history, antiparasitic history and potential for access to anticoagulant rodenticides should always be assessed.
- ○ In younger animals, a history of unexplained bleeding, prolonged bleeding after surgery, dental eruption, minor wounds or at oestrus may raise a suspicion of bleeding diathesis.
- Physical examination in dogs with epistaxis should always include
  - ○ Careful palpation of the nasal, incisive, maxilla and frontal bones for deformation, asymmetry, swelling and pain.
  - ○ Observation of the nares and nasal planum, especially for quantity and nature of discharge, crusting and erosion, depigmentation and protruding mass lesions or foreign material. Airflow can be assessed by means of vibration of cotton-wool fibres held over the nares sequentially or by condensation on a glass slide, but is of questionable utility since it does not help distinguish between solid and liquid obstructions and evaluation should always include both nasal cavities in any case.
  - ○ Careful observation of facial and ocular symmetry and for ocular discharge. It is also useful, provided that ocular disease is not suspected, to gently retropulse the globes, especially if retro-orbital pathology is suspected.
  - ○ Inspection of the oral cavity, paying close attention to the dentition (and possibility of nasal discharge related to apical tooth abscess), the hard palate and the mucous membranes for evidence of haemorrhage. Pain/discomfort on jaw opening should be noted.
  - ○ Palpation of regional lymph nodes.
  - ○ Close inspection of other body areas for evidence of haemorrhage, petechiation or ecchymoses. Petechiation is most commonly appreciated along the gingival margins, inner pinnae, ventral abdomen and inguinal region.
  - ○ A complete general physical examination.

3. **What are the principle differential diagnoses for epistaxis in the dog? From the information available, which of these would be most likely?**

Epistaxis

The most common causes of epistaxis in the dog are

- Trauma
- Sinonasal aspergillosis
- Nasal neoplasia
- Leishmaniasis and monocytic ehrlichiosis (in areas where they are endemic)

However, this list is not exhaustive and it is appropriate to consider epistaxis to be due to either a locally destructive process with resulting local haemorrhage or bleeding due to a systemic bleeding tendency (or diathesis). Bleeding diatheses may be due to

- Disorders of primary haemostasis (platelet number, platelet function or von Willebrands' factor).
- Disorders of secondary haemostasis (altered amount or function of coagulation factors).
- Disorders causing enhanced fibrinolysis.
- Diseases primarily affecting the vasculature (vasculopathies, systemic hypertension).

Additionally, any process that involves local inflammation or damage to nasal turbinates and mucosa may result in epistaxis, including inflammatory rhinitis, foreign bodies (in situ or penetration), dental disease and extending oral tumours. It is extremely unlikely that epistaxis is due to a bacterial infection and routine antibiotic administration in these patients represents a probable misuse of antimicrobials and delays diagnosis. Interestingly, although epistaxis is often a feature of systemic hypertension in man, this appears to be very rarely the case in dogs or cats.

Given the progressive nature, the presence of epistaxis, pain, ventral nasal depigmentation and lack of travel to *Leishmania*-endemic areas, a diagnosis of sinonasal aspergillosis would be most likely in this case.

3. **What investigations would you recommend?**

The diagnostic approach for most dogs with epistaxis should involve

(a) An initial diagnostic consideration of whether localised or systemic disease is likely to be present. This can often be ascertained by a pertinent history and physical examination, though in the event of the latter or where significant doubt exists then diagnostic testing to assess the possibility of a bleeding tendency should precede evaluation for local disease.

(b) Some form of diagnostic imaging of the nasal chambers and frontal sinuses.

(c) Some form of direct visualisation of the nasal chambers (and, if possible, the frontal sinuses) accompanied by biopsy.

Diagnostic approach recognising cost-constraints

One must apply 'common sense' and wise utilisation of financial resources in investigation of epistaxis. It behoves clinicians not to adopt a financially wasteful 'protocol'-based approach to epistaxis but to pick the tests that most adequately answer the clinical questions proffered whilst taking into account the cost of treatment. For instance, it would be totally inappropriate to embark upon expensive assessment of individual coagulation factors unless evaluation implicated a secondary coagulopathy. Therapy for both of the two most common differential diagnoses can be costly and involved. It is therefore sensible to discuss clients' wishes in the eventuality of either sinonasal aspergillosis or nasal neoplasia first of all, before embarking on diagnostic tests. For instance, whilst cross-sectional imaging is required for planning radiotherapy in cases of nasal neoplasia, if client wishes preclude this treatment but diagnostic certainty is desired, radiography and rhinoscopy may achieve this diagnosis.

- **Haematological assessment**
  - A simple blood haemogram and examination of a fresh blood-smear allows evaluation for
    - Developing anaemia in those patients in which epistaxis has been prolonged/exuberant.
    - Evaluation of platelet number.
  - A buccal mucosal bleeding time is a simple but crude and highly variable global test for primary haemostasis but should be undertaken only if thrombocytopenia has been excluded.
  - Assessment of an activated clotting time (note that this requires an activating substrate not just a plain blood collection tube, or an automated cartridge-based system) or of prothrombin time (PT) and activated partial thromboplastin time (APTT) may be considered if secondary coagulopathy is considered.

- **Serological tests and fungal cultures for aspergillosis**
  - Agar gel immuno-/double diffusion (AGIDD), counter-immunoelectrophoresis (CIE) and ELISA-based tests are all available.
  - Whilst ELISA-based tests have been reported by some authors as being superior, in general all serological tests suffer from having only moderately good sensitivity, meaning that false negative test results are relatively common. Although false positive results are less common they may still occur.
  - For these reasons it is recommended that a diagnosis of sinonasal aspergillosis is neither made nor excluded on the basis of serological testing alone but that positive test results are viewed as 'corroborative evidence'.
  - Assessment of fungal culture of nasal swabs is not recommended except when used to determine the species of fungus involved in known mycotic rhinitis by direct sampling of fungal colonies. Positive fungal cultures have been found in normal dogs and in dogs with non-mycotic nasal pathology such as neoplasia.
- **Other laboratory tests**
  - In endemic areas for ehrlichiosis and leishmaniasis, biochemical evaluation that might identify hyperglobulinaemia and detection of evidence of organism exposure or active infection by serology, PCR or direct organism identification should be undertaken.
- **Diagnostic imaging**
  - Radiography, computed tomography (CT) and magnetic resonance imaging (MRI) have all been used to evaluate dogs with epistaxis and with nasal disease.
  - Radiography is both more widely available and much less costly than cross-sectional imaging techniques such as CT or MRI. The principle disadvantages of radiography over cross-sectional imaging tests is the degree of superimposition of nasal structures and the associated reduction in anatomical acuity, the relatively poor definition of soft tissue changes and the inability to distinguish between soft-tissue and fluid opacities.
  - In the diagnosis of sinonasal aspergillosis, radiography has been shown to have a diagnostic sensitivity of 72% versus 88% for CT.
  - Both CT and MRI have been demonstrated to have similar diagnostic sensitivity with CT having greater utility in demonstrating the extent of bony pathology/involvement and MRI having superior soft tissue resolution and being of more use where pathology (e.g. neoplasia) is extending within the cranial vault.
  - A practical decision is often made depending on availability of both the equipment, and most importantly the expertise in interpretation, of different diagnostic imaging modalities and cost.
  - Radiography is likely to remain the most cost-effective and widely available imaging technique to assess nasal disease in dogs.

Diagnostic imaging positioning in epistaxis

When radiographs are performed it is essential that symmetrical and carefully positioned views are obtained without superimposition of mandible, tongue, endotracheal tube or other structures over the region of interest. The most useful views are a dorsoventral occlusal view of the nasal chambers utilising non-screen film inserted orally and the rostrocaudal ('skyline') view of the frontal sinuses. Self-critical evaluation for image quality and symmetry are essential with repetition mandatory if perfect positioning is not obtained. Images should be systematically evaluated with particular reference to the presence, integrity and symmetry of the ethmoturbinates and the presence or absence of normal air lucency throughout the remaining nasal cavities and sinuses. The dentition should also always be examined. It should be remembered that soft tissue and fluid are isodense on radiographs. It is sensible to take thoracic radiographs (or if CT is used, for the thorax to be included), due to the potential for pulmonary metastatic disease with nasal neoplasia, though most nasal neoplasms are characterised more by their local invasiveness.

In the majority of dogs with chronic nasal disease and epistaxis, one of three broad radiographic diagnoses may be attainable:

(a) Presence of symmetrical present ethmoturbinate structures with largely normal air-lucency throughout the nasal chambers (which may be partly attenuated) is usually consistent with a non-destructive inflammatory rhinitis.

(b) Presence of ethmoturbinate destruction with a concurrent increase in the extent of the normal air-lucency is consistent with mycotic rhinitis, most commonly due to sinonasal aspergillosis.

(c) Presence of ethmoturbinate destruction with a concurrent decrease in the extent of the normal air-lucency and replacement with a soft tissue/fluid opacity is consistent with nasal neoplasia.

However, in some instances a diagnosis is not clear and, in particular, the presence of large amounts of intranasal discharge in cases of sinonasal aspergillosis may mimic nasal neoplasia (see **Figure 21.2**).

- **Rhinoscopy and biopsy**
  - Rhinoscopy must be performed under general anaesthesia and a systematic approach adopted.
  - Use of an otoscope does not allow visualisation of most of the nasal chambers in dogs and endoscopic equipment is usually required.
  - Examination of the nasopharynx by retrograde passage of a flexible endoscope is usually performed initially, followed by anterograde assessment of both nasal chambers, examining the least affected side first.
  - When performing anterograde rhinoscopy both rigid lens-based endoscopes and flexible fibreoptic endoscopes may be employed, with the former being preferred due to greater visual acuity.
  - Thorough revision of nasal endoscopic anatomy, performance of rhinoscopy in a systematic manner, recording of findings and an appreciation of anatomical 'blindpsots' are all mandatory prior to performing rhinoscopy.
  - The nasal mucosa is delicate, friable and prone to small amounts of haemorrhage even with very gentle manipulation and this may severely impair examination. It is therefore recommended that prior to anterograde rhinoscopic examination
    - The patient's airway is protected both by a cuffed endotracheal tube and by use of a 'throat pack' with the head tipped downwards.
    - That sterile saline is irrigated anterograde either through the channel of the endoscope sheath or alongside it to provide an 'underwater' view with constant flushing away of haemorrhage (**Figure 21.3a**).

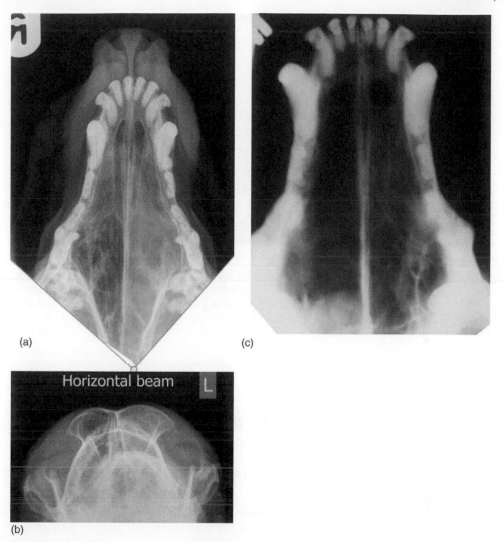

(a)

(c)

Horizontal beam   L

(b)

Figure 21.2 Dorsoventral occlusal views of the nasal chambers (a, c) and rostra-caudal frontal sinus view (b). In (a) and (b), loss of turbinate structure and replacement with soft tissue/fluid opacity is seen in both the left nasal cavity and left frontal sinus. The cause was an extensive epithelial neoplasm. (c) Extensive loss of turbinates on the right side is shown, with normal turbinate pattern on the left. There is normal gas (air) lucency on the right side consistent with the final diagnosis of aspergillosis.

- That the nasal meati are evaluated from ventral to dorsal and biopsies are taken only after thorough evaluation are also recommended to avoid diagnostic impairment by haemorrhage.

Systematic evaluation of nasopharynx, lower, middle, upper and common meati on both sides and finally biopsy should be undertaken.

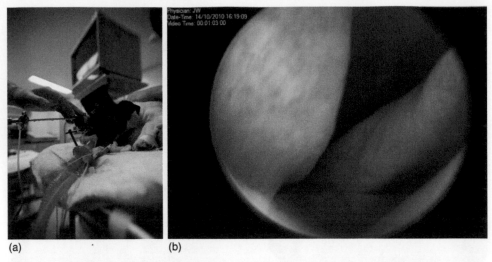

(a)   (b)

Figure 21.3 (a) Anterograde rhinoscopy being performed in a dog. Note that the rigid sheath around the endoscope includes side ports, through which fluid is irrigated to improve visualisation. (b) A typical endoscopic view of normal turbinates, which should be pink, slightly velvety and have interdigitating 'hills' and 'valleys' with an airspace in between.

Nasal biopsy

Endoscopic biopsy forceps are generally too small to provide adequate specimens and investing in ENT biopsy forceps is recommended. Biopsies should include mucosa and underlying turbinate and should involve careful cutting of the biopsy fragment by the forceps cups not 'dragging' mucosa from the turbinates. Haemorrhage induced by this may usually be controlled by topical packing with 'stick swabs' or application of vasoconstrictors such as topical adrenaline, phenylephrine or iced water for several minutes. After rhinoscopy the oropharynx should be carefully inspected and swabbed clear of any material and the throat-pack removed prior to extubation.

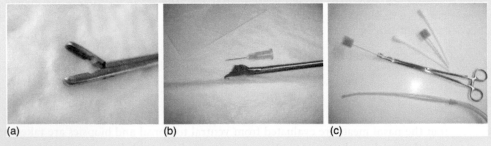

(a)   (b)   (c)

Figure 21.4 (a) Suitable ENT biopsy forceps, (b) a typical rhinoscopic biopsy specimen (impression cytology smears and histopathology may both be performed) and (c) a variety of stick-swabs and suction used to clear debris from the pharynx and apply topical pressure after biopsy.

Rhinoscopic examination will often yield unequivocal evidence of mycotic rhinitis (**Figure 21.5a**) or a mass lesion (**Figure 21.5b**), but biopsies of representative tissue should still be taken even if no obvious focal pathology is present. Cytological preparations are easy to perform from rhinoscopic biopsy of both neoplastic mass lesions and mycotic plaques. Cytology of aspergillosis is a very rapid and useful diagnostic aid (**Figure 21.5c**).

Diagnosis

In the dog reported in this case, the following investigation was performed:

- Haematology
  - Demonstrated a normal haematocrit and platelet numbers. A mild inflammatory leukogram was present.
- Computed tomography (CT) of the nose and thorax (**Figure 21.6**)
  - Thorax
    - Unremarkable lungs
  - Head (nose to retropharyngeal lymph nodes)
    - Marked cavitation in the rostral right nasal chamber, with loss of turbinates, destruction of the nasal septum rostrally and thinning of the maxillary recess.
    - Some soft tissue attenuating material between the remaining turbinates ventrally and within the entrance to the choana, and this extends to the area ventral to the cribriform plate, although there is no turbinate destruction here.
    - Small amount of destruction and some blunting of the turbinates in the left rostral nasal chamber, with some soft tissue material.
    - No involvement of the frontal sinuses.
  - *Conclusion:* destructive process in the rostral nasal chambers bilaterally – more severely destructive on the right, more recent/active inflammation on the left.
- Rhinoscopy (**Figure 21.7**)
  - Demonstrated destructive rhinitis, predominantly on the right side, with clear loss of normal turbinate structure and increase in the nasal airspaces.
  - Areas of 'cottage-cheese'-like material were seen to be accumulated over areas of turbinate destruction.
  - Samples of this material were collected for
    - Cytology, which demonstrated neutrophilic inflammation and numerous fungal hyphae, consistent with (but not diagnostic of) *Aspergillus fumigatus*.

  Fungal culture, which yielded profuse growth of *Aspergillus fumigatus*.

- **A final diagnosis of nasal aspergillosis was made.**

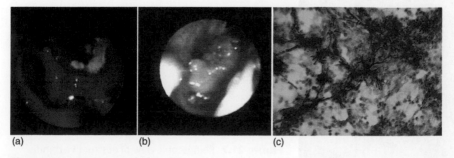

Figure 21.5 (a) Mycotic rhinitis, (b) nasal carcinoma and (c) aspergillosis.

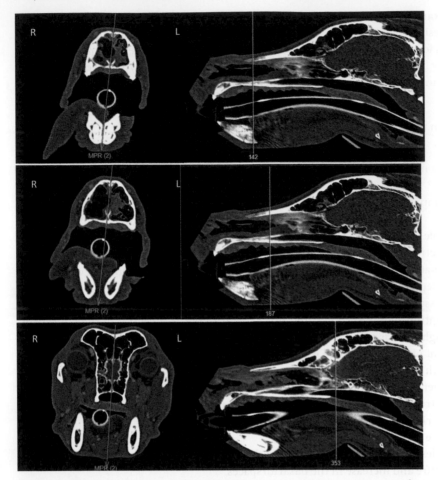

Figure 21.6 Transverse (left image) and sagittal (right image) CT image sections from rostral to caudal through the nose of the dog presented. Destructive rhinitis can be seen with turbinate loss predominantly on the right side. The yellow line represents the level at which the transverse image is positioned.

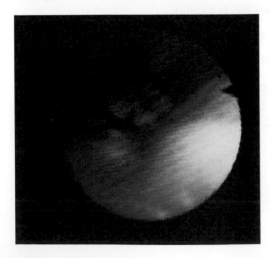

Figure 21.7 Rhinoscopic view of destructive rhinitis and mycotic plaque.

Treatment (Figure 21.8)

The dog was treated by topical instillation of a fungicidal solution followed by instillation of a depot of fungicidal cream. Briefly, after surgical skin preparation the frontal sinuses were trephined and 50–100 ml of sterile saline flushed anterograde to ensure patency of the nasofrontal ostium by witnessing fluid egress from the ipsilateral nares. Then 50 ml of 1% clotrimazole solution (Canestan solution, Bater) was used to irrigate each side over 5 minutes and 20 g/side of 1% clotrimazole

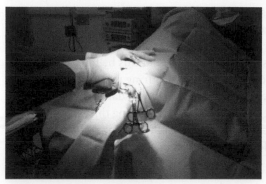

Surgical trephination of frontal sinuses

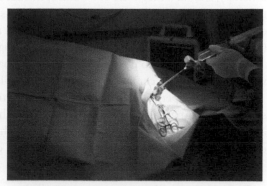

To ensure patency of the nasofrontal ostia, 50–100 ml of sterile saline is flushed anterograde

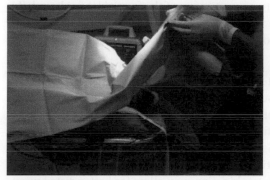

Inspection of egress of saline from ipsilateral nares

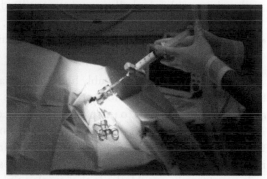

After irrigation with 1% clotrimazole solution, 20 g/side of 1% clotrimazole cream is instilled into both frontal sinuses

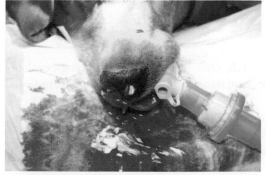

Some cream can be seen leaching down through the nasal cavities to exit at the nares

Figure 21.8 The treatment procedure.

cream (Canestan cream, Bayer) was instilled into the frontal sinus. The small incisions were sutures and the dog received appropriate analgesia provided post-operatively.

Discussion

Prior to undertaking investigation for epistaxis due to local disease it is essential to discuss likely treatment options and differential diagnoses with clients since the outcome of this may, in part, dictate the most appropriate clinical approach. For example, if clients are unwilling to pursue radiotherapy, should a diagnosis of a nasal epithelial tumour be made, but are desirous of a diagnosis, then the increased expense associated with cross-sectional imaging with CT or MRI in order to document the extent of the mass lesion and plan radiotherapy may not represent value for money (when a diagnosis can be achieved through radiography and rhinoscopy/biopsy).

It is also sensible to plan for therapy of sinonasal aspergillosis should this be found, since it is very common that a confident diagnosis of this disorder can be made during rhinoscopy.

Sinonasal aspergillosis is most successfully treated with topical fungicidal agents. Although systemic antifungal agents have been employed, their success rate in eradicating this mycosis is disappointing, though newer 'azole' antifungals such as posaconazole and voriconazole have not been evaluated. Topical treatment with enilconazole, clotrimazole or bifonale have all been reported. The agent may be delivered

- Daily via indwelling catheters, surgically inserted into the frontal sinuses.
- As a non-invasive 'soak' whereby the agent is infused through catheters placed into the nasal chambers, with foley balloon catheters utilised to prevent egress of the fungicidal fluid caudally via the nasopharynx or rostrally via the nares.
- As a combination of a lavaging fungicidal liquid followed by a depot of fungicidal cream delivered by trephination of the frontal sinuses.

All methods have a reasonably high success rate (in the region of 60–90%), although therapeutic failure is unfortunately not uncommon and is suspected to be largely due to failure of adequate distribution of fungicide to infected areas or lack of prolonged contact time to achieve fungal 'kill'. Although in this case disease appeared largely confined to the nasal cavities, it is sensible to assume that some frontal sinus involvement is present in most cases of aspergillosis. Non-invasive soak methods may not be effective if the nasofrontal ostia are obstructed by fungal material/secretions/inflammatory change. Methods that employ sinus trephination may allow for better distribution of fungicide and the ability, if needed, to surgically debride fungal colonies, and it is thought that depot cream preparations may result in prolonged contact time. A significant minority of patients nonetheless will require more than one treatment to achieve a clinical cure.

Further reading

Pomrantz, J.S., Johnson, L.R., Nelson, R.W. & Wisner, E.R. (2007) Comparison of serologic evaluation via agar gel immunodiffusion and fungal culture of tissue for diagnosis of nasal aspergillosis in dogs. *J Am Vet Med Assoc* **230**, 1319–1323

Saunders, J.H., van Bree, H., Gielen, I. & de Rooster, H. (2003) Diagnostic value of computed tomography in dogs with chronic nasal disease. *Vet Radiol Ultrasound* **44**, 409–413

Sharman, M.J. & Mansfield, C.S. (2012) Sinonasal aspergillosis in dogs: a review. *J Small Anim Pract* **53**, 434–444

Cardiovascular

Canine Internal Medicine: What's Your Diagnosis? First Edition. Jon Wray.
© 2018 John Wiley & Sons Ltd. Published 2018 by John Wiley & Sons Ltd.

Cardiovascular

Clinical presentation

A 10 year-old male-neutered Golden Retriever (**Figure 22.1**) is presented with a recent history of lethargy, exercise intolerance and increase in abdominal size. On physical examination the abdomen is distended with a palpable fluid thrill of ascites. Heart rate is 140/min and on auscultation the normal heart sounds are muffled bilaterally. Peripheral pulse quality is poor and appears to vary in quality from beat-to-beat but the rhythm is regular. On clipping the area of the jugular furrow prior to venepuncture, spontaneous jugular venous distension is noted (**Figure 22.2**).

Questions

1. What is the problem list for this dog and what is the significance of the physical examination findings?
2. What differential diagnoses would you consider?
3. What diagnostic tests would you perform to distinguish between them?

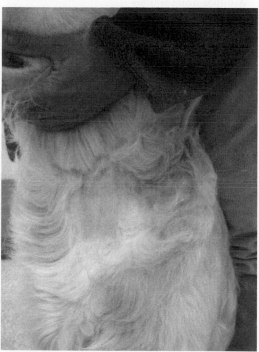

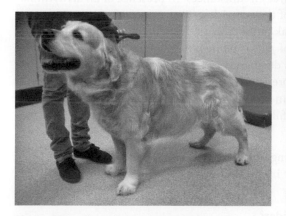

Figure 22.1 The patient at presentation.　　**Figure 22.2** Jugular venous distension.

Canine Internal Medicine: What's Your Diagnosis? First Edition. Jon Wray.
© 2018 John Wiley & Sons Ltd. Published 2018 by John Wiley & Sons Ltd.

Answers

1. What is the problem list for this dog and what is the significance of the physical examination findings?

This patient's problem list would be

- Exercise intolerance
- Ascites
- Muffled heart sounds
- Weak and variable pulse quality
- Jugular venous distension

Whilst the heart rate of 140 bpm is within the normal canine reference range of 60–160/min, a mid-sized breed such as a Golden Retriever would be expected to have a heart rate under normal circumstances of <120/min or so and unless the dog was very excitable this might be interpreted as a 'relative' tachycardia in this breed.

Ascites

Indicates fluid accumulation in the abdomen, which may be a pure transudate, modified transudate, exudate (either sterile or septic), blood, urine, chyle or bile.

Muffled heart sounds

Occurs due to attenuation of transmission of normal sounds from their source (the cardiac valves) to the thoracic wall. This is usually due to the presence of fluid, either within the pleural space or the pericardial sac, but may also occur in the presence of excessive fat or the presence of a mass lesion, consolidated lung tissue or a viscus between the heart and the thoracic wall.

Poor and variable peripheral pulse quality

Pulse quality represents the difference between systolic and diastolic pulse pressure and depends primarily on stroke volume and arterial stiffness. Variation of pulse quality from beat-to-beat is unusual and usually occurs in three circumstances: (i) presence of an arrhythmia and variation in the diastolic filling time of the ventricles, (ii) presence of *pulsus alternans*, which describes alternating strong and weak pulse pressures usually in animals with severe left ventricular failure and (iii) presence of *pulsus paradoxus* whereby pulse pressure falls cyclically during inspiration and increases during expiration. This occurs where combined ventricular filling is limited either by the presence of pericardial effusion or by constrictive pericardial disease, such that the increase in venous return to the right ventricle during inspiration restricts left ventricular diastolic filling volume.

Jugular venous distension

This either represents increased 'back' filling of the jugular veins due to obstruction of venous return (due to extramural, mural or intramural obstruction) or reflects elevation in right-sided cardiac filling pressure.

2. What differential diagnoses would you consider?

'Beck's triad'

The presence of muffled heart sounds, poor pulse quality and jugular venous distension is commonly known as **'Beck's triad'** and is considered a hallmark feature of cardiac tamponade due to **pericardial effusion**. However, jugular venous distension, ascites and muffled heart sounds may also be encountered in patients with right-sided congestive heart failure and accumulation of fluid in both the pleural and peritoneal spaces.

Right-sided congestive heart failure is less commonly encountered in dogs than left-sided failure and causes may include

- Cardiac tamponade due to pericardial effusion or constrictive pericardial disease.
- Tricuspid valve dysplasia.
- Severe elevation in right ventricular outflow pressure or pulmonary arterial pressure due to
  - Pulmonic stenosis.
  - Pulmonary arterial hypertension (either primary or acquired secondary to other diseases).
  - Heartworm disease caused by *Dirofilaria immitis* (which is not endemic to the United Kingdom)*

usually when these are combined with some degree of insufficiency in the tricuspid valve apparatus.

3. **What diagnostic tests would you perform to distinguish between them?**

Identify the cause of ascites before treating

The key is to determine the underlying cause of ascites *prior* to instituting therapy. It is all too common for ascites in dogs to be treated with agents such as loop diuretics (e.g. furosemide) before either the nature of the ascites or its underlying cause has been determined and this can lead to placing patients at undue risk of iatrogenic complications. Ascites is very seldom an emergency that requires immediate alleviation in advance of determining the underlying cause.

Abdominal paracentesis

In cases where the likely cause of ascites is not apparent from the rest of the physical examination, the initial step in determining its aetiology is to perform abdominal paracentesis to obtain a sample of the fluid. This can either be performed under ultrasound guidance (which has the advantage that if fluid 'pockets' are present, these may be accurately sampled and limits the risk of floating falciform fat becoming entrapped in the sampling needle and frustrating collection) or more commonly 'blind'. When performing a blind paracentesis the patient is gently restrained in the left lateral recumbency (which will allow the spleen to 'fall' to the dependent side, reducing the risk of accidental penetration of it) and a site approximately 2 fingers' breadth caudal to the umbilicus (to avoid falciform fat) is clipped and aseptically prepared. Using an aseptic approach, a 21G needle of length dependent on patient size and attached to a 2–5 ml syringe is gently introduced through the midline with the needle bevel angled so that it is *'en face'* to the abdominal contents to reduce the risk of inadvertent laceration of any abdominal viscera (which is a very rare occurrence). *Gentle* aspiration of ascitic fluid is then performed. Fluid produced should be analysed for protein

---

* *Angiostrongylus vasorum*, which is endemic in the UK, has been reported in association with pulmonary hypertension.

content, cellularity and a cytological examination should be performed on a fresh sample. Should an infectious aetiology (i.e. septic peritonitis) be suspected then the fluid should be cultured. If uroperitoneum, chyloperotoneum or biloperitoneum are suspected then fluid creatinine, trigyceride and bilirubin levels may be compared with serum levels of the same analyte and the diagnosis supported by finding peritoneal levels exceeding those in serum. Similarly high concentrations of peritoneal fluid lipase may support the presence of pancreatitis. It should be noted that assessment of glucose concentration in peritoneal effusions is unreliable for the diagnosis of septic peritonitis. A summary of peritoneal effusion findings and their aetiologies is given in **Table 22.1**.

> In this case the principle differential diagnoses are of pericardial effusion versus other causes of right-sided congestive heart failure and thoracic radiography and echocardiography are the two diagnostic tests of choice.

Radiography

It is of course important to obtain orthogonal thoracic views. In the presence of a pericardial effusion it is expected to find an enlarged and 'globoid' cardiac silhouette in which the normal subtle

Table 22.1 Characteristics of different types of abdominal effusion

	Pure transudate	Modified transudate	Exudate	Other
Pathogenesis	Extravasation of low-protein fluid due to decreased vascular colloid oncotic pressure (usually in hypoalbuminaemic states) *or* Extravasation of fluid within the pre-hepatic portal circulation due to increased intravascular hydrostatic pressure and leakage of protein-/cell-poor fluid	Extravasation of fluid principally from increased hydrostatic pressure in abdominal vessels due to right-sided congestive heart failure, tamponade and obstruction of the caudal vena cava However, modified transudates may also be neoplastic in origin or represent local fluid production from organ torsion, vasculitis and infarctions	The most common cause is inflammation, which may be septic or non-septic. Common causes of septic effusion include bowel perforation, dehiscence of enterotomy sites. Causes of non-septic exudates commonly include pancreatitis, gall bladder rupture, urinary tract rupture	Other considerations are: • Chyle • Bile • Blood • Urine Specific analysis of fluid including cytology, triglyceride content compared with serum (chyle) and creatinine content compared with serum (urine) may help distinguish these
Fluid protein	<20 g/l	20–50 g/l	>30 g/l	
Fluid nucleated cell count	<1500/µl	<5000/µl	>5000/µl	
Common aetiologies	Severe hypoalbuminaemia, portal vein hypertension	Commonly right-sided congestive heart failure and cardiac tamponade	Pancreatitis Septic peritonitis	

distinctions in outline where chambers meet are lost. Because normal thoracic radiographs involve a certain amount of movement 'blur' due to the rapidly pulsatile nature of the cardiac structures, where the heart is surrounded by a relatively fixed volume of fluid contained within the pericardium, this movement blur is no longer an issue and the globoid cardiac outline will frequently appear 'crisp' and well-defined compared with the normal situation (**Figure 22.3**). In the case of both pericardial effusion and with other causes of right-sided congestive heart failure, pleural effusion may be present.

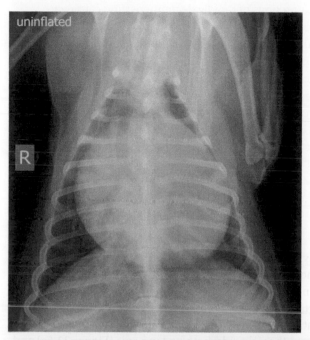

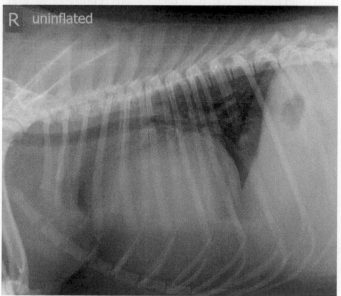

Figure 22.3 Dorsoventral and right lateral recumbent thoracic radiographs of a dog with a pericardial effusion. Note the generalised globoid cardiomegaly with absence of indentation of the outline distinguishing between chamber borders and the very 'crisp' outline to the cardiac silhouette. A small amount of pleural effusion is present and partly effaces the cranioventral and caudoventral borders of the cardiac outline.

Echocardiography (Figure 22.4)

Even in the hands of an operator who is relatively unskilled in echocardiography, cardiac ultrasound can be used to evaluate for presence of pericardial effusion, examine for possible aetiology and to direct therapy. A few basic principles should be remembered when performing echocardiography in this situation.

Echocardiography in pericardial effusion

In animals that are not collapsed or exhibiting signs of rapidly decompensating cardiovascular status, it is preferable to obtain echocardiographic images prior to drainage of any pericardial effusion. The presence of relatively hypoechoic or anechoic fluid effectively provides additional 'contrast' between soft tissue structures and the pericardium, which may aid in the diagnosis of cardiac neoplasia. Echocardiography should *always* be performed from both left and right parasternal approaches. In the presence of pericardial effusions especially it should be remembered that a common aetiology is cardiac haemangiosarcoma and that these tumours have a site of predilection in the right atrium and right auricle. Since left-sided structures are best imaged from the right and vice versa, these areas are best imaged from a left-sided approach. Specifically the left cranial parasternal short-axis view of the heart is the only view from which the right auricular appendage can be satisfactorily viewed in most dogs.

When examining by echocardiography take care to avoid making rapid 'snap' judgements based on one initial view. In particular, sometimes the presence of an enlarged left atrium with distended left auricular appendage can result in the auricular appendage 'hooking' over and down the left ventricular free wall such that, from certain views, it may look as though a fluid-filled structure with a thin wall is sitting outside the left ventricle, which could be mistaken for pericardial effusion.

In the presence of pericardial effusion from the right side, both on long-axis (**Figure 22.5a**) and shortaxis (**Figure 22.5b**) views, hypoechoic to anechoic fluid should be visible contained within the

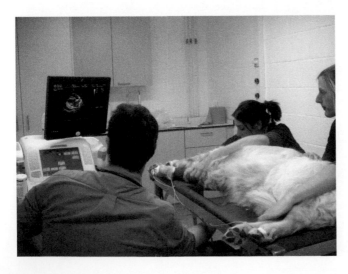

Figure 22.4 Echocardiography.

hyperechoic pericardial sac, as can be seen in the images from this patient. Where cardiac tamponade is occurring (due to intrapericardial pressure exceeding the diastolic intracardiac pressure) this is visible as diastolic sinuous indentation of the right atrial (and sometimes right ventricular) free wall (Figure 22.5a: arrow). From the left cranial parasternal short-axis plane, the right atrium and right auricle can be imaged (**Figure 22.5c**) and in this patient no mass lesion is identified in this area.

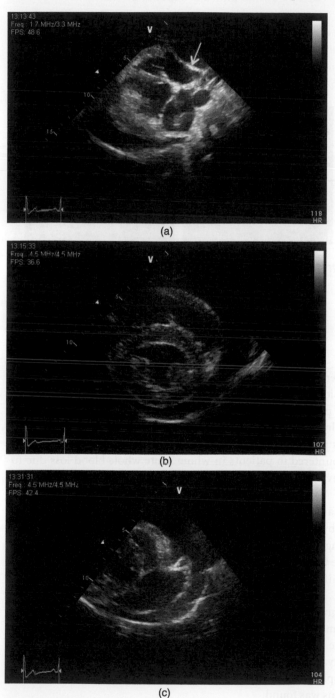

(a)

(b)

(c)

Figure 22.5 Right parasternal four-chamber long axis (a), right parasternal short axis at level of papillary muscles (b) and left cranial parasternal right atrium/right ventricle (c) echocardiographic views in the patient prior to drainage of pericardial effusion.

Echocardiographic identification of cardiac neoplasia

In patients with cardiac neoplasia the site of predisposition of some cardiac tumours may help provisional diagnosis in the absence of tissue biopsy. Cardiac haemangiosarcoma commonly occurs in association with the right atrium/auricular appendage and whilst large tumours may be visualised from the right parasternal long-axis (RPLAx) view (**Figure 22.6a**), smaller masses may only be seen on a left cranial parasternal short-axis (LCrSAx) view (**Figure 22.6b**). Heart base masses, commonly paraganglioma, tend to occur in a 'triangle' bordered by the roof of the left atrium, the pulmonary artery and the aorta (**Figure 22.6c**), seen best on a right parasternal short-axis (RPSAx) view.

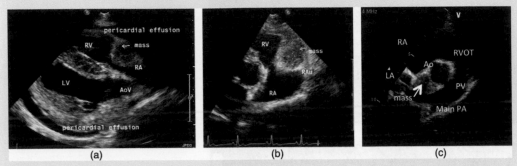

Figure 22.6 (a) RPLAx right atrial mass, (b) LCrSAx view and (c) RPSAx heart base.

Further diagnostic tests

In general, laboratory tests such as haematology and serum biochemistry are unhelpful in (a) distinguishing between pericardial effusion and other forms of right-sided congestive heart failure and (b) determining the aetiology of pericardial effusions. In animals with ascites of unknown aetiology, the presence of profound hypoalbuminaemia may, however, be a helpful diagnostic finding. Where pericardial effusion is present, the finding of concurrent anaemia and panhypoproteinaemia is most commonly encountered in patients in whom acute whole blood loss due to haemorrhagic neoplasia is seen. However, this is not present in the majority of cases, even when a neoplastic aetiology is present.

Electrocardiography is not necessary to diagnose pericardial effusion, though a suspicion of pericardial effusion may be generated by the finding of *electrical alternans* (**Figure 22.7**). Although the term '*alternans*' suggests alternating changes from beat-to-beat, this in fact indicates a more cyclical alteration in the amplitude of the QRS complexes, which occurs in the presence of pericardial fluid and which is thought to reflect shifting in the heart's electrical axis as it 'swings' to-and-fro in the fluid-filled pericardial sac.

There is a high incidence of malignant cardiac neoplasia associated with pericardial effusion in dogs and cardiac haemangiosarcoma often occurs as a 'concurrent' primary tumour in association with haemangiosarcoma of the liver and spleen. It is therefore sensible to critically review thoracic radiographs for the possibility of metastatic disease given this possibility and perform an abdominal ultrasound review of the spleen and liver for suspect neoplastic lesions. In this patient no evidence of splenic or hepatic lesions was found.

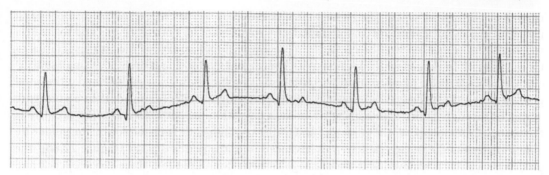

Figure 22.7 *Electrical alternans* in the patient described above with pericardial effusion. Lead II, 50 mm/s, 1 cm = 1 mV. Note the variation in amplitude of the QRS complexes.

Diagnosis

A diagnosis of an 'echo negative' pericardial effusion is made in this dog. Provisional diagnosis is of idiopathic pericardial effusion, but such a diagnosis must be 'under review' (and this should be discussed with owners) since some neoplastic causes of pericardial effusion, notably mesothelioma, may not initially be detectable with echocardiography.

Treatment

Given the echo negative findings, drainage of the pericardial effusion to relieve the tamponade is indicated as an urgent procedure. No medical treatment is effective in alleviating cardiac tamponade; it is essentially a 'mechanical' problem with a similarly 'mechanical' solution (i.e. drainage of the effusion). In particular, administering diuretics to animals with pericardial effusion is not only unhelpful but is likely to cause intravascular volume contraction and potentially exacerbate the effects of tamponade.

Ultrasound-guided or 'blind' pericardiocentesis?

Pericardial effusion may be drained 'blind' or under ultrasound-guidance (where this is available the author believes that it is easier and safer to drain effusions with ultrasound guidance, but it is not an absolute requirement for performing pericardiocentesis if unavailable). It is convention to drain pericardial effusions from the right side since risk of iatrogenic damage to coronary arteries and penetration of the high-pressure left ventricle is minimised by this route of approach (though neither should be a risk if suitable care is taken). The landmarks for approach is to penetrate just cranial to a rib (avoiding the caudal neurovascular bundle) the right 'cardiac notch' – the region of intercostal space 4–6 at the level of the costochondral junction, aiming the drainage catheter towards the opposite elbow if performing 'blind'.

In this dog, an initial bolus of 20 ml/kg of a crystalloid solution was initially given. After pre-medication with 0.3 mg/kg of butorphanol given intravenously slowly and diluted in 10 ml of 0.9% NaCl, this patient was administered oxygen at 2 l/min by facemask held close to the muzzle and then 0.5 mcg/kg dexmedetomidine given, again dilute in 10 ml or 0.9% NaCl, very slowly to effect over 10 minutes. Equipment needed for pericardiocentesis was set out (**Figure 22.8a**). The right hemithorax was clipped and surgically prepared and after assessment of the heart by ultrasound from the right 'cardiac notch' (the region of intercostal space 4–6 at the level of the costochondral junction), the thoracic skin was drawn cranially by an assistant (to both tense this and to create a subcutaneous 'tunnel' upon release in order to prevent pneumothorax) and the area just cranial to the adjacent rib infiltrated with lidocaine. With concurrent monitoring of an ECG, a small stab incision was made with a number 11 scalpel blade and using the Seldinger technique and ultrasound guidance a needle was advanced slowly until the pericardium was penetrated; then a guidewire advanced through it until approximately 5 cm of it lay within the pericardial sac. The needle was then carefully removed over the guidewire and whilst keeping gentle back-tension on the guidewire a multi-fenestrated drainage catheter was advanced in to the pericardial sac (**Figure 22.8b**). The guidewire was then removed and the drainage catheter connected to a three-way stopcock and extension set and drainage performed (**Figure 22.8c**). During drainage it is important to regularly review the fluid for the presence of clotting.

Discussion

Unless circulatory collapse has occurred due to tamponade and immediate pericardiocentesis is needed in order to stabilise the patient, a thorough diagnosis should precede definitive treatment. Pericardial effusion and tamponade is a mechanical problem with a mechanical solution (drainage) (see **Figures 22.8 and 22.9**). Because of the highly variable prognosis it is sensible to discuss with owners, prior to drainage of pericardial effusions, their wishes in the situation where a mass lesion is discovered.

Overall, approximately two-thirds of dogs with pericardial effusions have 'echo negative' disease and the majority of these have idiopathic pericardial effusion. In approximately one-third of cases echocardiographic abnormalities other than the effusion are identified and the majority of these dogs have cardiac neoplasia as an underlying cause of the effusion. Haemangiosarcoma is by

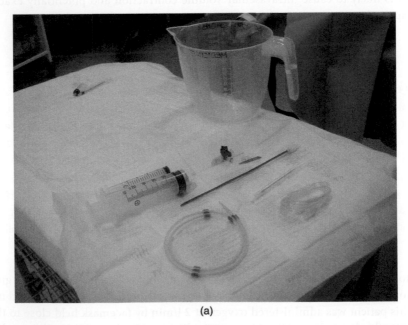

(a)

Figure 22.8a Equipment needed for pericardiocentesis, comprising a 20 ml syringe, three-way stopcock or one-way drainage valve set, pericardiocentesis catheter and Seldinger needle/ wire set and extension tube and collection vessel.

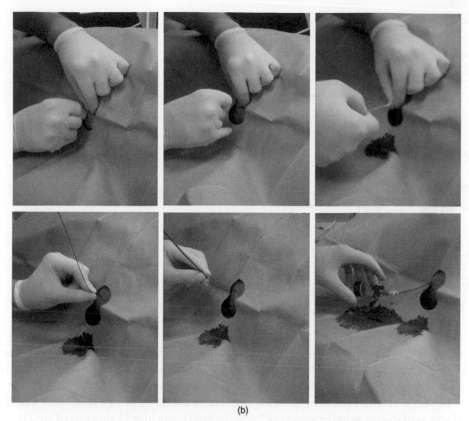

(b)

Figure 22.8b (L to R from top row) A stab incision is made with a number 11 scalpel blade and a needle is advanced into the pericardial sac (fluid, usually sanguinous, will emerge at this point). The Seldinger guidewire is then advanced into the sac, the needle removed over the wire and, applying gentle backtension on the wire, the drainage catheter is advanced over the wire and into the sac. A gentle to-and-fro twisting motion on the catheter during advancement aids passage through the subcutaneous tissues. The syringe and three-way stopcock are then attached.

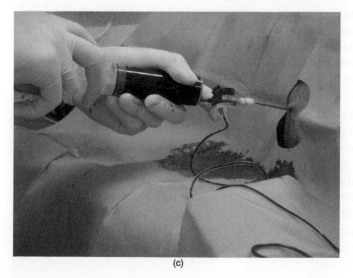

(c)

Figure 22.8c Drainage of the effusion is performed. Approximately 400 ml of sanguinous fluid was removed, entirely draining the pericardial effusion.

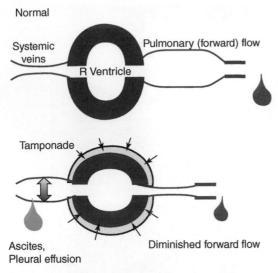

Normal

Systemic veins

Pulmonary (forward) flow

R Ventricle

Tamponade

Ascites, Pleural effusion

Diminished forward flow

Figure 22.9 Pathogenesis of cardiac tamponade.

far the most common tumour associated with pericardial effusion in dogs and because of the generally very poor associated prognosis, it is sensible to gauge an owner's wishes should unequivocal evidence of cardiac neoplasia consistent with haemangiosarcoma be found prior to drainage since (a) it may be reasonable to consider euthanasia without drainage in this circumstance and (b) the beneficial effects of drainage in the setting of haemangiosarcoma may be short-lived (and if there is a lot of haemorrhage from a tumour, very rapid deterioration, even with drainage, might be seen). However, haemangiosarcoma is not the only neoplastic condition that may be associated with pericardial effusions and heart base tumours; mesothelioma, lymphoma and a variety of other tumour types may also be encountered, though with lesser frequency than haemangiosarcoma. Since cytological assessment directly from the tumour is often not practical, the tumour type is often inferred by its location should a mass lesion be identified. Haemangiosarcomas usually, but not exclusively, occur within the right atrium or right auricular appendage and the finding of mass lesions here, especially if of a 'complex' echotexture, is highly suggestive of haemangiosarcoma. Heart base tumours are usually located in a triangle between the aorta, the pulmonary artery and the left atrium, and scanning dorsally to the heart base is mandatory to detect them. Mesotheliomas are frequently not visualised with echocardiography.

Analysis of fluid from pericardial effusions has, frustratingly, not been shown to be helpful in distinguishing malignant from benign/idiopathic effusions, though it is still sensible to perform cytology and chemical analysis on fluid so removed. Occasionally animals presenting with infectious pericardial effusions and those with pericardial effusion due to lymphoma will be detected in this way.

In cases of pericardial effusion that recur, development of 'constrictive pericarditis' often occurs, whereby the pericardial sac becomes progressively thickened and 'leathery' and can afford progressively less distension before intrapericardial pressure increases and tamponade occurs. For this reason it is recommended to perform pericardiectomy in those patients with pericardial effusions that do occur. There is some debate as to whether to 'permit' a specific number of recurrences

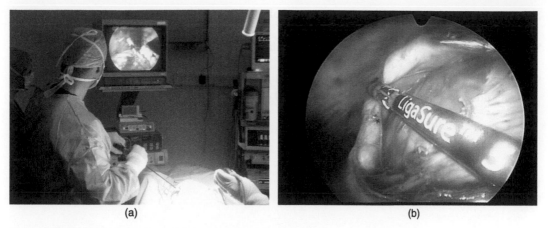

(a)

(b)

Figure 22.10 Thoracoscopic pericardiectomy being performed.

before making this recommendation, though it is the author's preference for this to be performed in any dog with recurrence since (a) it is very unlikely that only one recurrence will occur, (b) if the parietal pericardium becomes progressively thicker and more adherent to the visceral pericardium, removal may be more difficult and more traumatic and (c) it allows histological and surgical evaluation for occult neoplasia. An exception may be practical in those patients who are very aged at the time of initial diagnosis and who present with a recurrence only after a very prolonged period of time. Pericardiectomy may also be considered as a palliative procedure in those patients with cardiac tumours causing tamponade due to effusion, but the benefits of this are mostly seen in patients with heart base masses, which tend to be slow growing and in which tamponade due to effusion, rather than wide metastatic disease, tends to be the process most impacting on quality of life.

Subtotal pericardiectomy may be performed thoracoscopically (**Figure 22.10**) or by thoracotomy. Whilst some advocate performing a limited pericardial 'window' to aid drainage, the author believes that as much pericardial tissue as possible should be resected and this should always be submitted for histopathology. A proportion of animals undergoing subtotal pericardiectomy will develop recurrent pleural effusions that may require future drainage. This might be either because occult mesothelioma is present or because enough effusing pericardial tissue remains that the fluid produced overwhelms the capacity of thoracic vessels and lymphatics to absorb it. Post-operative administration of corticosteroids is advocated by some in an attempt to prevent this but clinical studies to document efficacy of this are lacking.

Surgical removal of right auricular appendage haemangiosarcomas may be attempted in carefully selected cases but peri-operative morbidity is high and median survival times, both with and without adjuvant chemotherapy, are poor and in many cases it may be inadvisable to attempt such surgery given the poor outcomes.

Further reading

MacDonald, K.A., Cagney, O. et al. (2009) Echocardiographic and clinicopathologic characterization of pericardial effusion in dogs: 107 cases (1985–2006). *J Am Vet Med Assoc* **235** (12), 1456–1461

Shaw, S P. and Rush, J.E. (2007) Canine pericardial effusion: pathophysiology and cause. *Compend Contin Educ Vet* **29** (7): 400–403; quiz 404

Shaw, S.P. and Rush, J.E. (2007) Canine pericardial effusion: diagnosis,treatment, and prognosis. *Compend Contin Educ Vet* **29** (7), 405–411

Stafford Johnson, M., M. Martin, M. et al. (2004) A retrospective study of clinical findings, treatment and outcome in 143 dogs with pericardial effusion. *J Small Anim Pract* **45** (11), 546–552

Clinical presentation

A 4 year-old female-neutered Boxer (**Figure 23.1**) is presented for a second opinion for investigation of shifting lameness, a heart murmur and lethargy. The dog has previously had investigation at another practice for a heart murmur, which has been noted since the dog was a puppy. Although no documentation is available, the owners report that a cardiologist has determined that the dog had valvular aortic stenosis of a mild gradient and had not recommended any therapy.

Three weeks ago the dog developed lameness of the left hindlimb. She was afebrile at this time and the dog's previously reported heart murmur was described at this time as grade II/VI, systolic and left-sided. A traumatic injury was suspected and a non-steroidal anti-inflammatory drug prescribed. Initial improvement was seen but the dog then re-presented with bilateral hindlimb lameness and fever of 40 °C. The heart murmur was reported again of similar amplitude. Antibiotic treatment with potentiated amoxycillin and further NSAID was prescribed and the dog appeared to improve again before re-presenting one week later. At this time the dog was no longer febrile but was reluctant to walk, being now lame on the left hind and right forelimb. The heart murmur

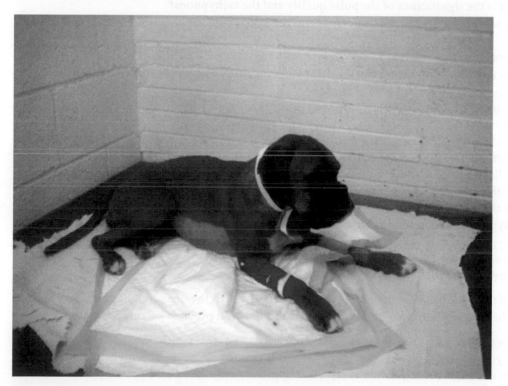

Figure 23.1 The patient at presentation.

Canine Internal Medicine: What's Your Diagnosis? First Edition. Jon Wray.
© 2018 John Wiley & Sons Ltd. Published 2018 by John Wiley & Sons Ltd.

is reported to have increased in amplitude and duration and the dog had developed tachypnoea. The owners report loss of body condition in the last 3 weeks and though the dog is still eating her appetite has decreased.

On physical examination the dog is very depressed, is in slightly poor body condition (body condition score 2/5) and has resting tachypnoea of 36/min with a restrictive (choppy) respiratory pattern. The dog walks with a stiff/stilted gait and appears uncomfortable when trying to lie or stand up and appears particularly lame on the left hindlimb and right forelimb. Manipulation of the left stifle and the right carpus appear to cause discomfort. Auscultation determines enhanced bronchovesicular sounds bilaterally and a grade V/VI systolic left basilar murmur with a grade III/VI diastolic left basilar murmur concurrently giving a continuous murmur sound. Heart rate is 140/min and the rhythm is regular. Femoral pulses are synchronous with the heart rate and are hyperdynamic in quality. Rectal temperature at this time is 39.6 °C.

Questions

1. **What is the problem list for this dog based on the history and physical examination findings?**
2. **What are the possible causes of persistent/recurrent pyrexia in the dog?**
3. **What are the possible causes of the heart murmur?**
4. **What is the significance of the pulse quality and the tachypnoea?**
5. **How would you investigate this case further?**

Answers

1. **What is the problem list for this dog based on the history and physical examination findings?**
    A problem list for this patient might be
    - Shifting lameness (currently involving left stifle and right carpus).
    - Pyrexia.
    - Tachypnoea further characterised as having a choppy/restrictive respiratory pattern and enhanced bronchovesicular sounds on auscultation.
    - A heart murmur, which was originally grade II/VI and systolic and which is now continuous with a peak intensity of grade V/VI and is described as having a point of maximal intensity at the left heart base.
    - Hyperdynamic femoral pulses.
    - Hyporexia.
    - Weight loss.
    - Depression/lethargy.

    Of these the heart murmur, the shifting lameness, the tachypnoea and the pyrexia are probably the most useful/pivotal problems upon which to base a problem-solving approach.

2. **What are the principle causes of persistent/recurrent pyrexia in the dog?**
    Hyperthermia is a raise in core body temperature above an acceptable normal upper reference limit (in dogs often accepted as approximately 39.3 °C). Fever or pyrexia defines hyperthermia that is due to 'resetting' of the anterior hypothalamic thermoregulatory centre 'set point' (or thermostat). This is distinct from those causes of hyperthermia that result in impaired heat dissipation or mechanical heat generation such as occurs in heat stroke, laryngeal paralysis, hypocalcaemic tetany, seizure activity, etc., and in which rapid external cooling (as well as attention to the underlying disease process) is necessary. Pyrexia may be initiated by exogenous pyrogens (infectious agents and their products, immune complexes,

products of inflammation, drugs) and endogenous pyrogens, which are substances elaborated by cells of the repertoire of the immune system; both are capable of altering the hypothalamic set-point.

When to investigate pyrexia of unknown origin

'Pyrexia (or fever) of unknown origin' (PUO) describes a situation of unremitting fever, without an immediately obvious cause, that is persistent. Whereas in human medicine PUO is often defined by the presence of fever lasting more than 3 weeks, no such universally accepted definition exists in veterinary medicine and descriptive studies performed in dogs list varying definitions of PUO (two descriptive studies of PUO patients at UK referral hospitals define as fever >40 °C on more than one occasion, or fever >39.7 °C mentioned as a reason for investigation). It is notable that in two large studies from the UK a diagnosis for a cause of fever was not made in approximately 1 in 5 patients and in one of these studies, of those patients in whom no diagnosis was made, fever resolved spontaneously about half of the time. The differential diagnosis for PUO is extensive and, in cases without localising signs on physical examination or history to proffer clues to aetiology, investigation can be lengthy and very costly. The author would always advise open and honest discussion with owners of animals with dogs with PUO in which the possibility of costly investigations coupled with a possibility of no diagnosis being made/spontaneous resolution of the inciting cause is candidly discussed. When to begin the investigation (rather than allowing observation time for spontaneous resolution in the setting of an ultimately self-limiting disease) can be a difficult clinical judgement and must be based on a degree of common-sense and serial assessment of the animal's physical examination status rather than be provoked by anxiety on the part of owner or veterinary surgeon, since injudicious investigation of such broad possibilities may expose animals to overly intrusive investigation that is ultimately unnecessary.

Those patients with PUO in whom a diagnosis is most easily and rapidly achieved are usually those whose physical examination or history proffers clues that localise the site of disease. For instance, animals with meningitides (who will usually have identifiable neck pain) or those with polyarthopathies (who usually exhibit pain and reluctance to move) will often allow a more rapid and targeted diagnostic approach. Where more broad-based investigation is necessary, if there are no localising signs, it is preferable to proceed in a logical and stepwise manner utilising those tests with least intrusiveness/patient impact first (see Further reading for a description of the investigative approach). The institution of empirical therapy such as antibiotic treatment or anti-inflammatory drugs is also a problematic decision since on the one hand (in the case of self-limiting fevers) this may hasten recovery but on the other hand one study demonstrated a prolongation of time to ultimate diagnosis in those patients who received treatment prior to definitive investigation. Certainly the author would advise against institution of therapy with corticosteroids if need for further investigation could be reasonably anticipated and would be desired by owners, since such treatment may delay some diagnostic efforts and obscure some differential diagnoses.

Common causes of PUO are listed in **Table 23.1**. In UK-based studies the two most common diagnoses made in cases referred for investigation of fever are of immune-mediated polyarthritis (IMPA) and inflammatory CNS disease/meningitides.

Table 23.1 *Common* differential diagnoses in PUO (based on two retrospective studies in the UK, Dunn and Dunn (1998) and Battersby and others (2006); also see Further reading). This list is not exhaustive and it is important to bear in mind that the differential diagnosis will be influenced, particularly in the case of infectious diseases, by regional and geographical variations. Transmissible infectious diseases are rather uncommon in the UK (those not found endemically are in parentheses) domestic animal population compared with many areas of the world.

Disease group	Approximate proportion of cases of PUO		Examples
	Dunn and Dunn (1998) ($n = 101$)	Battersby et al. (2006) ($n = 66$)	
Immune-mediated	22%*	33.3%	• Inflammatory CNS disease
			• Immune-mediated polyarthritis
			• Panniculitis
			• Masticatory muscle myositis
			• Immune-mediated haemolytic anaemia
			• Immune-mediated thrombocytopenia
			• Immune-mediated neutropenia
			• Uveitis
			• Pyogranulomatous inflammation
			• Systemic lupus erythematosus (SLE)
			• Vasculitis
Bone marrow	22%	Not reported**	• Myelodysplastic syndrome
			• Leukaemias
			• Multiple myeloma
Infectious	16%	27.2%	• Localised bacterial infections especially
			○ Lower urinary tract infection
			○ Prostatitis
			○ Pyelonephritis
			○ Pyometra
			○ Discospondylitis
			○ Cholecystitis
			○ Bronchopneumonia
			○ Endocarditis
			○ Pyothorax
			○ Osteomyelitis
			○ Septic arthritis
			○ Periodontal abscessation
			• Systemic bacterial infections especially
			○ Bartonellosis
			○ Leptospirosis

| Disease group | Approximate proportion of cases of PUO | | Examples |
	Dunn and Dunn (1998) ($n = 101$)	Battersby et al. (2006) ($n = 66$)	
			○ Mycobacteriosis
			○ Brucellosis
			○ L-form bacteria
			• Protozoal infections with
			○ *Toxoplasma gondii*
			○ *Neospora caninum*
			○ *Babesia* spp.
			○ (*Leishmania infantum*)
			• Fungal infections with
			○ *Aspergillus* spp. (both sinonasal and systemic infections)
			○ *Cryptococcus neoformans*
			○ *Pneumocystis jiroveci*
			○ *Candida* spp.
			○ (*Histoplasma capsulatum*)
			○ (*Coccidioides* spp.)
			○ (*Blastomyces dermatitidis*)
			• Rickettsial diseases
			○ Ehrlichiosis
			○ Anaplasmosis
			○ (Salmon poisoning disease)
			○ (Rocky mountain spotted fever)
Neoplastic	9.5%	7.5%	• Leukaemia
			• Lymphoma
			• Gastric neoplasia
			• Pulmonary neoplasia
			• Vertebral neoplasia
			• Bone metastases
			• Hypertrophic osteopathy secondary to pulmonary neoplasia
			• Metaphyseal osteopathy
			• Panosteitis
			• Shar pei fever
			• Bone infarction/necrosis

Disease group	Approximate proportion of cases of PUO		Examples
	Dunn and Dunn (1998) (*n* = 101)	Battersby et al. (2006) (*n* = 66)	
Miscellaneous	11.5%*	9%**	• Pancreatitis • Lymphadenitis • Pansteatitis • Intervertebral disc disease
Cause undetermined	19.5%	22.5%	

*In this study, 'meningitis' (3 cases) was included in the 'miscellaneous' grouping rather than immune-mediated, which was the designation in the later study.

**In this study, no separate designation for bone marrow disease was included and 2 cases of myelodysplatic syndrome are included in the 'miscellaneous' designation. Cases of leukaemia were included in the 'neoplastic' group in this study but in the 'bone marrow' group of Dunn and Dunn (1998).

3. What are the possible causes of the heart murmur?

Continuous heart murmurs

A continuous murmur is one that has both systolic and diastolic components with seemless progression between the two. Continuous murmurs are relatively uncommon in dogs and are usually reflective of either a communication between the arterial and venous systems or a valvular pathology that involves concurrent valvular stenosis and regurgitation.

Of the former, patent ductus arteriosus (PDA) is the most common cause of a continuous murmur and the murmur is usually harsh and has a 'machinery' timbre to it, having a point of maximal intensity at the left heart base. More rarely other types of arteriovenous fistula may create a continuous murmur.

Concurrent valvular stenosis and regurgitation is uncommon. Dysplasia of the atrioventricular valves may be characterised by both stenosis and regurgitation, especially mitral valve dysplasia. Stenosis of the AV valves may cause a diastolic murmur with a point of maximal intensity at the left or right cardiac apex (mitral and tricuspid stenosis respectively) though such murmurs are usually very soft if they are appreciated at all. A harsher systolic murmur of mitral or tricuspid insufficiency is more typically heard at the same sites.

Pulmonic stenosis and insufficiency may be present in congenital pulmonary valvular stenosis though the diastolic murmur of pulmonic insufficiency is rarely appreciated unless significant pulmonary hypertension is present. Diastolic murmurs originating from the aortic valve are usually most appreciated when significant aortic regurgitation due to valvular endocarditis is present. Such lesions often cause a degree of valvular stenosis, causing a harsh systolic ejection murmur of aortic stenosis, and a continuous murmur formed by these two components may be detected.

In this case the continuous murmur is described as having a point of maximal intensity at the heart base. The cardiac structures located in this region are the aortic and pulmonic valves and the arteries in which they are situated. Both PDA and aortic valvular endocarditis would cause continuous murmurs in this area but the dog has not been described as having a continuous murmur before, but has been evaluated as having mild aortic stenosis previously. The dog also has constitutional signs of illness (weight loss, pyrexia, hyporexia) as well as a change in the murmur intensity, all of which make aortic valvular endocarditis more likely than previously undiagnosed PDA.

4. **What is the significance of the pulse quality and the tachypnoea?**

'Hyperdynamic' pulses

Pulse quality is a reflection of the pulse pressure. Note that this is not a measure of arterial blood pressure but reflects the difference between systolic and diastolic blood pressure. Hyperdynamic pulses may be detected in some physiological and pathological states of high cardiac output such as exercise, fever, sepsis and hyperthyroidism and may also be detected when there is significant diastolic 'run-off' of blood during ventricular ejection. This may be present in patent ductus arteriosus (diastolic run-off occurs into the pulmonary circulation) and with significant aortic regurgitation (diastolic run-off occurs into the left ventricle).

The tachypnoea may be a reflection of the pyrexia and discomfort associated with lameness but should also alert the clinician to the possibility that, especially with the possibility of significant aortic regurgitation, the patient may be developing congestive heart failure.

5. **How would you investigate this case further?**
The shifting lameness is suggestive of a polyarthropathy and for discussion of differential diagnosis of polyarthritis and investigation of this the reader is referred to **Case 9** in this book.

However, in the setting of an intensifying heart murmur with continuous profile at the left heart base, fever and constitutional signs of illness, bacterial endocarditis of the aortic valve should be suspected. A suggested investigation might be

- Performance of haematology and serum biochemistry to detect inflammatory leukogram and potentially septic foci in other organs.
- Echocardiography.
- Thoracic radiography, principally to determine whether congestive heart failure is occurring.
- Blood cultures.
- Urine culture (by cystocentesis) since concurrent urinary tract infection caused by the same organism may be detected in endocarditis.
- Radiography of affected joints and synoviocentesis.

Blood cultures

Blood culture is important in trying to identify the causative organism of bacterial endocarditis though unfortunately negative cultures are reported in 42–70% of patients. Prior antimicrobial therapy and infection with *Bartonella*, an organism that is highly fastidious, may contribute to false negative cultures. Ideally 3–4 samples should be collected by aseptic venepuncture of surgically prepared sites, taken at least 30 min to 1 hour apart and preferably when the dog is pyrexic. Adequate volumes of blood (5–10 ml) should be collected and directly inoculated in a sterile manner into an appropriate culture medium for aerobic and anaerobic blood cultures. Bartonella is usually detected by identifying serum titres >1:1024 or by positive PCR, though false negatives are common with the latter.

Diagnosis

In this patient, haematology demonstrated a mild inflammatory leukogram only and serum biochemistry was essentially normal. Echocardiography demonstrated a very abnormal aortic valve with a 'shaggy/ragged' appearance due to vegetative lesions (**Figure 23.2**). A very large degree of aortic regurgitation was seen during diastole and severe aortic stenosis due to the valvular vegetative lesions was seen with a peak trans-stenotic pressure gradient of 88 mmHg (**Figures 22.3 and 23.4**). End-diastolic left ventricular dimensions were increased. No valvular lesions of the mitral valve, pulmonic valve or tricuspid valve were identified and mitral insufficiency was not appreciated.

Thoracic radiographs demonstrated no evidence of congestive heart failure. Radiographs of the carpi and stifles demonstrated absence of erosive changes and mild joint effusions of the right carpus and left stifle. Synoviocentesis samples from these joints demonstrated an increased white cell count of approximately 5400/µl (<1000) with a predominance of non-degenerate neutrophils. Joint fluid culture was negative.

Blood cultures yielded a pure growth of *Enterococcus faecium* from two samples with widespread sensitivity against a variety of antimicrobial agents, in particular most beta-lactam antibiotics, cefalosporins and fluoroquinolones, but resistance to trimethoprim sulphonamide. Serology for *Bartonella* spp. was negative.

A diagnosis of bacterial aortic valvular endocarditis with either reactive (Type II) immune-mediated polyarthritis or bacterial polyarthritis was made.

Treatment and outcome

Therapy was instituted with intravenous potentiated-amoxycillin and enrofloxacin whilst pending blood culture results.

Unfortunately 48 hours after commencement of therapy the dog developed acute onset rapidly progressive neurological signs comprising altered consciousness, decerebrate rigidity and subsequent cardiorespiratory arrest from which resuscitation was not successful. Septic or non-septic thromboembolisation of the CNS was suspected to be the cause of this event.

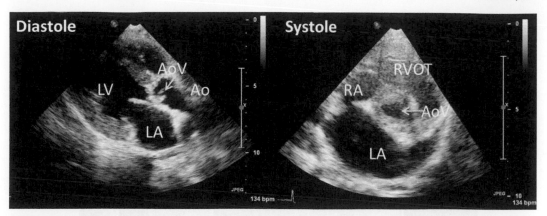

Figure 23.2 Right parasternal long-axis view of left ventricular outflow (left) and right parasternal short-axis view at level of aortic valve (right). The valve (arrows, AoV) can be seen to be thickened and irregular and on the systolic short-axis view the lumen of the aorta is reduced in size. LV = left ventricle, LA = left atrium, RA = right atrium, AoV = aortic valve, RVOT = right ventricular outflow tract.

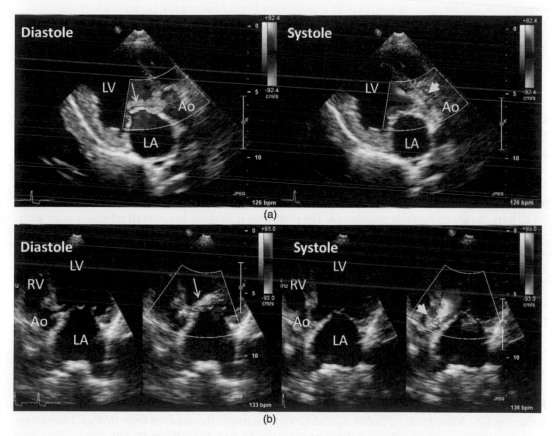

Figure 22.3 Top row: right parasternal long-axis view of left ventricular outflow tract showing diastolic aortic regurgitation (arrow, left image) and systolic aortic stenosis (arrowhead, right image). Bottom row: left caudal parasternal 5 chamber inflow–outflow view showing diastolic aortic regurgitation (arrow, left image) and systolic aortic stenosis (arrowhead, right image).

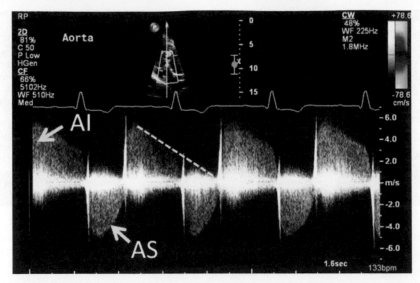

Figure 23.4 Continuous wave (CW) Doppler of aortic valve from a subcostal site. Severe aortic stenosis (AS) and aortic insufficiency (AI) profiles are seen, which are the causes of the systolic and diastolic component of the continuous heart murmur respectively. The slope of the aortic insufficiency (dashed line) abruptly decreases, reflecting a rapid rise in the diastolic left ventricular pressure and subsequent decrease in the pressure gradient across the aortic valve during diastole due to the severe aortic insufficiency.

Discussion

Bacterial endocarditis is uncommon in dogs but may be underrecognised as clinical signs may be highly variable. The mitral and aortic valves are most commonly affected and predisposing factors include presence of congenital valvular heart disease, especially aortic stenosis. The most common bacterial isolates are *Staphylococci* and *Streptococci*, though a variety of bacteria have been associated with endocarditis and the importance of *Bartonella* spp., which are uncommonly identified on culture, has been recently recognised. The prognosis is variable but overall relatively poor with a reported mortality rate of 56% and median survival time of 54 days; nonetheless, long-term survival, especially with mitral valve endocarditis, is possible. Severe aortic valve endocarditis often carries a poor prognosis and heart failure due to severe aortic insufficiency commonly develops. Septic and non-septic embolisation to other organs and development of concurrent immune-mediated disease, especially immune-mediated polyarthritis and immune-mediated glomerulonephritis and subsequent protein-losing nephropathy, are commonly reported complications. CNS embolisation may cause acute deterioration in some patients and post-mortem studies in dogs that have succumbed to infective endocarditis have shown a high prevalence of suppurative meningitis and vasculitis.

References

Battersby, I.A., Murphy, K.F., Tasker, S. et al. (2006). Retrospective study of fever in dogs: laboratory testing, diagnoses and influence of prior treatment. *J Small Anim Pract* **47**, 370–376

Dunn, K.J. & Dunn, J.K. (1998) Diagnostic investigations in 101 dogs with pyrexia of unknown origin. *J Small Anim Pract* 39, 574–580

Further reading

Flood, J. (2009) The diagnostic approach to fever of unknown origin in dogs. *Compendium Cont Educ* **31**, 14–20; quiz 20–11, E11–13

Macdonald, K. (2010) Infective endocarditis in dogs: diagnosis and therapy. *Vet Clin North Am Small Anim Pract* **40**, 665–684

Miller, M.W., Fox, P.R. & Saunders, A.B. (2004) Pathologic and clinical features of infectious endocarditis. *J Vet Cardiol* **6**, 35–43

Peddle, G. & Sleeper, M.M. (2007) Canine bacterial endocarditis: a review. *J Am Anim Hosp Assoc* **43**, 258–263

Sykes, J.E., Kittleson, M.D., Pesavento, P.A., Byrne, B.A., MacDonald, K.A. & Chomel, B.B. (2006) Evaluation of the relationship between causative organisms and clinical characteristics of infective endocarditis in dogs: 71 cases (1992–2005). *J Am Vet Med Assoc* **228**, 1723–1734

Sykes, J.E., Kittleson, M.D., Chomel, B.B., Macdonald, K.A. & Pesavento, P.A. (2006) Clinicopathologic findings and outcome in dogs with infective endocarditis: 71 cases (1992–2005). *J Am Vet Med Assoc* **228**, 1735–1747

Wall, M., Calvert, C.A., Greene, C.E. (2002) Infective endocarditis in dogs. *Compend Contin Educ Vet* **24**, 614–625

Urology and Nephrology

Canine Internal Medicine: What's Your Diagnosis? First Edition. Jon Wray.
© 2018 John Wiley & Sons Ltd. Published 2018 by John Wiley & Sons Ltd.

Clinical presentation

A 4 year-old female-neutered Boxer (**Figure 24.1**) is presented for investigation of azotaemia due to findings on laboratory testing preceding any such suspicion. The current owners obtained the dog, already neutered, as a 'rescue' two years previously and report that she has always been in a very thin body condition and has had a variable appetite with more recent episodic vomiting. The dog's exercise tolerance remains very good. The owners feel that the dog has always drunk and urinated copiously but no episodes of dysuria or incontinence have been reported. A colleague examined the dog the previous week after an acute onset left hindlimb lameness occurring during vigorous exercise and suspected to be due to cranial cruciate ligament rupture. A blood sample had been taken prior to proposed surgical treatment of this and shows the following:

Haematology

Parameter	Value	Units	Range
RBC	**3.1**	$\times 10^{12}$/l	(5.5–8.5)
Haemoglobin	**7.4**	g/dl	(12.0–18.0)
Haematocrit	**0.24**	l/l	(0.37–0.55)
Mean cell volume	**78**	fl	(60–77)
Mean cell haemoglobin concentration	30.6	g/dl	(30.0–38.0)
Mean cell haemoglobin	23.9	pg	(19.5–25.5)
Total white cell count	6	$\times 10^9$/l	(6.0–15.0)
Neutrophils	4.3	$\times 10^9$/l	(3.0–11.5)
Lymphocytes	**0.8**	$\times 10^9$/l	(1.0–4.8)
Monocytes	0.4	$\times 10^9$/l	(0.2–1.4)
Eosinophils	0.5	$\times 10^9$/l	(0.1–1.2)
Basophils	0	$\times 10^9$/l	(0.0–0.1)
Platelets	314	$\times 10^9$/l	(200–500)
Film comment:		Anaemia appears to be normocytic, normochromic	

Canine Internal Medicine: What's Your Diagnosis? First Edition. Jon Wray.
© 2018 John Wiley & Sons Ltd. Published 2018 by John Wiley & Sons Ltd.

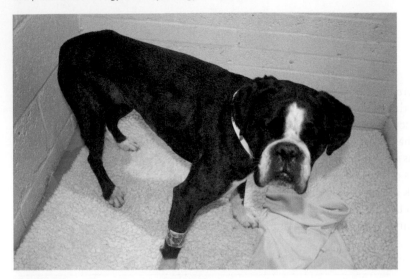

Figure 24.1 The patient at presentation.

Biochemistry

Parameter	Value	Units	Range
Total protein	59	g/l	(54–77)
Albumin	25	g/l	(25–40)
Globulin	34	g/l	(23–45)
Urea	**61**	mmol/l	(2.5–7.4)
Creatinine	**890**	mmol/l	(40–145)
Potassium	5	mmol/l	(3.4–5.6)
Sodium	149	mmol/l	(139–154)
Chloride	105	mmol/l	(105–122)
Calcium	2.2	mmol/l	(2.1–2.8)
Magnesium	–	mmol/l	(0.62–0.90)
Inorganic phosphate	**5.2**	mmol/l	(0.60–1.40)
Glucose	5	mmol/l	(3.3–5.8)
ALT	83	IU/l	(13–88)
AST	44	IU/l	(13–60)
ALKP	99	IU/l	(14–105)
GGT	5	IU/l	(0–10)
Bilirubin	2	mmol/l	(0–16)
Cholesterol	**9.6**	mmol/l	(3.8–7.0)
Triglyceride	1.1	mmol/l	(0.56–1.14)
Creatine kinase	167	IU/l	(0–190)

On physical examination the dog is in poor body condition (condition score 2/5) but is very bright and interactive and 2/10 lame on the left hindlimb palpation, which demonstrates some mild articular swelling of the stifle joint. Mucous membranes are pale pink with normal moistness and capillary refill of <2 seconds. Heart rate is 96/min with normal sinus rhythm, no abnormalities of auscultation and with synchronous peripheral pulses of normal quality. Abdominal palpation is unremarkable; it is not possible to discern normal renal structures on palpation.

Questions

1. Where is the likely source of this dog's medical problem and is it likely to be acute or chronic?
2. What is the most likely differential diagnosis and how could this be confirmed?
3. What are the likely consequences of the primary problem that should be medically addressed and how would you treat this patient?

Answers

1. **Where is the likely source of this dog's medical problem and is it likely to be acute or chronic?**

   The principle laboratory findings are of a severe azotaemia and moderate normocytic normochromic anaemia. The relative proportion of increase in the urea is similar in proportion to the elevation in creatinine.

Azotaemia

Azotaemia (elevation in urea, creatinine or both due to decreased glomerular filtration rate, GFR) may be described as pre-renal, renal or post-renal. It should be distinguished from uraemia, which is a clinical syndrome of ill-health resulting from advanced kidney disease. Pre-renal azotaemia is most commonly associated with decreased renal blood flow most commonly due to hypovolaemia and the physical examination is key in determining this likelihood; in this case the patient is normocardic and has no evidence of dehydration. Furthermore, pre-renal azotaemia is usually characterised by a greater proportional increase in the magnitude of elevation of urea versus creatinine, since the former is reabsorbed in the proximal tubule in states of diminished renal blood flow. It would also be somewhat unusual for creatinine to be elevated to such a degree in such circumstances. Post-renal azotaemia is usually caused by obstructive disease and the lack of clinical signs of lower urinary tract disease (such as dysuria, pollakiuria) makes this less likely. An intrinsic renal problem is therefore suspected. Contemporaneous assessment of urine specific gravity should, wherever possible, accompany assessment of urea and creatinine in order to elucidate further. Specific gravity varies considerably from hour-to-hour in the dog. It is a common cause of misapprehension that there really is no such thing as a 'normal' urine specific gravity and that specific gravity merely reflects renal tubular ability to respond to antidiuretic hormone. It is more pertinent to consider in the context of whether it is appropriate for the patient's physiological fluid-balance circumstances at the time of assessment. In the dog, urine SG in the range <1.008 indicates hyposthenuria, 1.008–1.012 represents isosthenuria, 1.013–1.029 represents the range of minimal concentration and ≥1.030 represents adequate concentrating ability.

Hyperphosphataemia is most commonly caused by decreased urinary phosphate excretion (though it can also be seen in intoxication with vitamin D products, in acidosis and where acute shifts from the intracellular to extracellular compartment arise) and may be seen in the setting of most causes of azotaemia whether acute or chronic. However, commonly persistent and marked elevations tend to be seen in animals with long-standing reduction in glomerular filtration rate. Similarly, a normocytic, normochromic anaemia, if related to renal disease, most commonly is due to chronic kidney disease.

Lastly, interpretation of laboratory abnormalities must *always* be undertaken in the context of the history and physical examination. Here the patient is 'constitutionally' well and has been noted to be in a thin condition over a long period of time, rather than presenting with sudden weight loss and signs of inappetence. Were such a magnitude of azotaemia to have developed suddenly, common-sense would dictate that the patient ought to be considerably less well.

A chronic, intrinsic renal problem is therefore most likely.

2. **What is the most likely differential diagnosis and how could this be confirmed?**

In addition to stating that the condition is likely to be chronic (commonly defined as having been in existence >3 months) we might reasonably surmise that if the patient has been in a thin body condition since being obtained 2 years previously that the underlying condition may have been present at least as long.

Furthermore, whilst anaemia of chronic kidney disease may develop in dogs with advanced disease, this generally takes a prolonged time to develop.

Chronic kidney disease is often identified only at a stage where the process initiating primary kidney injury is no longer identifiable. Histologically, the most common pathologic findings in biopsies from canine patients with chronic kidney disease is tubulointerstitial nephritis, but this is a pathological consequence, not a disease entity in its own right. Causes of chronic kidney disease are listed in **Table 24.1**.

Given the time-course of clinical signs and the well-compensated status of the patient, **juvenile kidney disease (JKD) of the boxer** is the most likely cause.

Investigation should include

- Urinalysis and culture with assessment of urine protein:creatinine.
- Assessment of renal architecture by diagnostic ultrasound examination.

Further investigations to exclude contributory causes and to stage the extent of both the primary problem and its sequelae, such as *Leptospira* spp. serology, measurement of systemic blood pressure, skeletal and abdominal radiography and measurement of parathyroid hormone, may all be justified but are unlikely to contribute to determining the cause of the chronic kidney disease.

Renal biopsy is, by definition, directly injurious to the diseased kidney(s) and undertaking of a biopsy must be considered in the context of the likelihood of information gained being directly beneficial to the patient by informing therapeutic decisions. In the case of juvenile kidney disease, renal biopsy may not distinguish ultrastructural changes from those of other end-stage kidney diseases and diagnosis on the basis of ultrasound and signalment is generally considered acceptable.

3. **What are the likely consequences of the primary problem that should be medically addressed and how would you treat this patient?**

A number of effects/sequelae to chronic kidney disease (of any aetiology) may be predicted and in some cases such changes may also represent independent risk factors for progression of the underlying disease (see **Table 24.2**).

Table 24.1 Differential diagnosis of chronic kidney disease (CKD) in dogs

Familial or congenital renal disease	Renal dysplasia (may be seen in any breed)
	• Juvenile kidney disease (JKD) of the Boxer
	• Familial in the Golden Retriever, Shih Tzu, Lhasa Apso, Elkhound, Chow Chow, Standard Poodle, Alaskan Malamute
	Amyloidosis in the Shar Pei, Foxhound, Beagle
	Polycystic kidney disease in the Cairn Terrier, English Bull Terrier, West Highland White Terrier
	Hereditary nodular dermatofibrosis/renal cystadenocarcinoma syndrome in German Shepherd Dogs
	Telangiectasia in the Pembroke Welsh Corgi
	Fanconi syndrome in the Basenji
	Familial glomerulonephropathy
	• Soft-coated Wheaten Terrier, English Cocker Spaniel, Rottweiler, Dobermann Pinscher, Samoyed, Bull Terrier, Bull Mastiff, Bernese Mountain Dog, Beagle, Brittany Spaniel
Acquired	Infectious
	• Bacterial
	○ Chronic pyelonephritis
	○ Leptospirosis
	• Protozoal
	○ Leishmaniasis
	• Mycotic
	Hypercalcaemia-induced
	Sequel to chronic obstruction
	• Obstructive nephro- or ureterolithiasis
	• Bladder urothelial carcinoma
	• Spay granuloma
	Proteinuric renal disease
	• Amyloidosis
	• Primary glomerulonephropathies
	• Secondary glomerulonephropathies
	Chronic nephrotoxin exposure
	• Prescribed drugs, e.g. NSAIDs
	• Poisoning
	Neoplasia
	• Renal cell carcinoma
	• Nephroblastoma
	• (Lymphoma – usually acute renal failure)
	As part of/sequel to
	• Sequel of acute renal failure
	• Polysystemic immune-mediated disease
	• Chronic renal ischaemia

Table 24.2 Consequences of chronic kidney disease

Predictable or frequent consequences of chronic kidney disease
• Uraemia
• Uraemic gastropathy
• Renal secondary hyperparathyroidism
• Metabolic acidosis
• Hypertension
• Proteinuria
• Chronic anaemia
• Vulnerability to urinary tract infections

As part of the initial assessment of all patients with chronic kidney disease it is recommended by the International Renal Interest Society (IRIS) that the following are undertaken in order to 'stage' both the severity and consequences of chronic kidney disease (**Figure 24.2**):

- Blood urea nitrogen, creatinine and phosphate
- PCV or haematocrit
- Systolic blood pressure
- Urinalysis including biochemistry, sediment examination, urine protein:creatinine ratio and culture

For an in-depth discussion of management of chronic kidney disease see the website of the International Renal Interest Society (IRIS) http://www.iris-kidney.com/:

- Nutritional therapy to reduce uraemia and perhaps retard progression of disease
    - Efficacy has been shown in randomised controlled clinical trials in IRIS stage II and III
        - Risk of uraemic crisis reduction by 75% compared with dogs eating a maintenance diet

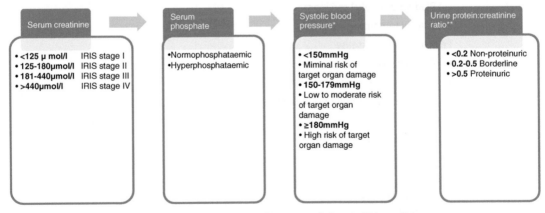

Figure 24.2 International Renal Interest Society (IRIS) staging of chronic kidney disease.

* Systolic blood pressure should always be evaluated after evaluation for extrarenal evidence of target organ damage such as hypertensive retinopathy. It is very common for hypertension to be overdiagnosed in anxious, unacclimatised canine patients and it is essential that strict guidelines are followed in diagnosis of hypertension, that a self-critical technique is employed and that findings are unequivocally shown to be reproducible, persistent and invariable before treatment decisions are made. Inappropriate treatment of normotensive patients with antihypertensive drug therapy may be just as deleterious to renal function as not treating hypertensive renal patients.

** Should always be interpreted in the light of examination of urine sediment.

- Median symptom-free survival of 615 days in dogs fed a renal diet versus 252 days for dogs fed an adult maintenance diet
- Limiting dietary protein reduces waste products of protein catabolism contributing to uraemia. It has not been demonstrated that protein-restriction *per se* limits progression of chronic kidney disease (and for that matter it should not be considered that feeding a 'normal' protein diet worsens kidney disease more rapidly).
- Reduction in dietary phosphorus (most of which is protein-derived) reduces phosphate retention and renal secondary hyperparathyroidism, maintains calcitriol and reduced renal mineralisation. Some evidence to support that dietary phosphate restriction retards progression of CKD.
- Omega-3 polyunsaturated fatty acid supplementation has been shown to reduce glomerulosclerosis, proteinuria, interstitial inflammation and tubulointerstitial fibrosis in dogs and most diets formulated for chronic kidney disease are supplemented with Omega-3 PUFA.
- Whilst not thought to be a major contributing uraemic toxin, blood urea nitrogen, since it is produced by protein turnover, is a reasonable barometer of dietary compliance in dogs fed renal diets (though gastrointestinal haemorrhage may contribute to elevations in this).

Important rules of thumb to bear in mind when introducing renal diets

- This should never be done hurriedly if the patient is inappetent or suffering effects of uraemic gatropathy. Not only are the beneficial effects of renal diets realised over months, rather than days, but injudicious attempts to introduce renal diets – *which are the single measure shown to impact on life-expectancy to a greater extent than any other medical measure* – may potentially dissuade both patient and owner from future feeding of such a diet. It is always therefore better to wait until animals are eating well before introducing a change of diet and to do so gradually.
- It is incumbent on the clinician not to cease attempts at dietary therapy simply because the first diet chosen is rejected.
- Conversely, reduction in dietary intake that causes loss of lean muscle mass contribute to uraemia and acidosis and must be assiduously avoided – it is better for a patient to receive a normal maintenance adult diet than a specific renal diet that is only consumed in quantities that result in protein malnutrition.

- Management of uraemic gastropathy (**Figure 24.3**)
  - Reduced appetite, nausea, vomiting, stomatitis and ulcer-induced gastrointestinal upset may result from both the effects of uraemic toxins and perhaps gastrointestinal effects of reduced gastrin excretion and effects of soft tissue mineralisation in severely hyperphosphataemic animals.
  - Evidence of gastric hyperacidity in dogs with chronic kidney disease is sparse and gastrointestinal ulceration is more often suspected rather than proven.
  - Management of uraemic gastropathy with H2 antagonists such as famotidine, ranitidine or cimetidine combined with an antiemetic (metoclopramide or maropitant are most frequently used) has been recommended, and mucosal barrier agents such as sucralfate may be useful.

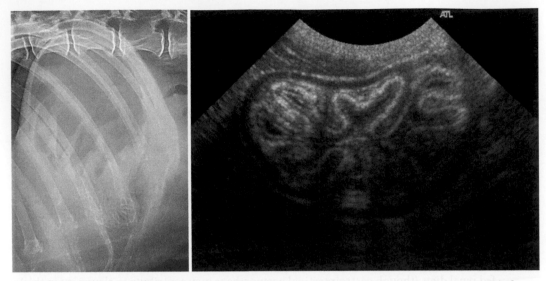

Figure 24.3 Lateral abdominal radiograph (left) and abdominal ultrasound (right) showing gastric calcification in a dog with uraemic gastropathy.

- ○ Uraemic stomatitis may be managed with dilute chlorhexidine-based oral preparations.
- • Hyperphosphataemia and renal secondary hyperparathyroidism
  - ○ Retention of phosphorus by declining glomerular filtration rate and proximal reabsorption is initially compensated for by decreased phosphorus reabsorption in surviving nephrons and the phosphaturic effects of PTH and fibroblast growth factor 23.
  - ○ Calcitriol (activated vitamin D, produced by hydroxylation of 25-hydroxycholecalciferol in renal tubular cells under the activity of 1α hydroxylase) levels decline early in renal disease, 1α hydroxylase activity is inhibited by FGF-23 and phosphorus retention and calcitriol production is further decreased by loss of renal tubular cells.
  - ○ PTH (which promotes 1α hydroxylase activity and formation of calcitriol) becomes elevated (calcitriol normally inhibits this) but this activity, which initially maintains calcitriol at the expense of elevated PTH, becomes exhausted quickly.
  - ○ Renal osteodystrophy with demineralisation of the bones of the skull and mandible is seen infrequently in dogs with chronic kidney disease and is seen most frequently in juvenile animals with congenital kidney disease.
  - ○ Elevated serum phosphate has been shown to be predictive of mortality in dogs with CKD and minimising phosphorus retention appears to prolong survival in CKD.
  - ○ When phosphorus elevations are marked and the product of calcium and phosphorus exceeds 6 mmol/l, calcium hydrogen phosphate (brushite) precipitation in proton-secreting organs such as the stomach and kidneys may occur.
  - ○ Initially dietary phosphate restriction is the most valuable means of reducing phosphate retention. Addition of phosphate 'binders' can also be considered, which is best achieved in conjunction with dietary therapy and given at times of feeding. Aluminium hydroxide and calcium carbonate or acetate-containing products are effective in binding phosphate, but the former are increasingly elusive to obtain and care must be taken with calcium-containing products that calcium absorption so resulting does not contribute to secondary soft tissue mineralisation, especially when calcitriol (see below) is also given. Newer agents

such as lanthanum salts and sevelamer hydrochloride have advantages of not inducing hypercalcaemia but reduction in vitamin K levels is a theoretical risk.

- o Some authorities recommend oral supplementation with calcitriol in an attempt to ame-liorate calcitriol level decline and resultant hyperparathyroidism (**Figure 24.4**). Propo-nents cite improved clinical demeanour and activity in calcitriol-treated dogs and there is evidence in the human field for a beneficial effect of calcitriol administration; objective peer-reviewed data supporting its use in veterinary medicine is currently lacking.

- Metabolic acidosis
  - o Metabolic acidosis appears to occur infrequently in dogs and cats with compensated stage II and III renal disease but is more common in those patients with overt signs of uraemia.
  - o Most renal diets are either neutral or alkalinising in terms of their acid effect and feeding such diets may be helpful in reducing the incidence of acidosis.
  - o Oral sodium bicarbonate or potassium citrate administration may be helpful with a target or maintaining serum bicarbonate levels between 18 and 25 meq/l, but treatment goals, thresholds to introduce treatment and beneficial outcome data are lacking.

- Management of hypertension
  - o Approximately 60% of dogs with chronic kidney disease have systemic hypertension.
  - o The mechanism by which this develops is obscure but may include inappropriate afferent arterial vasodilation, increased renin–angiotensin–aldosterone secretion and diminished sodium excretion.
  - o End-organ damage to the eyes (hypertensive retinopathy), heart (ventricular hypertro-phy) and CNS (haemorrhagic stroke) may result but hypertension is also an independent risk factor for progressive renal disease.
  - o For guidelines on measurement of blood pressure in dogs, see the ACVIM consensus statement in Brown et al. (2007).
  - o Many texts advocate the use of angiotensin converting enzyme (ACE) inhibitors such as benazepril for the management of hypertension but clinical experience in both dogs and cats would suggest that this is largely ineffective in restoring normotension in genuinely hypertensive patients.

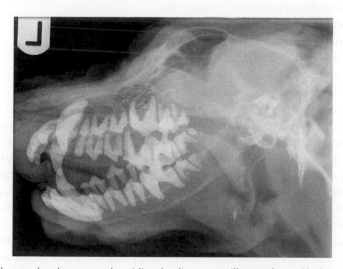

Figure 24.4 Renal secondary hyperparathyroidism leading to maxillary and mandibular osteopenia.

- ○ The dihydropyridine calcium-channel blocker amlodipine, given at a dose of 0.1–0.2 mg/kg p/o SID, increasing up to 0.5 mg/kg p/o BID to effect, is much more effective in management of hypertension in dogs.
- Proteinuria
  - ○ Presence of proteinuria has been shown to be an independent risk factor for progression of chronic kidney disease and signifies reduction in glomerular 'permselectivity'. It is essential that assessment of urine protein is undertaken in conjunction with sediment examination as lower urinary tract inflammation will increase urine protein. Significant proteinuria is frequently seen in dogs with untreated hyperadrenocorticism and with immune-mediated polyarthritis and presence of either of these conditions should mandate reassessment of urine protein after treatment.
  - ○ The mainstay of therapy aimed at reducing proteinuria has been combining renal diets with use of ACE inhibitors. The preferential efferent arterial dilatation of the glomerulus by angiotensin II reduction may be one mechanism in which glomerular filtration pressure and subsequent proteinuria is reduced but effects of ACE inhibitors on downstream aldosterone production may also be beneficial in retarding progression of local vascular and interstitial remodelling in renal injury.
  - ○ Whilst studies in veterinary medicine documenting the benefits of ACE inhibitors are sparse, those studies (which primarily evaluate severe proteinuria in glomerulonephritis) performed show a modest reduction in proteinuria, which is more marked with more severe proteinuria. Clinical experience would suggest that significant variability in proteinuria may exist from day to day in patients with chronic renal disease, which makes objective assessment of therapeutic efficacy difficult, and that similarly very modest effects on proteinuria are expected rather than resolution.
  - ○ There is increasing interest in combining ACE inhibitors with angiotensin receptor blocking agents since angiotensin production through non-ACE-dependent means (e.g. local chymase activity) may occur.
- Anaemia
  - ○ Anaemia in chronic kidney disease may be multifactorial and may be contributed to by
    - Lack of erythropoietin production by diseased kidneys
    - Blood loss through uraemic gastropathy
    - Iron deficiency
    - Hyperparathyroidism causing
      - -- Eyrthropoeitin resistance
      - -- Decreased red blood cell lifespan
      - -- Myelofibrosis of bone marrow
    - Increased red blood cell osmotic fragility
  - ○ Whilst it is common to detect a mild normocytic normochromic non-regenerative anaemia of haematocrit 0.28–0.37 l/l in dogs with chronic kidney disease it is somewhat less common to detect moderate or severe anaemias. When seen, these are usually in animals with long-standing compensated chronic kidney disease such as due to congenital dysplasia or juvenile nephropathies. In adult-acquired chronic kidney disease, signs of uraemia are usually so severe by the time clinically impactful anaemia develops that euthanasia due to the former is undertaken.
  - ○ When anaemia is profound enough to be associated with clinical signs, usually in dogs with CKD at haematocrits <0.20 l/l or so, direct therapy may be considered. In less severe anaemia and where clinical signs associated with reduced tissue oxygen delivery are not seen, and considering the inherent drawbacks of direct therapy, treatment is usually not recommended.

- Assessment for and speculative treatment of uraemic gastropathic bleeding is usually undertaken with a combination of sucralfate and antacid therapy. Iron deficiency may be treated with ferrous sulphate at a dose of 200 mg/dog/day p/o.
- Blood transfusion with type-compatible packed red blood cells or whole blood may be undertaken.
- Hormone replacement therapy may be undertaken with either
  - Recombinant human erythropoietin (Eprex) at a dose of 100 units/kg s.c. three times weekly or
  - Darbepoietin (Aranesp) at a dose of 1.5 µg/kg s.c. once weekly

Iron supplementation should be undertaken with hormone replacement therapy and regular monitoring of haematocrit and systolic blood pressure undertaken to avoid complications of polycythaemia and hypertension respectively. Restoration of haematocrit to low normal values usually takes 4–8 weeks.

Darbepoietin is preferred over erythropoietin due to the risk of antierythropoietin antibodies developing and subsequent worsening of anaemia with the latter. The risk of cross-reactive antibody development with darbepoietin therapy is not well established in veterinary medicine.

Diagnosis and treatment
- Urinalysis in this patient was undertaken from a cystocentesis sample:

Urinalysis

Parameter	Value	Units	Range
Appearance	Clear, very pale yellow		
Chemistry			
Specific gravity	1.010		
pH	6		
Protein	I I		
Nitrite	Negative		
Blood/Hb	Negative		
Glucose	Negative		
Ketones	Negative		
Bilirubin	Negative		
Urobilinogen	Negative		
Cytology			
Red cells	0	/hpf	(0–2)
White cells	0	/hpf	(0–2)
Epithelial cells	1	/hpf	(0–5)
Casts	Small numbers of hyaline casts		
Crystals	Negative		
Bacteria	Negative		
Other			
Quantitative protein			
Urine protein:creatinine	**2.6**	Ratio	<0.5

- ◦ Urine was isosthenuric and the small number of hyaline casts represent protein of renal origin. A urine protein:creatinine of 2.6 in the absence of an inflammatory urine sediment is significant and suggests decreased renal glomerular 'permselectivity'.
- ◦ Urine culture was negative.
- Orthogonal abdominal radiographs demonstrated lack of peritoneal detail due to reduced body composition and neither renal outline could be determined on either a VD or right lateral projection.
- Abdominal ultrasound (**Figure 24.5**) demonstrated both kidneys to be small (left kidney 3.6 cm in length and right kidney 6 cm in length) with lack of corticomedullary definition, bilateral pyelectasia and loss of normal architecture with bands of hyperechoic cortical echogenicity interspersed with more hypoechoic areas.
- Serial systolic blood pressure assessments were undertaken with oscillometry with a cuff of >40% of the limb circumference in width placed on the left antebrachium, which was at the level of the right atrium. Three sets of measurements with six measurements/set were performed over the course of one day with a variability between the highest and lowest measurements of 12%. Average systolic pressure was 174 mmHg.
- Renal biopsy was not performed.

A presumptive diagnosis of either **renal dysplasia** or **juvenile kidney disease (JKD) of the Boxer** was made.

The patient received the following treatment:

- In light of the recent vomition, a presumptive diagnosis of uraemic gastropathy was made and treatment instituted with
  - ◦ Famotidine 0.8 mg/kg p/o BID.
  - ◦ Metoclopramide 0.5 mg/kg p/o TID.
- Once the patient was eating her normal diet consistently, gradual change to a renal diet (Purina NF canned) with a dry matter content of protein 20.3%, fat 26.6%, carbohydrate 46.7%, calcium 0.66%, phosphate 0.28% and total omega-6 PUFA 4.34%.
- Benazepril was introduced at a dose of 0.4 mg/kg p/o SID due to both proteinuria and hypertension.

Re-evaluation of blood pressure and proteinuria was scheduled after 2 weeks and restaging of serum biochemistry, serial systolic blood pressure and urinalysis every 3 months thereafter.

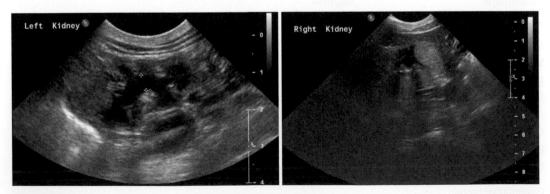

Figure 24.5 Ultrasound of the left and right kidneys in the patient.

Discussion

Both kidneys were small, dysplastic and end-stage in this patient and biopsy was not undertaken since it was viewed that the risk of renal decompensation versus the lack of likely information that would alter therapeutic options was too high.

A syndrome of renal disease in juvenile Boxers with onset of clinical signs of uraemia below 5 years of age (median 2 years in one study) identified with bilateral small, architecturally distorted end-stage kidneys has been reported mainly in the UK and in Scandinavia. Cases are principally identified due to onset of clinical signs of uraemia or due to finding of azotaemia as an incidental finding on a blood sample taken for other purposes. Previously renal dysplasia has been reported in young Boxer puppies (Hoppe and Karlstam 2000). Renal dysplasia is characterised histologically by the presence of persistent metanephric ducts and other foetal or immature ultrastructural components surrounded by primitive mesenchyma. In more recent studies in older juvenile boxers in the UK, though renal histopathology findings were reported in only a minority of cases, findings were not consistent with renal dysplasia but with pericapsular and interstitial fibrosis, mononuclear inflammation, tubular dilatation and sclerotic glomeruli (Chandler et al. 2007). However, in a pathological study of seven Boxer dogs in Norway presenting at a similar age and with similar clinicopathological findings, lesions consistent with some features of renal dysplasia were present in all kidneys in addition to sharply demarcated areas of cortical fibrosis, abundant narrow, hyperplastic small arteries and tubular atrophy with abundant tubular or glomerular microcysts. However, an additionally diffuse interstitial mononuclear inflammation was seen in all kidneys and pelvic luminal pus containing tubular polymorphonucleocyte casts was identified in 4 cases (Kolbjornsen et al. 2008). The authors of this latter study concluded that the pathological findings in these Norwegian dogs were most similar to 'reflux nephropathy with segmental hyperplasia' (so-called Ask-Upmark kidney) in man and proposed that a chronic atrophic non-obstructive pyelonephritis was the underlying cause. Vesicoureteral reflux, which predisposes to pyelonephritis in man, is difficult to ascertain in dogs, but it is interesting to note that in the paper by Chandler and others, over half the affected dogs had a history of urinary incontinence felt to be due to urethral sphincter mechanism incompetence. It is currently unknown whether this disorder is inherited in origin but 6 of the 7 Norwegian dogs studied had a genetic relationship.

Until the aetiology of this disorder is better understood, the term 'juvenile kidney disease' (JKD) of the Boxer is probably a suitable term. Prognosis appears to be highly variable and in the 37 dogs reported by Chandler and others two patients were still alive 5 years after diagnosis. Of dogs that had been euthanased prior to the study median survival time was five months.

Management of dogs with JKD is as described for chronic kidney disease but the addition of antibiotic therapy, in the light of the Norwegian findings, may also be appropriate.

References

Brown, S., Atkins, C., Bagley, R., Carr, A., Cowgill, L., Davidson, M., Egner, B., Elliott, J., Henik, R., Labato, M., Littman, M., Polzin, D., Ross, L., Snyder, P., Stepien, R. & American College of Veterinary Internal Medicine (2007) Guidelines for the identification, evaluation, and management of systemic hypertension in dogs and cats. *J Vet Intern Med* **21**, 542–558

Hoppe, A. & Karlstam, E. (2000) Renal dysplasia in boxers and Finnish harriers. *J Small Anim Pract* **41**, 422–426

Chandler, M.L., Elwood, C., Murphy, K.F., Gajanayake, I. & Syme, H.M. (2007) Juvenile nephropathy in 37 boxer dogs. *J Small Anim Pract* **48**, 690–694

Kolbjornsen, O., Heggelund, M. & Jansen, J.-H. (2008) End-stage kidney disease probably due to reflux nephropathy with segmental hypoplasia (Ask-Upmark kidney) in young Boxer dogs in Norway. A retrospective study. *Vet Pathol* **45**, 467–474

Further reading

de Morais, H.S., DiBartola, S.P. & Chew, D.J. (1996) Juvenile renal disease in golden retrievers: 12 cases (1984–1994). *J Am Vet Med Assoc* **209**, 792–797

Greco, D.S. (2001) Congenital and inherited renal disease of small animals. *Vet Clin North Am Small Anim Pract* **31**, 393–399, viii

Lucke, V.M., Kelly, D.F., Darke, P.G. & Gaskell, C.J. (1980) Chronic renal failure in young dogs – possible renal dysplasia. *J Small Anim Pract* **21**, 169–181

Miyamoto, T., Wakizaka, S., Matsuyama, S., Baba, E., Ohashi, F., Kuwamura, M., Yamate, J. & Kotani, T. (1997) A control of a golden retriever with renal dysplasia. *J Vet Med Sci* **59**, 939–942

Clinical presentation

A 3 year-old female-neutered Miniature Schnauzer is presented with a history of pollakiuria, dysuria, dyschezia and gross haematuria. On physical examination firm abnormal structures can be felt in the region of the urinary bladder and urolithiasis is suspected. Lateral and ventrodorsal radiographs are taken and are shown in **Figure 25.1** and an ultrasound examination is also performed (**Figure 25.2**).

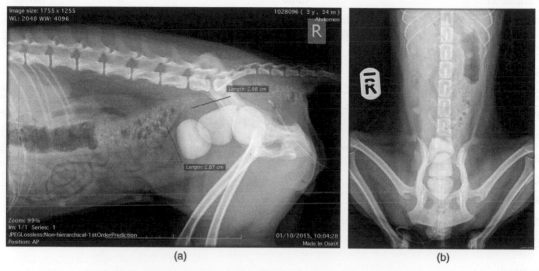

(a) (b)

Figure 25.1 (a) Right lateral abdominal radiograph and (b) dorsoventral radiograph.

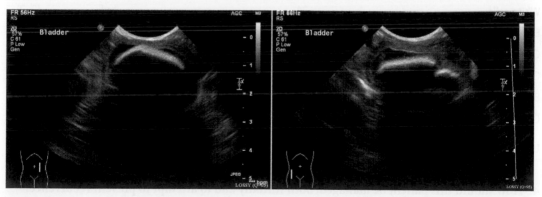

Figure 25.2 Ultrasound images of the bladder. Note that the number of uroliths present is much more apparent radiographically than with ultrasound examination.

Canine Internal Medicine: What's Your Diagnosis? First Edition. Jon Wray.
© 2018 John Wiley & Sons Ltd. Published 2018 by John Wiley & Sons Ltd.

Questions

1. Describe the radiographic and ultrasound findings. Based on the radiographic appearance alone, what is the most likely type of urolith present?
2. What other factors may be taken into account to allow the clinician to make an informed assessment of the likely composition of a canine urolith?
3. Look at the urinalysis results from this case. Does this support the same urolith type and if so what is the most likely reason for formation of this?

Urinalysis (cystocentesis sample)

Parameter	Value	Units	Range
Appearance	Turbid, port-wine coloured		
Chemistry			
Specific gravity	1.026		
pH	7.6		
Protein	++		
Nitrite	+		
Blood/Hb	+++		
Glucose	−		
Ketones	−		
Bilirubin	−		
Urobilinogen	−		
Cytology			
Red cells	>50	/hpf	(0–2)
White cells	24	/hpf	(0–2)
Epithelial cells	−	/hpf	(0–5)
Casts	−		
Crystals	Plentiful magnesium ammonium phosphate (MAP)		
Bacteria	Plentiful gram negative rods		
Other			
Urine culture: Profuse growth of *Proteus mirabilis*			

4. How should this patient be managed, both initially and to attempt to prevent recurrence?

Answers

1. **Describe the radiographic and ultrasound findings. Based on the radiographic appearance alone, what is the most likely type of urolith present?**

   The lateral radiograph shows 3 large smoothly faceted pyramidal cystouroliths present within the urinary bladder. These are very large, being just under 3 cm in maximal dimensions, and are radiodense, having a density similar to the skeletal structures. The caudal-most urolith, and by implication (though it cannot be clearly visualised) the part of the urinary bladder that contains it, is intrapelvic in location. The colon and rectum contains plentiful faecal material, which appears to taper and narrow at a site between the dorsal urinary bladder and the L7 vertebra and sacrum before widening again caudal to this point. A urinary catheter appears to be placed within the caudodorsal part of the urinary bladder. On the dorsoventral view the uroliths appear to be more obviously smoothly faceted and pyramidal in shape and there is a flattened area of contact between the middle and caudal-most of the uroliths.

The ultrasound images show very bright curvilinear echogenic bands arising from the surface interface of the calculi nearest the transducer. Distal 'acoustic shadowing', a radiating fan of signal-void representing an area of non-penetrance of ultrasound, is seen in the far-field below these echogenic signals. Note that in the first image only one urolith can be determined and in the second only two. Whilst ultrasound is relatively sensitive for detection of cystouroliths, especially those that are not radiodense, determination of the number may not be accurate, particularly where a large surface contour of a sizeable urolith prevents assessment of any structures distal to it.

Radiographic appearance in aiding assessment of urolith composition

Knowledge of urolith type is essential to effective management, but in the absence of compositional analysis of a spontaneously voided or removed urolith (which is the only definitive means of assessing this), clinical features must be used to make a best 'educated guestimate' of the urolith type. Radiographic features such as radiodensity, size, number, shape and surface contour may be useful. Uroliths of mineral composition with a higher effective atomic number (Z_{eff}) will attenuate incident X-rays to a greater extent than those in which Z_{eff} is lower and will appear more radiodense. Generally speaking, calcium-containing uroliths have the highest Z_{eff}, silicates, cystine and struvite (magnesium ammonium phosphate) are intermediate and urate-containing uroliths have a relatively low Z_{eff}, making them frequently radiolucent. A comparison of radiographic features is shown in **Table 25.1**.

Table 25.1 Radiographic features of different uroliths

Urolith	Radiodensity	Size	Shape	Usual number	Surface
Calcium oxalate (monohydrate)	++++	2–7 mm	Round	<20	Smooth
Calcium oxalate (dihydrate)	++++	1–15 mm	Rosette	Single to >5	Rough
Calcium phosphate	++++	2–6 mm	Round to cuboidal	Few to many	Smooth

Urolith	Radiodensity	Size	Shape	Usual number	Surface
Silicate	+++	2–10 mm	Spoked/'jackstone'	One or many	Spokes are smooth-edged
Cystine	- to ++	2–10 mm	Round	Few to many	Smooth
Magnesium Ammonium Phosphate (struvite): Infection	+ to +++	5–>20 mm	Round, faceted, pyramidal	Often many	Smooth
Magnesium Ammonium Phosphate (struvite): Sterile	++ to +++	5–15 mm	Round to oval	1–3	Smooth or slightly roughened
Urate	– to ++	1–15 mm	Round to oval	Few to large numbers of sandy debris	Smooth
Xanthine	– to ++	1–4 mm	Round to oval	Few to many	Smooth

As can be seen from the table, the urolith type, which most commonly displays a pyramidal shape and which is often >20 mm in diameter, is magnesium ammonium-phosphate (struvite). In fact, the finding of uroliths >10 mm in diameter correlates with a final compositional diagnosis of MAP 90% of the time.

2. **What other factors may be taken into account to allow the clinician to make an informed assessment of the likely composition of a canine urolith?**

   The breed and sex of the patient should also be taken into account and also the pH of the urine (since some uroliths will form more avidly at certain urinary pH), the presence and type of crystalluria and the presence of medical conditions that may predispose to urolith formation (such as urinary tract infection, systemic hypercalcaemia, hepatic dysfunction or portosystemic shunting) and the administration of medications that may predispose to urolith formation.

Crystalluria is not the same as urolithiasis!

Note that the presence of crystalluria is not synonymous with macroscopic stone formation (it merely represents supersaturation of urine with that mineral type and an environment that might support stone formation) and that crystalluria may form *in vitro* with sample analysis delay; stone formation may occur without identifiable crystalluria or of a type not predicted by the crystalluria present. **Table 25.2** compares known predisposing factors to a number of commonly identified stone types.

Table 25.2 Use of signalment, urine pH and co-morbid conditions to 'guesstimate' urolith composition

Urolith	Breed	Sex	Age	Urine pH	Co-morbid conditions	Predisposing medications
Calcium oxalate	Miniature and Standard Schnauzer, Lhasa Apso, Bichon Frise, Shih Tzu, Miniature Poodle	>71% are male	Most 5–11 years	Acid to neutral	May be associated with hypercalcaemia	Excessive vitamin C or vitamin D
Calcium phosphate	Miniature Schnauzer, Lhasa Apso, Shih Tzu, Yorkshire Terrier	Slight male predisposition	Bimodal age distribution in very young and old	Alkaline to neutral	May be associated with hypercalcaemia	
Silicate	GSD, Miniature Schnauzer, Cocker Spaniel, Labrador, Shih Tzu	>93% are male	Most 3–10 years	Acid to neutral		
Cystine	Newfoundland, English Bulldog, Dachshund, Staffordshire Bull Terrier, Mastiff	>98% are male	Most 1–7 years	Acid to neutral	Associated with renal tubular defect, often familial	
Magnesium ammonium phosphate (struvite)	Miniature Schnauzer, Shih Tzu, Bichon Frise, Miniature Poodle, Cocker Spaniel, Lhasa Apso	>85% are female	Most are 2–9 years	Alkaline to neutral	Most are infection-induced, with bacteria producing urease	
Urate	Dalmatian, Miniature Schnauzer, Yorkshire Terrier, Shih Tzu, English Bulldog	>90% are male	Most are 1–4 years	Acid to neutral	Usually associated with defective urate transport or presence of hepatic dysfunction or porto-systemic shunt. Infection with urease producers may contribute but probably does not initiate	
Xanthine				Acid to neutral		Treatment with allopurinol

3. **Look at the urinalysis results from this case. Does this support the same urolith type and if so what is the most likely reason for formation of this?**

This patient has alkaline urinary pH and evidence of a urinary tract infection with a urease-producing organism. Bacterial urease hydrolyses urea to form ammonia and carbon dioxide and the ammonia consequently spontaneously reacts with water to form ammonium and hydroxyl ions, which further alkalinise urine. Free phosphate is released from hydrogen phosphate dissociating in the alkaline environment.

Plentiful magnesium ammonium phosphate crystals were present in the urine sample. A diagnosis of infection-induced magnesium ammonium phosphate (MAP, struvite) is supported. Struvite stones may form rapidly (can form within 2–5 weeks) after a urinary tract infection.

4. **How should this patient be managed, both initially and to attempt to prevent recurrence?**

Small uroliths may be removed by anterograde voiding urohydropulsion; clearly in this case the large size of the uroliths precludes this approach. Magnesium ammonium phosphate (struvite) stones may be surgically removed, either by standard cystotomy or by per-endoscopic entrapment and fragmentation with laser lithotripsy, or medical dissolution may be performed.

Canine struvite uroliths are, for the most-part, infection-associated/induced

Since most struvite stones in dogs are infection-induced, appropriate antibiotic therapy should be given for the duration of medical dissolution (and for one month beyond radiographic resolution given the low sensitivity for radiography in detecting uroliths <3 mm in size) and in advance of any surgery.

Medical dissolution using a combination of an appropriate antibiotic and an acidifying diet will accomplish resolution of struvite uroliths in an average of 2–3 months. Regular evaluation of urinalyses for attainment of a target pH <6.3 and absence of crystalluria and bacteriuria should be assiduously performed. There is a slight risk of urethral obstruction occurring as uroliths decrease in size, though this risk is very small in female dogs in whom obstruction is rare. In this case the stones were associated with significant clinical signs and surgical removal was considered the most expedient way of resolving these (**Figure 25.3**).

Based on predicted culture and sensitivity data and informed subsequently by these results, clavulanate-amoxycillin was administered starting 24 hours prior to surgery and for 3 weeks afterwards. A urine culture performed 5 days after discontinuation of the antibiotic therapy was negative.

Since most struvite stone formation in dogs is infection-induced, long-term strategies to prevent a recurrence should emphasise surveillance for urinary tract infections and identification of possible predisposing causes (such as structural bladder abnormalities or co-morbid conditions such as hyperadrenocorticism) rather than dietary therapy per se.

Discussion

Urolithiasis (the presence of stones formed by precipitation of excretory metabolites in the urinary tract) has been reported to occur in 0.24–1% of dogs in Germany and Sweden, with struvite and calcium oxalate being the most common. Whilst analysis of uroliths submitted for analysis to the Minnesota Urolith Center between 1981 and 2007 has shown a decrease in the proportion

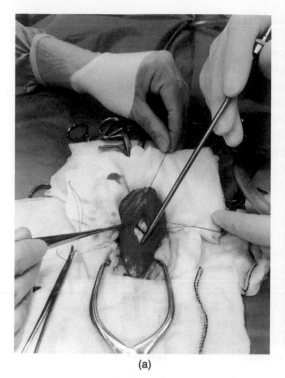

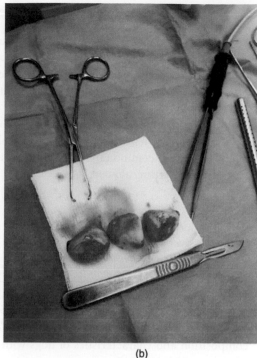

(a)   (b)

Figure 25.3 (a) Intraoperative view of cystotomy and (b) removed cystouroliths.

of struvite and an increase in the proportion of calcium oxalate over this time, a study of 14 008 uroliths (99.6% from the lower urinary tract) submitted from the UK over a 10-year period (1997–2006) showed the relative proportion of struvite uroliths (overall 49.5% of submissions) to remain fairly constant over the 10 year period. By contrast to this and overall submissions to the Minnesota Urolith Center, the proportion of calcium oxalate uroliths submitted from UK dogs fell from 37% to 25% over this time (Roe and others 2012). The same study showed, by comparing stone submission rates with a database of insured dogs, an increased odds ratio for struvite urolithiasis in some breeds, including the Border Collie, Miniature Poodle, Pekingese, Shih Tzu, English Bull Terrier, Bichon Frise, Miniature Schnauzer, Schnauzer, Scottish Terrier, Pug, Lhasa Apso, Yorkshire Terrier, Cavalier King Charles Spaniel, Norfolk Terrier, Tibetan Terrier and Jack Russell Terrier.

In most instances urinary tract infection precedes and causes struvite stone formation in dogs. Urease-producing bacteria, especially *Staphylococcus* spp., but also (less commonly) *Proteus* spp. account for the majority of infections causing struvite uroliths in dogs. Other urease-producing bacteria such as *Klebsiella* spp. and *Pseudomonas* spp. are not as commonly associated.

Small stones (<5 mm diameter) may be retrieved by voiding urohydropulsion in female dogs but this technique is not suitable for animals with urethral obstruction (usually male dogs) since for this to occur the stone is invariably larger than the smallest urethral diameter through which it would have to pass anterograde. Stones entrapped within the urethra may be passed retrograde to the bladder for removal by cystotomy via retrograde urohydropulsion (see Further reading for descriptions of both techniques).

In this case the large size of the stones precluded non-surgical removal and this, coupled with the associated clinical signs and expected time-course for medical dissolution, dictated surgical removal as the preferred course of action. Extracorporeal shock wave lithotripsy (ESWL) is not available in the United Kingdom for pets.

Prevention of a recurrence of infection-induced struvite urolithiasis relies on eradication of urease-producing organisms, correction of structural or functional disorders of the urinary tract that may predispose to infection recurrence or persistence and avoidance of those factors that may predispose to development of infection. Intermittent surveillance for asymptomatic urinary tract infections is sensible in patients with a history of infection-induced struvite uroliths. Dietary management (restriction of magnesium and phosphorus, acidifying diets) may be helpful but are not as important as infection prevention. By contrast, although sterile struvite urolithiasis is uncommon in dogs (being most common in spaniels) acidifying diets restricted in magnesium and phosphorus are useful in preventing a recurrence.

Reference

Roe, K., Pratt, A., Lulich, J., Osborne, C. & Syme, H.M. (2012) Analysis of 14,008 uroliths from dogs in the UK over a 10-year period. *J Small Anim Pract* **53**, 634–640

Further reading

Bartges, J.W., Osborne, C.A., Lulich, J.P., Kirk, C., Allen, T.A. & Brown, C. (1999) Methods for evaluating treatment of uroliths. *Vet Clin North Am Small Anim Pract* **29**, 45–57, x

Low, W.W., Uhl, J.M., Kass, P.H., Ruby, A.L. & Westropp, J.L. (2010) Evaluation of trends in urolith composition and characteristics of dogs with urolithiasis: 25,499 cases (1985–2006). *J Am Vet Med Assoc* **236**, 193–200

Osborne, C.A., Lulich, J.P., Polzin, D.J., Allen, T.A., Kruger, J.M., Bartges, J.W., Koehler, L.A., Ulrich, L.K., Bird, K.A. & Swanson, L.L. (1999) Medical dissolution and prevention of canine struvite urolithiasis. Twenty years of experience. *Vet Clin North Am Small Anim Pract* **29**, 73–111, xi

Osborne, C.A., Lulich, J.P., Kruger, J.M., Ulrich, L.K. & Koehler, L.A. (2009) Analysis of 451,891 canine uroliths, feline uroliths, and feline urethral plugs from 1981 to 2007: perspectives from the Minnesota Urolith Center. *Vet Clin North Am Small Anim Pract* **39**, 183–197

Palma, D., Langston, C., Gisselman, K. & McCue, J. (2013) Canine struvite urolithiasis. *Compend Contin Educ Vet* **35**, E1; quiz E1

Clinical presentation

A 9 year-old male-entire Munsterlander (**Figure 26.1**) is presented with a history of gross haematuria which has waxed and waned for the preceding 6 weeks. The owner reports an increase in the frequency of urination and mild stranguria. The colour of the urine is reported to vary between normal, dark 'port-wine' coloured and crimson and more noticeable haematuria is noted at the end of urination. The dog received a 7-day course of oral clavulanate-amoxycillin for a presumed urinary tract infection when signs were first noted, but with no apparent effect. No dyschezia is noted and the dog is otherwise bright and happy, retains a normal appetite, thirst, body condition and exercise tolerance.

Physical examination was essentially unremarkable, including per-rectal palpation of the prostate and pelvic urethra, examination of the penis/prepuce/testes and abdominal palpation.

Question

1. What are the most common causes of gross haematuria in the dog?
2. How can the history and physical examination help determine the most likely cause?
3. What further investigation would you recommend?

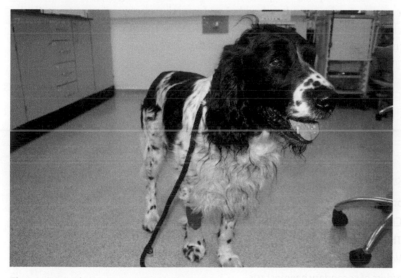

Figure 26.1 The patient at presentation.

Canine Internal Medicine: What's Your Diagnosis? First Edition. Jon Wray.
© 2018 John Wiley & Sons Ltd. Published 2018 by John Wiley & Sons Ltd.

Answers

1. What are the most common causes of gross haematuria in the dog?

Not all discoloured urine is haematuria

It is usual to assume, and is most commonly the case, that grossly red-discoloured urine represents haematuria, but bear in mind that haemoglobinuria and myoglobinuria may have a similar appearance.

- These can be differentiated from haematuria by
  - Centrifugation (1500 rpm for 5 minutes) of a grossly pigmented urine sample, which in the case of haematuria will result in a 'pellet' of erythrocytes at the base of the spun tube (whereas in haemoglobinuria and myoglobinuria the urine will remain discoloured throughout with no 'pellet'). Myoglobinuria may be differentiated from haemoglobinuria by the ammonium sulfate myoglobin solubility test.
  - Microscopic examination of the urine sediment showing plentiful erythrocytes.
- True haematuria may be due to bleeding within the urogenital tract because of
  - Systemic coagulopathy or
  - More commonly localised disruption in epithelial or endothelial integrity.
  - The latter is most conveniently considered as being from the upper urinary tract (kidneys and ureters), lower urinary tract (bladder and urethra) or the genital tract. Common causes of true haematuria in dogs are listed in **Table 26.1**.

Lower urinary tract and genital causes are generally more common than upper urinary tract and bleeding disorders as causes of haematuria. Maintain an open mind as to the differential diagnoses possible.

Table 26.1 Differential diagnosis of haematuria

Bleeding disorders	Disorders of primary haemostasis
	• Critical thrombocytopenia
	• Thrombocytopathia
	• Von Willebrand's disease
	Disorders of secondary haemostasis
	• Congenital coagulopathies (e.g. haemophilia A and B)
	• Acquired coagulopathies
	◦ Vitamin K antagonist rodenticides
	◦ *Angiostrongylus vasorum*-induced coagulopathy
	◦ Hepatic failure
	◦ Disseminated intravascular coagulation
	◦ Neoplasia
	◦ Anticoagulant drug treatment

Renal and ureteric	Trauma
	Neoplasia
	Calculus
	Renal telangiectasia of the Welsh corgi
	Benign idiopathic renal haematuria
	Renal vascular malformations
	Nodular dermatofibrosis/renal cystadenocarcinoma syndrome of GSD (**Figure 26.2**)
	Infarction
	Cystic disease
	Glomerulonephritis
	Pyelonephritis
	Haematoma
	Dioctophyma renale in endemic areas
	Dirofilaria immitis microfilaraemia in endemic areas
	Capillaria plica in endemic areas (**Figure 26.3**)
Bladder and urethra	Bacterial urinary tract infection (UTI)
	Calculus
	Trauma
	Neoplasia
	Polypoid cystitis
	Urethritis
	Capillaria plica in endemic areas
	Cyclophosphamide therapy
	Fungal infection
Genital tract	Female
	• Oestrus
	• Trauma
	• Neoplasia
	• Polyps
	• Foreign body
	Male
	• Preputial/penile trauma
	• Urethral prolapse
	• Foreign body
	• Preputial/penile neoplasia
	• Testicular trauma/neoplasia
	• Prostatic disease
	○ Benign prostatic hyperplasia (BPH)
	○ Prostatic neoplasia
	○ Prostatitis
	○ Prostatic cyst or abscess

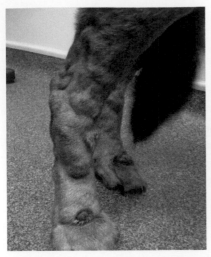
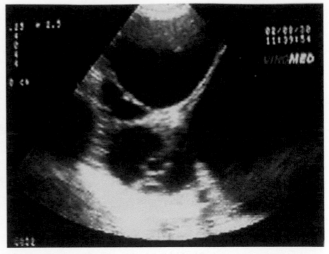

Figure 26.2 Distal hindlimbs of a 4 year old FN German Shepherd with nodular dermatofibrosis /renal cystadenocarcinoma, a genodermatosis, and (right) an ultrasound image of the severe cystic transformation of the kidneys.

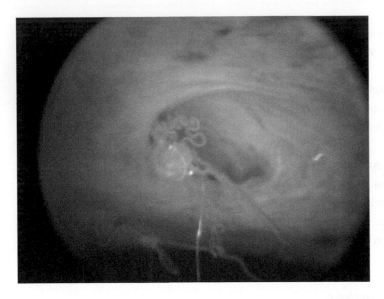

Figure 26.3 Endoscopic view of the ureterovesicular junction (UVJ) of a dog infested with *Capillaria plica* and presenting with haematuria. The parasite commonly colonises the ureters and may be an underdiagnosed cause of haematuria in dogs, especially in rural environments.

2. **How can the history and physical examination help determine the most likely cause?**

Pertinent historical clues

Review of the anamnesis, discussion of diet, environment, travel and access to medication and drugs prescribed for humans as well as intoxicants (especially anticoagulant rodenticides – see **Figure 26.4**).

- History of evidence of bleeding elsewhere (particularly of petechiation/ecchymoses, haematomata, melaena, epistaxis, haemoptysis, haematemesis or prolonged bleeding after prior surgery or oestrus) may give rise to the suspicion of a systemic bleeding disorder.

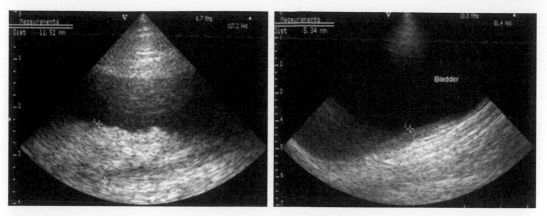

Figure 26.4 Sagittally orientated bladder ultrasound before (left) and after (right) treatment for anticoagulant rodenticide (Brodifacoum) toxicity in a dog. Note that very marked intramural haemorrhage, resolved by the second study, mimics irregular bladder wall infiltrative disease such as neoplasia in this patient.

- The presence of normal urination should be established as dysuria strongly implicates a source of blood loss within the lower urinary tract (though occasionally dysuria may result from large clots of blood dwelling within the bladder from an upper urinary tract source).
- The presence of dyschezia in an animal with haematuria may suggest pathology causing 'mass-effect' within the pelvic canal to affect both urinary and gastrointestinal tracts (such as is commonly reported with gross prostatomegaly).

The timing of gross haematuria may be helpful, though some caution is advised in interpretation of this as there may be considerable overlap between causes.

- *Typically* gross haematuria seen at the beginning of urination originates in the lower urinary or genital tracts.
- Gross haematuria seen only at the end of urination originates from the upper urinary tract.
- Dripping of blood from the external genitalia at times other than urination usually indicates a source distal to the bladder and is most commonly encountered in dogs with prostatic disease.

The physical examination should include

- Examination of the external genitalia (including retraction of the prepuce and inspection of the penis, which may be done under sedation or anaesthesia in fractious/uncomfortable patients but should always be done).
- Palpation of the kidneys (for size, shape, symmetry, firmness and pain).
- Palpation of the bladder (for size, thickening, irregularity, masses and pain) – this should be performed in the context of knowing when the animal last urinated.
- Digital examination per-rectum (of urethra, for intrapelvic mass lesions and of the prostate shape, size, symmetry, texture and comfort in male dogs).
- Digital examination per-vaginum in female dogs.
- Careful inspection of the rest of the body for evidence of bleeding, for evidence of constitutional signs of excessive blood loss and for dermal nodules of dermatofibrosis.

3. **What further investigation would you recommend?**

The decision to treat empirically with antibiotic therapy in the case of simple lower urinary tract infection is a rational and often cost-effective one. In this case it was also useful in that the complete lack of any response made a simple UTI unlikely.

Further investigation might include

- Urinalysis with cytological examination of sediment and bacterial culture.
- Evaluation of a complete blood count, especially for evidence of anaemia consequent to haematuria and thrombocytopenia, that may indicate a cause.
- Assessment of urea and creatinine in conjunction with urine specific gravity to assess renal function – this may conversely highlight primary renal disease or may indicate post-renal obstruction due to ureteral disease, ureterovesicular junction obstruction or urethral obstructive problems.

Although a urine sample obtained by cystocentesis is ideal for microbiological evaluation, where lower urinary tract neoplasia is a differential diagnosis, caution should be undertaken since seeding of neoplastic tissue down the needle tract of cystocentesis has been reported in this situation.

- Evaluation of coagulation status, should the platelet count be normal or insufficiently low to provoke spontaneous haemorrhage (though if diagnostic imaging of the urinary tract is to be performed, it might be argued that the results of this be evaluated prior to assessing coagulation status since the discovery of primary urinary tract pathology would render a concurrent systemic coagulopathy much less likely). Of course, these may not be mutually exclusive as in the example above (**Figure 26.4**).
- Diagnostic imaging of the urinary tract
  - The author is of the opinion that radiography and ultrasonography offer complementary information to each other in this setting.
  - It should be emphasised that thorough imaging evaluation of the ureters and urethra are commonly overlooked in favour of the kidneys and bladder, and this error of omission should be assiduously guarded against.
  - Where urinary tract neoplasia is suspected, or subsequent to its diagnosis, thoracic radiographs (or CT) should be performed in order to gauge whether pulmonary metastasis has occurred in advance of any further treatment.
  - Ultrasound
    - Is especially helpful in evaluating the urinary bladder, prostate, female genital tract and kidneys.
    - Requires a systematic approach and should include imaging of structures in all standard planes.
  - Plain radiography
    - Is helpful in evaluating renal size, shape, position and radiodensity.
    - Is helpful in evaluating ureteroliths.
    - Is helpful in documenting radiodense urocystoliths.
    - Is helpful in documenting prostatic disease, especially if calcification has occurred.
    - Is helpful in documenting radiodense urethroliths provided that the whole urethra is imaged.
  - Contrast radiography
    - Intravenous urography is helpful in evaluating the kidneys and ureters.
    - Retrograde urethrocystography is essential to evaluate the urethra and is helpful in evaluating the bladder (especially for documenting urocystoliths).

The often-neglected urethra: why urethrography is so important

The urethra (with the exception of those portions that are visible trans-abdominally and those sections that are accessible to superficial ultrasound) is poorly visualised by plain radiography and ultrasound. Localised pathology within the urethra with associated haemorrhage may therefore easily be missed. It is essential to consider performing imaging studies that may fully evaluate the entire urethra and this may be by contrast urethrogram (or urethroscopy if facilities and familiarity with this technique are available). Contrast urethrography is simple to perform and diagnostically useful, yet is often neglected in the author's experience, even when efforts have been made to perform radiographic contrast studies of the urinary bladder.

In the example below (**Figure 26.5**) a Staffordshire Bull Terrier was presented with persistent haematuria and bleeding from the penis between urinations (upper left panel). Ultrasound evaluation and fine needle aspiration cytology of the prostate demonstrated benign prostatic hyperplasia but despite castration and a marked reduction in prostatic size (upper centre and right panels), episodes of gross haematuria persisted. Contrast urethrography (lower left and centre panels) subsequently demonstrated a filling defect within the penile urethra representing a benign vascular malformation (lower right panel) which was the source of the haemorrhage.

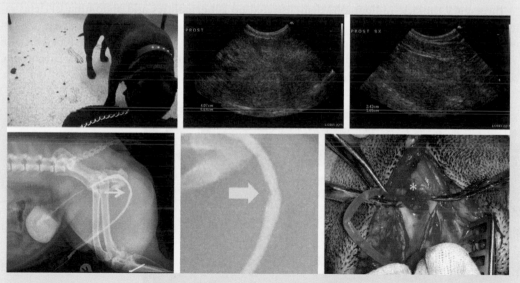

Figure 26.5 Persistent dripping of blood from the prepuce of the patient (upper left) and prostatic ultrasound before (upper centre) and after (upper right) castration. Contrast urethrography (lower left) and magnified (lower centre) demonstrated a filling defect in the proximal penile urethra (arrows). At surgery (urethrotomy on lower right) a benign vascular malformation (asterisk) was discovered, which was successfully resected (a urinary catheter is seen extending into the urethra proximal to the incision).

- Where the equipment and expertise is available, endoscopy of the genitourinary tract may be helpful
  - In evaluating the preputial fornix of male dogs and the vagina of female dogs.
  - In evaluating the urethral papilla.
  - In evaluating the urethra – in male dogs the size of the urethra as it runs through the groove of the os penis is a size-limiting area and small-sized flexible endoscopes are needed to achieve access to the proximal urethra.
  - In evaluating the bladder trigone area, uretrovesicular junctions (and especially viewing the nature of urine coming from these in the case of renal or ureteral haemorrhage).
  - In evaluating the bladder.

Diagnosis

In this case a urine sample demonstrated macro- and microscopic haematuria but no cytological evidence of infectious agents was seen and the urine culture was negative. A blood sample demonstrated no evidence of anaemia or thrombocytopenia and the dog was not azotaemic. Thrombin time and partial thromboplastin time were normal. An abdominal ultrasound demonstrated the presence of an irregularly marginated, broad-based, vascular, 2-cm thick soft tissue lesion within the region of the bladder neck (**Figure 26.6**). This mass was seen to intermittently 'plug' the transition point to the urethra but no direct urethra involvement was seen and no ureteric obstruction or pyelectasia was demonstrated. The upper urinary tract and prostate appeared normal and no lymphadenomegaly or evidence of distant nodular disease was seen.

Three-view thoracic radiographs demonstrated no abnormalities and abdominal/skeletal radiographs demonstrated no bony metastatic disease. A catheter suction biopsy was taken (see below), which yielded both cytological material and solid tissue for histopathology, both of which on analysis were compatible with a diagnosis of **urothelial (previously transitional cell) carcinoma**. Staging of bladder tumours is described in **Table 26.2**.

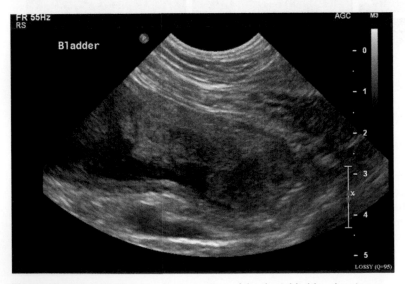

Figure 26.6 Sagittal ultrasound examination of the dog's bladder, showing an extensive broad-based mass.

Table 26.2 Staging of canine bladder tumours

T: Primary tumour

T_{is}	Carcinoma *in situ*
T_0	No evidence of gross tumour
T_1	Superficial papillary tumour
T_2	Tumour invading bladder wall
T_3	Tumour invading adjacent organs

N: Regional lymph nodes (internal and external iliac)

N_0	No regional lymph node involvement
N_1	Regional lymph node involved
N_2	Regional and more distant lymph node involved

M: Distant metastases

M_0	No metastasis
M_1	Distant metastasis

Urothelial carcinoma stage $T_2/N_0/M_0$ was the final diagnosis.

Treatment

The dog was placed on piroxicam at a dose of 0.3 mg/kg/day and mitoxantrone was planned to be administered at a dose of 5 mg/m^2 q21 days for 5 occasions. However, the patient developed gastro-intestinal toxicity related to the mitoxantrone administration (though tolerated piroxicam well) to an extent that the mitoxantrone was discontinued in favour of monotherapy with piroxicam alone. After a six week period of apparently improved clinical signs, progressive haematuria and dysuria developed and the patient was euthanased.

Taking a catheter suction biopsy

A flexible but stiff dog urinary catheter with side holes (usually size 6–8Fr is sufficient for most dogs) is lubricated with sterile gel and inserted in a sterile fashion into the urinary bladder with the patient anaesthestised or sedated. The urinary bladder is emptied of urine and the catheter is drawn back to the region of interest either under ultrasound guidance (sagittal plane) or after pre-measuring the catheter against patient radiographs to determine the required length. Suction of 5–10 cc is applied to the catheter with a 10–20 ml syringe to draw soft tissue from the mass within the lumen of the catheter through the side-holes; then the catheter is agitated back and forth by 2–3 cm to 'guillotine' off small fragments of tissue. Suction is then removed and the catheter withdrawn. Collected material is submitted for cytology (liquid component) and histopathology (solid tissue) and it may be necessary to cut the tip off the catheter and flush this material free anterograde.

Examples of material obtained are shown in **Figure 26.7**.

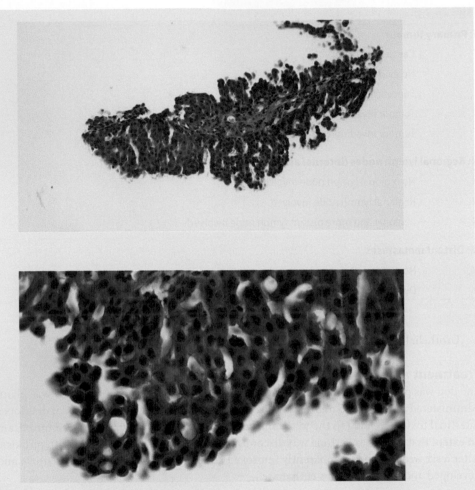

Figure 26.7 Above (×40 magnification) and below (×500 magnification) photomicrographs of tissue obtained from a urothelial carcinoma of the bladder by catheter suction biopsy. The histological features of transitional epithelial cells with moderate eosinophilic cytoplasm, moderate cellular and nuclear pleomorphism and formation of small papillae and microcysts typify urothelial carcinoma.

Prognosis and discussion

The cause of urothelial carcinoma is poorly understood and likely to be multi-factorial though the disease is more prevalent in some breeds such as the Scottish Terrier. Diagnosis requires staging the extent of the disease (since metastasis is present in approximately 14–16% of dogs at diagnosis), to visualise the relationship of the primary tumour with structures such as the urethra and the ureteral papillae and to directly sample the mass. Ultrasound-guided needle biopsy is not recommended due to the risk of tumour seeding. Collection of material for histopathology can very often be accomplished by catheter suction biopsy but direct visualisation and biopsy by urethrocystoscopy is required in some patients. Urine antigen tests are sensitive but blighted by lack of specificity and false positive diagnoses in the presence of other urinary tract pathology. Where catheter suction biopsy is not successful direct visualisation of the mass by cystoscopy (and directed biopsy) is needed (see **Figure 26.8**).

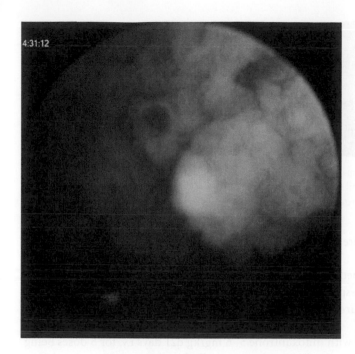

Figure 26.8 Cystoscopic view of a bladder urothelial carcinoma.

Surgical therapy of bladder urothelial carcinoma is generally not effective due to the extent and position of the mass, leading to lack of complete excision and/or unacceptable surgical trauma to the structures communicating with the bladder neck and trigone. Where urethral obstruction is occurring palliative urethral stent placement (**Figure 26.9**) can be effective for medium-term relief

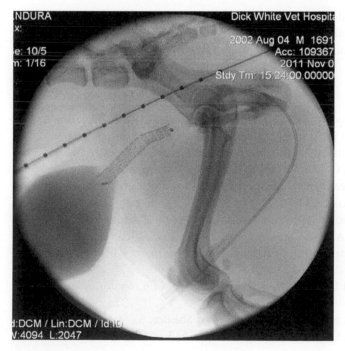

Figure 26.9 Fluoroscopic image of a urethral stent after deployment. The bladder is filled with dilute iodinated contrast agent. A radiographic marker catheter is positioned in the colon and a catheter for contrast injection is within the distal urethra.

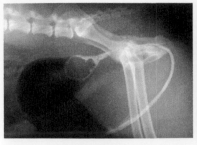
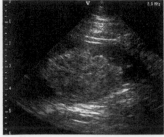
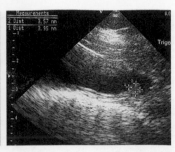

Figure 26.10 Bladder urothelial carcinoma in an 11 year old cross-bred dog before treatment shown by a double-contrast urethrocytogram (left) and sagittal ultrasound examination (centre). The same mass after 12 weeks of piroxicam therapy (right). A scale in cm of size is shown on the left of the ultrasound images.

and ureteral stents or subcutaneous ureteral bypass (SUB) can be accomplished for relief of ureteral obstruction in selected cases.

Medical therapy may be performed most simply with the COX-inhibitor piroxicam at a dose of 0.3 mg/kg/24 hours. An overall response rate of 17% is reported and a minority of cases may experience complete remission (**Figure 26.10**). Gastrointestinal side effects of piroxicam may be dose-limiting in some dogs.

Chemotherapy may be employed with mitoxantrone 5–6 mg/kg q21 days i.v. for 5 doses being the most commonly reported treatment to date, with an overall objective response rate of 35%. Other agents that may show some antitumour effects are carboplatin, vinblastine and gemcitabine. Use of any of these agents mandates clinical experience with their use, cogniscence of likely side effects and rational monitoring strategies. Because only a significant minority of patients will show measurable response to chemotherapy in our practice we will advise repeat tumour staging by ultrasound examination after 2–3 doses of chemotherapy and discontinue therapy if progressive disease is seen.

The median survival time of bladder TCC is dependent on tumour stage and severity of clinical signs, but broadly speaking median survival times of 2–3 months are reported with no treatment, 5–6 months with piroxicam alone and 8–11 months when cytotoxic chemotherapy is given additionally.

Further reading

Allstadt, S.D., Rodriguez, C.O., Jr, Boostrom, B., Rebhun, R.B. & Skorupski, K.A. (2015) Randomized phase III trial of piroxicam in combination with mitoxantrone or carboplatin for first-line treatment of urogenital tract transitional cell carcinoma in dogs. *J Vet Intern Med* **29**, 261–267

Blackburn, A.L., Berent, A.C., Weisse, C.W. & Brown, D.C. (2013) Evaluation of outcome following urethral stent placement for the treatment of obstructive carcinoma of the urethra in dogs: 42 cases (2004–2008). *J Am Vet Med Assoc* **242**, 59–68

Boria, P.A., Glickman, N.W., Schmidt, B.R., Widmer, W.R., Mutsaers, A.J., Adams, L.G., Snyder, P.W., DiBernardi, L., de Gortari, A.E., Bonney, P.L. & Knapp, D.W. (2005) Carboplatin and piroxicam therapy in 31 dogs with transitional cell carcinoma of the urinary bladder. *Vet Comp Oncol* **3**, 73–80

Cannon, C.M. & Allstadt, S.D. (2015) Lower urinary tract cancer. *Vet Clin North Am Small Anim Pract* **45**, 807–824

Henry, C.J., McCaw, D.L., Turnquist, S.E., Tyler, J.W., Bravo, L., Sheafor, S., Straw, R.C., Dernell, W.S., Madewell, B.R., Jorgensen, L., Scott, M.A., Higginbotham, M.L. & Chun, R. (2003) Clinical evaluation of mitoxantrone and piroxicam in a canine model of human invasive urinary bladder carcinoma. *Clin Cancer Res* **9**, 906–911

Knapp, D.W., Richardson, R.C., Chan, T.C., Bottoms, G.D., Widmer, W.R., DeNicola, D.B., Teclaw, R., Bonney, P.L. & Kuczek, T. (1994) Piroxicam therapy in 34 dogs with transitional cell carcinoma of the urinary bladder. *J Vet Intern Med* **8**, 273–278

Knapp, D.W., Ramos-Vara, J.A., Moore, G.E., Dhawan, D., Bonney, P.L. & Young, K.E. (2014) Urinary bladder cancer in dogs, a naturally occurring model for cancer biology and drug development. *ILAR J* **55**, 100–118

Mutsaers, A.J., Widmer, W.R. & Knapp, D.W. (2003) Canine transitional cell carcinoma. *J Vet Intern Med* **17**, 136–144

Norris, A.M., Laing, E.J., Valli, V.E., Withrow, S.J., Macy, D.W., Ogilvie, G.K., Tomlinson, J., McCaw, D., Pidgeon, G. & Jacobs, R.M. (1992) Canine bladder and urethral tumors: a retrospective study of 115 cases (1980–1985). *J Vet Intern Med* **6**, 145–153

Poirier, V.J., Forrest, L.J., Adams, W.M. & Vail, D.M. (2004) Piroxicam, mitoxantrone, and coarse fraction radiotherapy for the treatment of transitional cell carcinoma of the bladder in 10 dogs: a pilot study. *J Am Anim Hosp Assoc* **40**, 131–136

Rocha, T.A., Mauldin, G.N., Patnaik, A.K. & Bergman, P.J. (2000) Prognostic factors in dogs with urinary bladder carcinoma. *J Vet Intern Med* **14**, 486–490

Reproductive/Genital Tract

Clinical presentation

A 9 year 7 month-old male-entire Border Collie is presented with a 2 week history of intermittent dripping of blood from the penis. The blood has not been seen every day and though the owners have noted that on several occasions the urine stream has been interrupted and some straining has been noted on two or three occasions there has not been any polyuria, polydipsia or pollakiuria. Most of the time the owners feel that urination has been normal. Faeces have been normal in size, shape and frequency and no dyschezia has been noted. A course of clavulanate-amoxycillin for 10 days had been prescribed but did not result in reduction in the dripping of blood. There has been no history of trauma and the dog does not seem particularly irritated/uncomfortable in the genital region. His previous medical history is unremarkable, he is not receiving any medications other than the antibiotic course (which finished 3 days previously), has never travelled outside the UK and is up to date with vaccination and worming.

Physical examination in this dog demonstrated prostatomegaly, which was not particularly painful on palpation and the prostate had normal firmness. Prostatomegaly seemed to be bilateral but some subtle irregularity to the prostate could be determined. Remaining examination was normal; the dog did not appear ill and was not febrile. Renomegaly or caudal abdominal pain were not determined and no source of blood loss could be determined on retraction of and examination of the prepuce and penis. No other evidence of bleeding was found elsewhere. Palpation of the testes and scrotum was normal.

Questions

1. What differential diagnoses should be considered for dripping of blood from the penis in the dog?
2. What specific questions should be answered from the history in this case and what particular areas of physical examination should be emphasised?
3. What specific abnormalities should be felt for on a rectal examination in this dog and how should such abnormalities be interpreted?
4. What further diagnostic methods may be appropriate and how may these aid in diagnosis?

Answers

1. **What differential diagnoses should be considered for dripping of blood from the penis in the dog?**

   This is a very common clinical presentation and dripping of what appears to be fresh blood or dark thick blood from the penis *independent* of urinating should always make the clinician suspect prostatic disease, especially in an *entire* male dog. However, this presentation is not pathognomonic for prostatic disease and differential diagnoses include:

   - Local bleeding of the external penile genitalia (penis, penile urethra, prepuce) or from the from a single lesion due to
     - Trauma
     - Inflammatory lesions

- Foreign bodies (these will often lodge in male dogs at the preputial fornix, which is surprisingly deep in most dogs and difficult to fully examine whilst conscious) and which may be focal or encircling the penis of male dogs (e.g. string, rubber bands)
  - Neoplastic lesions
  - Paraphimosis
  - Urethral prolapse
- Bleeding into the urethra from testicular disease such as
  - Testicular neoplasia
  - Inflammatory and infectious testicular disease
  - Testicular torsion
  - Testicular trauma
- Prostatic disease
  - Benign prostatic hyperplasia (BPH)
  - Prostatic neoplasia
  - Prostatitis
  - Prostatic cyst or abscess
- Bleeding originating from the lower urinary tract (bladder and urethra) due to
  - Bacterial urinary tract infection (UTI)
  - Calculus
  - Trauma
  - Neoplasia
  - Polypoid cystitis
  - Urethritis
  - *Capillaria plica* in endemic areas
  - Cyclophosphamide therapy
  - Fungal infection
- Bleeding originating from the upper urinary tract due to
  - Trauma
  - Neoplasia
  - Calculus
  - Renal telangiectasia of the Welsh Corgi
  - Benign idiopathic renal haematuria
  - Renal vascular malformations
  - Nodular dermatofibrosis/renal cystadenocarcinoma syndrome of GSD (see **Figure 26.2**)
  - Infarction
  - Cystic disease
  - Glomerulonephritis
  - Pyelonephritis
  - Haematoma
  - *Dioctophyma renale* in endemic areas
  - *Dirofilaria immitis* microfilaraemia in endemic areas
  - *Capillaria plica* in endemic areas (see **Figure 26.3**)
- Bleeding from the upper urinary tract, lower urinary tract or genital tract due to systemic bleeding disorder

2. **What specific questions should be answered from the history in this case and what particular areas of physical examination should be emphasised?**

Given the observed clinical sign of blood dripping from the penis, initial history taking should exclude the possibility of recent observed trauma and that signs of bleeding in other body areas have been seen (which might suggest a bleeding disorder). A description of urinating behaviour, the association of blood loss with urination and whether dyschezia or alteration in faecal shape (specifically dorsoventral flattening of faeces) has been noted. Signs of systemic illness might indicate that infection is present that is severe enough to cause significant illness (which often occurs with acute bacterial prostatitis) or is associated with extension to the peritoneum or involves the kidneys. Constitutional signs may also be seen in those patients in whom post-renal obstruction is being caused (for instance due to prostatic or bladder mass lesions obstructing the ureters) and in patients with neoplasia with metastatic spread. Reproductive history and prior medical history (especially of previous urolithiasis) is essential.

Physical examination should emphasise thorough examination of the external genitalia including inspection and digital palpation of the vulva/vestibule in female dogs and retraction of the prepuce, inspection of the penis with the prepuce retracted in male dogs and testicular palpation. It is practically impossible to adequately examine the deep preputial fornix in most male dogs whilst conscious and re-evaluation should always be undertaken under sedation or anaesthesia. Careful longitudinal palpation of the penis and extrapelvic urethra from a distal to proximal direction should always be undertaken in male dogs. Per-rectal examination of the intrapelvic urethra in male dogs, palpation of the pelvic canal dorsolaterally for lymphadenomegaly and careful palpation of the prostate in all male dogs should be undertaken (see below). Careful general physical examination should highlight whether caudal abdominal pain, renomegaly or evidence of bleeding, petechiation or echymoses at other sites is identifiable.

3. **What specific abnormalities should be felt for on a rectal examination in this dog and how should such abnormalities be interpreted?**

The prostate should always be carefully palpated though in larger dogs for if the prostate is enlarged it may attain a position foreward of the pelvic brim, rendering just the caudal portion of it palpable per-rectum. Palpation can be aided by simultaneous per-abdominal palpation and moving the prostate dorsally and caudally to aid per-rectal palpation.

Notables of per-rectal prostatic palpation

The prostate should be evaluated for

- Size
- Regularity and symmetry
- Firmness/deformability
- Pain

This may aid in identification of the most common disorders of the prostate, in conjunction with the sexually intact status of the patient (**Table 27.1**).

4. What further diagnostic methods may be appropriate and how may these aid in diagnosis?

Diagnostic imaging of the prostate

Diagnostic imaging of the prostate both by radiography and trans-abdominal ultrasonography is the most useful means of further investigation and is described further in the case diagnosis and discussion. Briefly, diagnostic imaging characteristics of the major types of prostatic pathology are summarised in **Table 27.2**.

Means of sampling the prostate include collection of fluid of prostatic origin or direct sampling of prostatic tissue (either by direct ultrasound-guided aspiration or spring-loaded biopsy device, or by suction catheter biopsy – see below).

Sampling of the prostate
Fluid collection

Semen can be collected from entire male dogs. Of the three fractions of semen produced (first being clear 'presperm' of volume 0.2–2 ml, second being whitish 'sperm-rich' portion of up to 4 ml), the third ('prostatic') fraction, which is usually clear and voluminous and is released over 3–35 minutes post-ejaculation, is most suitable for analysis. Due to contamination by bacteria in the distal urethra it is recommended that quantitative culture results are interpreted with cytological evaluation.

Table 27.1 Differentiating prostatic disease based on palpable characteristics

	Size	Regularity/ symmetry	Firmness/ deformability	Pain	Intact/ neutered
Benign prostatic hyperplasia	Enlarged	Symmetrical	Usually firmer than normal but not 'hard'	Not usually painful	Intact males
Prostatic neoplasia	Enlarged	Usually irregular/ asymmetrical	Variable but usually firm. There may be areas of mineralisation interspersed with cystic areas causing variation in palpation features	Not usually painful unless concurrent prostatitis	Both, but there is increased risk in neutered dogs
Bacterial prostatitis/ prostatic abscess	Usually enlarged but some cases, especially chronic ones, prostate may be normal size	Variable and depends on extent and volume of abscessation if present	Usually normal to soft. Abscesses may be identified as fluctuant	Usually associated with pain, especially where prostatic abscess is present	Usually intact males in combination with urinary tract infection. May complicate prostatic neoplasia and BPH
Prostatic cyst	Usually enlarged	Usually asymmetrical unless very large cyst or centrally positioned	Usually soft and appreciably fluctuant except when mineralised where they may have a very hard/ solid feel	Usually not painful unless secondarily infected	Usually intact males but also reported in a small number of neutered males

Table 27.2 Radiographic and ultrasonographic characteristics of prostatic pathology

Prostatic disease	Radiography findings	Ultrasound findings
Benign prostatic hyperplasia (BPH)	Prostatomegaly, regular and symmetrical	Prostatomegaly, which is usually regular and symmetrical, generally slightly inhomogenous in echotexture and may contain small cystic structures. Architecture largely preserved but may lose normal bilobed appearance
Bacterial prostatitis	Prostatomegaly, usually regular and symmetrical unless abscessation accompanies. Localised loss of serosal detail may accompany serositis due to extension of infection	Variable appearance and may be symmetrical or asymmetrical, hyper- or hypoechoic and may contain small abscesses or even areas of gas production
Prostatic neoplasia	Prostatomegaly, which may appear radiographically symmetrical or asymmetrical. Irregular mineralisation may be seen and periosteal reactions on the ventral surface of lumbar and sacral vertebrae may be present. Enlarged local lymph nodes due to metastasis may cause deviation of adjacent structures	Variable appearance but characterised by irregularity and strikingly inhomogenous echotexture. Cystic structures may be present and mineralisation may be apparent within prostatic parenchyma
Prostatic cyst	Increase in size of the prostatic silhouette which may be indistinct from generalised prostatomegaly or may form a lobed appearance if asymmetric/paraprostatic. A number of prostatic cysts develop mineralised walls displaying an egg-shell-like appearance, which is not seen in other prostatic disease (see **Figure 27.3** later)	Cysts may be prostatic or paraprostatic and may be single or numerous. They are generally smooth-walled, rounded with anechoic contents. Membranous internal septations may be seen in larger cysts and those with wall mineralisation produce acoustic 'shadows' distal to mineralised segments

An alternative to semen collection is to perform prostatic massage and wash (see below). Prostatic massage and wash is especially helpful in cases of bacterial prostatitis and may also yield cytological evidence of prostatic neoplasia, especially in patients with carcinoma involving prostatic urethra

Prostatic massage and wash technique

This is usually best accomplished under sedation or general anaesthesia. After decontamination and cleansing of the prepuce and peri-preputial area, a sterile urinary catheter of size appropriate for the patient and with side holes is advanced into the urinary bladder, which is then emptied of urine and sterile saline is used to wash and then empty the bladder several times. The catheter is then retracted to a position just distal to the prostate, which may be felt trans-rectally for position or positioned using trans-abdominal ultrasound as a guide. The prostate is then digitally massaged per-rectum for 1–2 minutes before 5–10 ml of sterile saline is slowly flushed through the catheter whilst occluding the urethra distally around the catheter to prevent leakage. The catheter is then slowly advanced whilst aspirating to retrieve the prostatic cellular fluid produced.

Fluid from cystic structures may be aspirated under ultrasound guidance but caution is recommended if prostatic abscessation is possible (see Discussion).

Tissue collection

Cytological evaluation of the prostate may be performed from samples directly aspirated from the prostate gland under ultrasound guidance. It should be recognised that whilst this technique is generally safe, principle risks are of iatrogenic damage to the prostatic urethra and of potential 'seeding' of neoplastic cells from prostatic tumours along the needle tract. In the case of larger, solid prostatic pathology a spring-loaded biopsy device may be used with care under direct ultrasound guidance to sample the canine prostate.

In situations where prostatic pathology encroaches on or proliferates within the urethra, tissue for diagnosis may be obtained trans-urethrally by direct endoscopic biopsy using a cystourethroscope or by suction/traumatic catheter biopsy. This latter method is particularly simple and has high diagnostic yield for confirming the presence of prostatic neoplasia. Briefly, the initial steps as for the prostatic massage and wash technique (as above) are performed and indeed the two techniques can be combined; a catheter with side holes is essential. Rather than position the catheter tip distal to the prostate, however, when using this technique the catheter is positioned so that the side holes are within the prostatic urethra and then 4–5 ml of suction is applied to the catheter with a 20 ml syringe. This will draw any proliferative/intraluminal tissue within the lumen of the catheter through the side holes and whilst still maintaining suction to-and-fro movement of the catheter is performed to 'guillotine'-off tissue so entrapped. Suction is released and the catheter withdrawn, any tissue being submitted for histopathology and the tip then being cut off the catheter and sterile saline flushed through to dislodge remaining cellular contents, which can be used to form a cytology preparation. Some cellular material may also be obtained using a brush catheter rather than traumatic suction.

Other laboratory tests

A serine protease, canine prostate-specific esterase (CPSE), is a secretory protein produced within the prostate and which can be measured in serum. However, whilst levels in dogs with benign prostatic hyperplasia are elevated compared with dogs with no evidence of prostatic disease there has been shown to be considerable overlap in levels of serum CPSE in dogs with bacterial prostatitis and prostatic neoplasia compared with dogs with BPH. It is therefore not recommended as a diagnostic test as it may discriminate between these possibilities.

Diagnosis

The following investigation was undertaken:

- Haematology
  - Normal including a normal platelet count
- Assessment of serum urea and creatinine
  - Normal
- Abdominal radiography (see **Figure 27.1**)

Abdominal radiography demonstrated

- Two soft tissue structures in the caudal abdomen, which may have been an enlarged prostate and bladder or an enlarged prostate and paraprostatic cyst (but with no evidence of mineralisation).

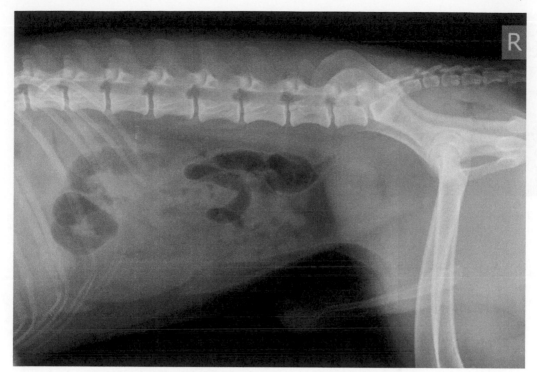

Figure 27.1 Right lateral abdominal radiograph.

- There were no bony changes or lymphadenopathy visible and the distal colon was empty, but it appears displaced dorsally by the prostate.
- Abdominal ultrasound (see **Figure 27.2**) was performed.

Fine needle aspiration cytology of the prostatic parenchyma was performed under ultrasound guidance and the cystic contents drained, yielding 20 ml of clear pink-tinged fluid. Results of analysis of these samples were:

- Fine needle aspiration cytology of prostatic parenchyma
  - ○ Low numbers of morphologically unremarkable prostatic epithelial cells are seen in the aspirates from the parenchyma. Here there is also evidence of macrophagic inflammation and mild chronic haemorrhage. There is no evidence of active inflammation or infection. Additionally there is a population of variably sized multi-nucleated cells whose origin is uncertain. Occasionally, these cells are larger and morphologically similar to osteoclasts and a possibility would be that these changes reflect an underlying osseous metaplasia.
- Analysis of cystic fluid
  - ○ One cytospin preparation is examined. The cellularity is high and the preservation is good. The background contains a small amount of blood. There are moderate numbers of activated macrophages. They have abundant and vacuolated cytoplasm and often contain haemosiderin or display erythrophagia.
  - ○ *Interpretation.* Macrophagic inflammation with evidence of mild chronic haemorrhage. Presence of frequent multinucleated cells of uncertain origin.
  - ○ Culture of cystic fluid
    - - Negative on aerobic and anaerobic culture

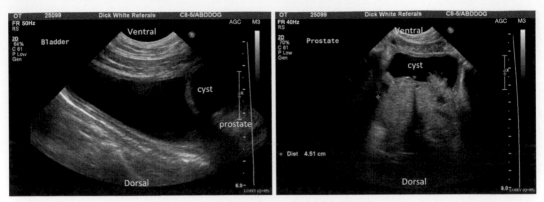

Figure 27.2 (left) Bladder ultrasound in the sagittal plane showing anechoic (urine) bladder contents and ventral bladder neck indented by the wall of the cystic lesion. (right) The prostate and cystic structure ventral to it imaged in transverse section. The prostate is enlared (7 × 4.5 cm) and heterogenous with multiple small cystic areas in addition to the larger cyst. The cystic lesion has anechoic content. Note that the prostate has retained its bilobed structure and is overall symmetrical, though small hypoechoic cystic lesions are present in the parenchyma. Non-mineralising immobile 'tree-like' proliferations were found at the margin of the cranioventral prostate and the cyst contents. A region of colon wall adjacent to the prostate appeared thickened. The remaining abdominal ultrasound was normal and no local lymphadenomegaly was detected.

- Prostatic massage fluid culture: negative
- Given the finding of a large inflammatory (apparently sterile) cystic lesion and unusual prostatic cytology, a provisional diagnosis of prostatic cyst with underlying benign prostatic hyperplasia, prostatitis or prostatic neoplasia was made. It was recommended that rather than pursue medical treatment that the patient undergo surgery to perform castration, resection and omentalisation of the prostatic cyst and submission of the cyst wall for histopathology and culture and prostatic biopsy.
  - At surgery a large paraprostatic cyst was identified but with multiple, apparently chronic, adhesions between the cyst wall and adjacent serosal surfaces including the colon.
  - A localised serositis was identified.
  - The cyst was subtotally resected and omentalised.
  - Castration and prostatic biopsy were performed.
  - The cyst wall and prostate were submitted for bacterial culture and the cyst wall, serosa and prostate were submitted for histopathology.
- Histological diagnosis was of
  - Benign prostatic hyperplasia.
  - Fibrosis, mild to moderate, multifocal, submitted tissues, peritoneum.
  - Peri-prostatitis and serositis, plasmacytic-lymphocytic to neutrophilic and histiocytic, chronic, multifocal to coalescing, marked with fibrosis, submitted tissues in the periprostatic region and cyst wall.
- Culture of tissues was negative.

Outcome
- Subsequent to surgery dripping of blood stopped and a repeat prostatic ultrasound 4 weeks after surgery showed marked reduction in the size of the prostate consistent with resolution of the benign prostatic hyperplasia.

- No consequences of the local serositis and adhesions have been noted and despite the changes apparent locally in the colonic wall, no clinical signs of colitis have developed.

Discussion

Whilst recognition of prostatic disease is not particularly challenging in dogs, provided that one maintains a high index of suspicion for it in appropriate presentations (and in particular in entire male dogs), differentiating different prostatic diseases can be challenging. Not only is it relatively common that more than one pathology may co-exist, as here, typically with cystic change or bacterial prostatitis complicating a pre-existing prostatic pathology, but diagnostic imaging of the prostate can be disarmingly difficult. Radiographs are helpful in determining prostatomegaly (on lateral radiographs occupation of more than 70% the pubic to sacral distance on the lateral view) but do not reliably distinguish between pathologies. The presence of mineralisation may be seen in prostatitis, benign prostatic hyperplasia, neoplasia and cysts though irregular prostatic mineralisation in a castrated dog is highly suggestive of neoplasia. Up to half of prostatic cysts have a mineralised ('egg-shell')-like appearance and when seen this is highly suggestive of a cyst (**Figure 27.3**).

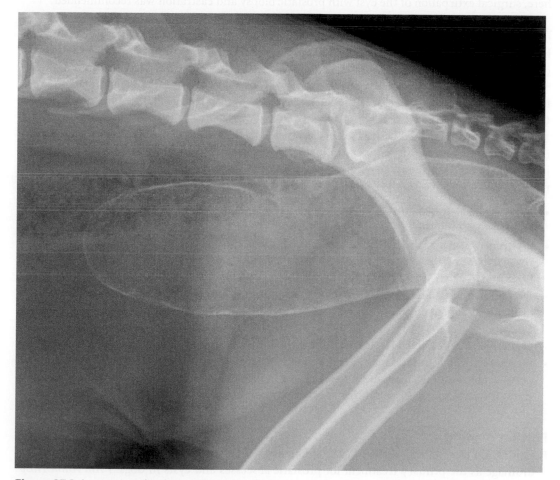

Figure 27.3 Large mineralised prostatic cyst in a dog.

There are various means of sampling prostatic tissue and prostatic cyst contents and all have advantages and disadvantages. Ultrasound-guided aspiration cytology has the advantage that with a skilled operator lesions can be specifically targeted. Potential disadvantages are that in the presence of a prostatic abscess localised distribution of infectious organisms could result in peritonitis (though practically most prostatic abscesses are walled off within the prostate and this risk should probably not be overstated, though it should also not be dismissed) and that prostatic neoplasia may be seeded down needle tracts. Pragmatically, since a surgical solution to prostatic neoplasia is not currently realised in dogs, this may be a more theoretical concern than one that negatively impacts on patients. Nonetheless, in cases where prostatic neoplasia is considered of high likelihood, initial attempts at obtaining a diagnosis by cytological analysis of urine or prostatic wash fluid (since these neoplasms are often exfoliative into urine and prostatic contribution to lower-urinary tract fluid content) and catheter suction biopsy should be first attempted. In this patient the anechoic and symmetrical nature of the cysts in a paraprostatic location made a cystic lesion more likely than an abscess.

Prostatic cysts may be safely drained percutaneously (as initially performed here) but recurrence and need for further drainage is seen in many patients. In older debilitated animals it may be reasonable to perform intermittent drainage and regular monitoring but since cystic change usually develops secondary to underlying prostatic disease and due to the unusual cytological changes here, surgical extirpation of the cyst with prostatic biopsy and castration was recommended.

Benign prostatic hyperplasia is a common disorder of intact male dogs with a prevalence of 80% in dogs over 5 years of age and 95% in dogs over 9 years of age. The normal prostatic cells undergo hyperplasia and hypertrophy under the influence of androgens (testosterone and dihydrotestosterone, DHT) and also of estradiol.

Castration is the most effective and rapid treatment for BPH and results in a decrease in prostatic volume by 50% in 3 weeks, with almost a complete return to normal size by 4 months (see **Case 26, Figure 26.5**).

Medical therapy may be desired in patients that are a poor anaesthetic risk, are used for breeding or where owner opposition to castration is intransigent. However, whilst effective in the majority of patients the response to medical therapy is variable, may be prolonged (often taking many months) and does not offer a permanent solution. Medical therapy options include

- Finasteride, a steroidal inhibitor of prostatic 5α-reductase (and so blocks production of DHT from testosterone).
- Oestrogens (such as diethylstilboestrol), which cause rapid reduction in testosterone via negative feedback on the hypothalamic–pituitary–testicular axis; their use is associated with risk of bone marrow toxicity and development of aplastic anaemia.
- Deslorelin and nafarelin, which are gonadotrophin-releasing hormone (GnRH) analogues, are available as subcutaneous sustained release implants, which induce downregulation of GnRH receptors.
- Osaterone acetate, which is a testosterone analogue that competitively inhibits DHT receptors.
- Gestagens, which include megoestrol acetate, medroxyprogesterone acetate and delmadinone acetate, are synthetic hormone analogues that induce negative feedback of the hypothalamic–pituitary–testicular axis, resulting in decreased androgen concentrations.

Further reading

Boland, L.E., Hardie, R.J., Gregory, S.P. & Lamb, C.R. (2003) Ultrasound-guided percutaneous drainage as the primary treatment for prostatic abscesses and cysts in dogs. *J Am Anim Hosp Assoc* **39**, 151–159

Bradbury, C.A., Westropp, J.L. & Pollard, R.E. (2009) Relationship between prostatomegaly, prostatic mineralization, and cytologic diagnosis. *Vet Radiol Ultrasound* **50**, 167–171

Freitag, T., Jerram, R.M., Walker, A.M. & Warman, C.G. (2007) Surgical management of common canine prostatic conditions. *Compend Contin Educ Vet* **29**, 656–658, 660, 662–653 passim; quiz 673

Krawiec, D.R. & Heflin, D. (1992) Study of prostatic disease in dogs: 177 cases (1981–1986). *J Am Vet Med Assoc* **200**, 1119–1122

Powe, J.R., Canfield, P.J. & Martin, P.A. (2004) Evaluation of the cytologic diagnosis of canine prostatic disorders. *Vet Clin Pathol* **33**, 150–154

Smith, J. (2008) Canine prostatic disease: a review of anatomy, pathology, diagnosis, and treatment. *Theriogenology* **70**, 375–383

Sirinarumitre, K. (2014) Benign prostatic hypertrophy and prostatitis in dogs. In *Kirk's Current Veterinary Therapy*, Vol. XV, eds J.D. Bonagura and D.C. Twedt, Elsevier Saunders, St Louis, pp. 1012–1015

Oncology

Clinical presentation

A 5 year-old male-neutered Standard Poodle is presented with a 2 week history of recurrent swelling of the left pelvic limb accompanied by mild lameness in the same limb. The swelling does not seem to be particularly painful and is not hot to the touch but is marked and impairs normal ambulation when present. It lasts generally for 24 hours before spontaneously resolving and has occurred six or seven times during this period, becoming more frequent. After careful palpation of the limb a small raised erythematous cutaneous nodular mass lesion approximately 1.5 cm in diameter is located on the lateral aspect of this limb (**Figure 28.1**). A fine needle aspiration cytology sample is taken from this mass and a photomicrograph of the resulting preparation is shown in **Figure 28.2**.

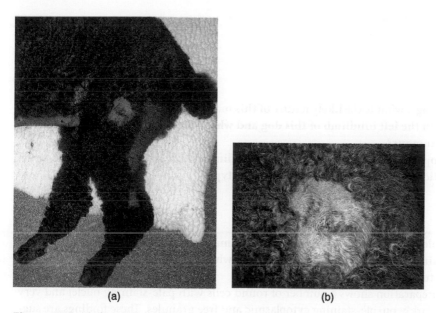

(a)   (b)

Figure 28.1 (a) The swollen left hindlimb of the patient and presentation and (b) inset of the cutaneous mass lesion.

Canine Internal Medicine: What's Your Diagnosis? First Edition. Jon Wray.
© 2018 John Wiley & Sons Ltd. Published 2018 by John Wiley & Sons Ltd.

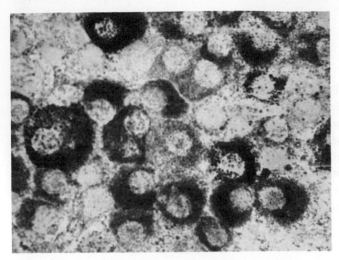

Figure 28.2 Photomicrograph of cytology of the cutaneous mass lesion (stained with haematoxylin and eosin).

Questions

1. **Based on the cytology, what is the likely nature of this mass lesion? Why might it have caused the swelling within the left hindlimb of this dog and what other systemic signs may be seen with this type of tumour?**
2. **What treatment options are recommended and what clinical features determine the prognosis and therapeutic recommendations in this tumour type?**

Answers

1. **Based on the cytology, what is the likely nature of this mass lesion? Why might it have caused the swelling within the left hindlimb of this dog and what other systemic signs may be seen with this type of tumour?**

   The cytology preparation shows a number of round cells with pale-staining nuclei and very large numbers of darkly purple-staining cytoplasmic and free granules. These findings are suggestive of a mast cell tumour.

   Local swelling and oedema formation in dogs with mast cell tumours is often attributed to periodic release of vasoactive substances such as histamine, heparin and other vasoactive amines.

   Other systemic signs of illness may include vomiting, haematemesis and melaena due to gastrointestinal ulceration. Dogs with mast cell tumours have increased plasma histamine and histamine release from mast cell tumour granules acts on H2 receptors of gastric parietal cells, resulting in increased secretion of hydrochloric acid (**Figure 28.3**).

2. **What treatment options are recommended and what clinical features determine the prognosis and therapeutic recommendations in this tumour type?**

   Mast cell tumours are both common (accounting for 16–21% of all skin neoplasms) and unpredictable in their behaviour. Nonetheless, the histological grade of mast cell tumours is the single most important prognostic factor in determining outcome as this, along with 'staging' the extent of the disease, is the basis for therapeutic decision making in mast cell tumours. The grade of

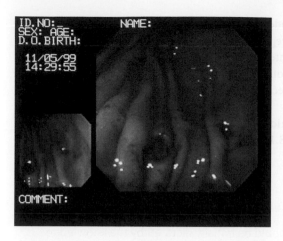

Figure 28.3 Endoscopic view of multiple deep gastric ulcers in a dog with a mast cell tumour.

tumour and thus likely biological behaviour cannot usually be reliably determined from cytology of fine needle aspirates (though highly pleomorphic cell distribution may raise suspicion of a high grade tumour), as useful as this technique is to diagnose mast cell tumour in the first place.

Importance of histological grading

Histopathology is the only reliable method to determine tumour grade but excision of mast cell tumours should be carefully planned as the success of the first surgery performed is the most important therapeutic factor in determining the long-term outcome. The histological grade is the single most important identifiable factor that loosely predicts likely behaviour of mast cell tumours; it should be performed in every case.

Some clinical features of mast cell tumours (such as rapid growth, local inflammation and poor demarcation from surrounding tissues, 'satellite' lesions and constitutional signs of illness) may suggest a higher grade, more aggressive tumour subtype. Additionally, some breed-types and anatomical locations are often associated with more behavioural malignant mast cell tumours.

The histological grade of mast cell tumours is often described by the Patnaik system in which tumours are described as grade I (well-differentiated), grade II (intermediately differentiated) or grade III (poorly differentiated). This system is most useful in the setting of grade I tumours, which generally have a low metastatic potential (around 10%) and are usually cured by surgery alone and in high grade (grade III) tumours that are typified by aggressive behaviour, a metastatic rate exceeding 80% and most of which result in death of the patient. A difficulty comes in predicting behaviour of intermediate-grade (II) mast cell tumours, which is highly variable. This has led to development of a 'two-tier' histological grading system (Kiupel) distinguishing high-grade tumours as having ≥7 mitotic figures per 10 high power fields, ≥3 multiucleated cells per 10 high power fields, ≥3 bizarre nuclear forms per 10 high power fields or the presence of karyomegaly. Recently a number of other markers have become popular and offered in attempts to clarify prognostication in intermediate-grade tumours, including the mitotic index, Ki-67 expression, argyrophilic nucleolar organiser regions (AgNORs) and proliferating cell nuclear antigen (PCNA). Care should be exercised in interpreting absolute values of these in an individual patient without an understanding that cut-off values commonly given are derived from 'best fit' levels shown to optimise sensitivity and specificity in papers describing limited numbers of subjects.

Distinct from histological grading, the clinical 'stage' of mast cell tumours has been previously described and is summarised in **Table 28.1**.

In most circumstances surgery is the most effective treatment for mast cell tumours

The therapeutic choice for mast cell tumours should be initially dictated by the knowledge that surgical excision is by some way the most effective treatment option for localised (non-metastatic) mast cell disease and that medical treatment options should only be considered in circumstances where this is not possible, or where systemic disease is present. The overall efficacy of medical therapy in mast cell tumours is disappointing and should only be considered where local disease control is not possible or unequivocal evidence of systemic disease risk is present.

The clinical questions that should be undertaken prior to planning treatment for MCT should be:

- Is wide excision possible?
- Is disease confined to a location(s) where local therapy is sufficient or is there evidence of systemic/distant involvement?
- What is the histological grade of the tumour?

The last of these is often answerable only after excision has been performed. A suggested approach to cytologically confirmed solitary cutaneous/subcutaneous mast cell tumour is displayed in Figure 28.4.

Table 28.1 Clinical staging of canine mast cell tumour

Stage	Description
Stage 0	One tumour incompletely excised from the dermis identified histologically
Stage 1	One tumour confined to the dermis without regional lymph node involvement
Stage 2	One tumour confined to the dermis with regional lymph node involvement
Stage 3	Multiple dermal tumours; large infiltrating tumours +/− regional lymph node involvement
Stage 4	Tumours with distant metastasis
Substage	(a) Without systemic 'constitutional' signs
	(b) With systemic 'constitutional' signs

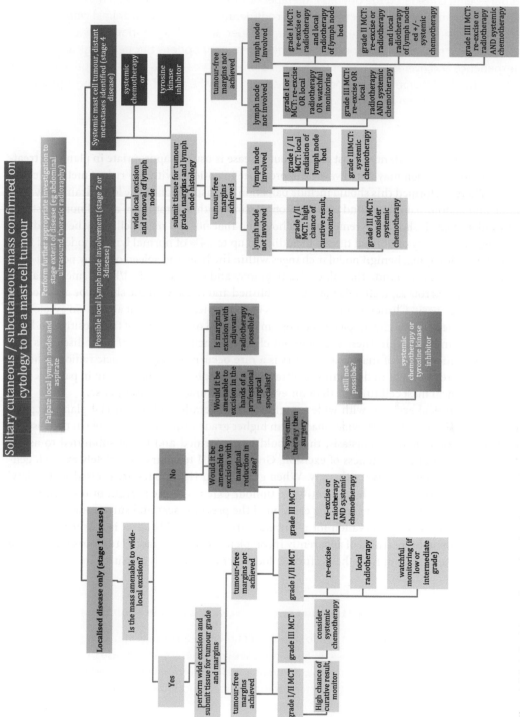

Figure 28.4 Decision making in localised mast cell tumours.

Explore all surgical options

Lack of surgical experience or presence of multiple cutaneous tumours should not preclude surgery being considered the optimum therapeutic option for most localised mast cell tumours. It is important that if it is a practical consideration, referral of an animal with a difficult-to-remove mast cell tumour to a surgical specialist colleague should always be considered preferable to undertaking medical treatment options through surgical inexperience and overestimation of the benefit of medical treatment. A further option is to institute medical therapy prior to performing surgery with the aim of 'downstaging' the size of the bulky mass to be excised.

Determining the extent of mast cell tumour disease is usually appropriate in planning treatment options, though may not always be appropriate in patients with low risk of metastatic disease. Where performed this should include palpation and aspiration of the local draining lymph node and abdominal ultrasound examination possibly with aspiration of any abnormal structures identified. It should be remembered, however, that normal mast cells may be found 'patrolling' in a variety of normal tissues including in up to 24% of normal lymph nodes and that, especially with aging, benign nodular changes within the liver and spleen of many normal dogs is identified on ultrasound. The value of radiography and haematological/buffy smear analysis and of bone marrow aspiration is not well established and need for these should be assessed on a case-by-case basis. Clinician preference varies in recommendations that aspiration cytology is routinely collected from liver, spleen and bone marrow and overall rates of true positive findings of mast cell infiltration in these sites without obvious concurrent signs of local disease is low. Pulmonary metastasis of mast cell tumours is a rare occurrence and thoracic radiographs are probably more of benefit in determining intracavitary lymph node enlargement in patients with thoracic truncal mast cell tumour than for evaluation for lung metastases per se.

Where surgical excision with wide margins (2 cm laterally and one fascial plane deep for grade I and II tumours, with wider margins in higher grade tumours) is possible in the absence of evidence of systemic metastasis, this should be performed and tissue submitted to assess tumour grade and completeness of excision. Grade I and II tumours, completely excised, generally do not require adjuvant therapy. When grade I and II tumours are excised with 'dirty' margins of excision in which an identifiable tumour extends to the margin of resected tissue, either further local treatment (en bloc excision of the previous scar and surrounding tissues or local radiotherapy) or observation for recurrence are options. This latter is reasonable in that only approximately one-third of apparently incompletely resected grade II tumours were shown to recur in one study, but nonetheless further local therapy is usually pursued.

Photographing mast cell tumours prior to excision is a good habit to get into

It is very helpful to routinely keep photographic documentation of such tumours prior to excision, especially if in difficult places, to plan subsequent therapy in the case of incomplete resection. It is very difficult for clinicians seeing mast cell tumour patients for re-excisional surgery or radiotherapy to know the extent of the original lesion when just faced with a post-operative scar. With the increased availability of easy digital photography and storage it is a very sensible habit to photograph mast cell tumours, along with some idea of scale, prior to any surgery.

Radiotherapy is generally not effective in the treatment of bulky disease but is of most use in the adjuvant setting where incomplete resection has occurred in a location where further surgery for en bloc local tissue resection may not be possible. This is most often true with mast cell tumours of the extremities.

Medical therapy with conventional cytotoxic chemotherapy or with receptor tyrosine kinase inhibitors (RTKIs, such as toceranib or masitinib) are undertaken in three circumstances:

1. To treat systemic/metastatic mast cell disease where local disease control alone would be ineffective,
2. In the neo-adjuvant setting to attempt to accomplish reduction in size ('down-staging') prior to surgery to make surgical excision more likely to be accomplished or
3. As a hopeful measure in the setting of likely residual microscopic disease after surgery where further surgery is not possible.

Systemic treatment is likely to be of most benefit in the setting of Stage 4 mast cell tumours, i.e. those with signs of systemic spread who are unlikely to benefit from local therapy. Those dogs with local grade III disease are also considered to benefit, with dogs with grade II disease that have markers of proliferation suggesting potential for aggressive behaviour also possibly benefitting. It is important to bear in mind that medical therapy should never be used in lieu of effective surgical treatment and that the overall measurable response rate/impact of medical treatments on mast cell tumours is generally low (usually less than a 50% objective response rate for most treatments evaluated to date). All medical options, including the use of newer RTKIs that target receptors for growth factors on the cell surface, involve a risk of side effects, including some that may on occasion be life-threatening. The most commonly used cytotoxic drug regimen uses vinblastine 2 mg/m² i.v. weekly for 4 weeks, then the same dose given fortnightly for 4 further occasions, accompanied by prednisolone at 2 mg/kg p/o SID for 1 week, then 1 mg/kg p/o SID for 2 weeks and then 1 mg/kg p/o every other day. Lomustine either alone at 60–70 mg/m² q21 days for 4 cycles or alternating (lower dose) with vinblastine at 2 mg/m², both given every 4 weeks alternating by 2 weeks apart, has also been reported. The RTKIs toceranib and masitinib have both been demonstrated to show a moderate response rate in dogs with recurrent grade 2 or grade 3 MCT, time to tumour progression and survival rate, but studies directly comparing the efficacy of conventional cytotoxic chemotherapy and RTKIs in these settings are only currently underway.

Further reading

Blackwood, L., Murphy, S., Buracco, P., De Vos, J.P., De Fornel-Thibaud, P., Hirschberger, J., Kessler, M., Pastor, J., Ponce, F., Savary-Bataille, K. & Argyle, D.J. (2012) European consensus document on mast cell tumours in dogs and cats. *Vet Comp Oncol* **10**, e1–e29

Dobson, J.M. & Scase, T.J. (2007) Advances in the diagnosis and management of cutaneous mast cell tumours in dogs. *J Small Anim Pract* **48**, 424–431

Govier, S.M. (2003) Principles of treatment for mast cell tumors. *Clin Tech Small Anim Pract* **18**, 103–106

London, C.A. & Seguin, B. (2003) Mast cell tumors in the dog. *Vet Clin North Am Small Anim Pract* **33**, 473–489

Misdorp, W. (2004) Mast cells and canine mast cell tumours. A review. *Vet Q* **26**, 156–169

Rogers, K.S. (2010) Mast cell disease. In *Textbook of Veterinary Internal Medicine*, 7th edn, eds S.J. Ettinger and E.C.Feldman, WB Saunders, St Louis, pp. 2193–2199

Welle, M.M., Bley, C.R., Howard, J. & Rufenacht, S. (2008) Canine mast cell tumours: a review of the pathogenesis, clinical features, pathology and treatment. *Vet Dermatol* **19**, 321–339

A 9 year-old female-neutered Labrador Cross (**Figure 29.1**) is presented with a history of mild weight loss and tachypnoea. The dog appears to develop worsening in its respiratory effort when trying to lie on the right side, becoming dyspnoeic when attempting to do so.

On physical examination the dog is in slightly poor body condition (body condition score 2/5) and has a mildly elevated respiratory rate of 36/min with a restrictive (choppy) respiratory pattern. Heart rate is 88/min and pulse rate is equal to this and of normal quality, mucous membrane colour and capillary refill is normal and the dog appears normally hydrated. Rectal temperature is normal and abdominal palpation and palpation of external lymph nodes is normal. On thoracic auscultation the cardiac sounds cannot be heard on the left side and bronchovesicular sounds are only audible caudally on the left. A cardiac apex beat can be appreciated displaced caudodorsally on the right and cardiac sounds can be auscultated here.

Dorsoventral and left lateral thoracic radiographs (due to positional dyspnoea in right lateral recumbency) are taken and are shown in **Figure 29.2**.

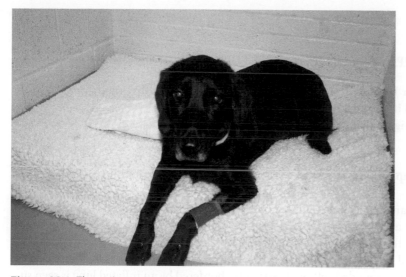

Figure 29.1 The patient at presentation.

Canine Internal Medicine: What's Your Diagnosis? First Edition. Jon Wray.
© 2018 John Wiley & Sons Ltd. Published 2018 by John Wiley & Sons Ltd.

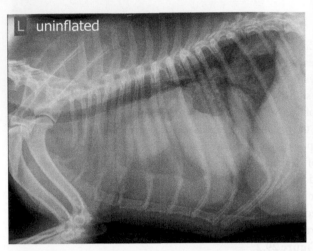
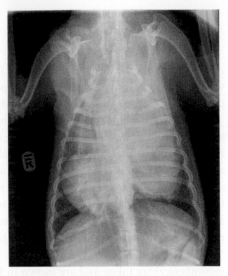

Figure 29.2 Left lateral and dorsoventral thoracic radiographs of the patient at presentation.

Questions

1. What do the radiographs show and what are the principle differential diagnoses for these findings?
2. Are haematological or biochemical findings likely to be helpful in distinguishing between these possibilities and if so in what way?
3. How would you investigate this patient further?

Answers

1. **What do the radiographs show and what are the principle differential diagnoses for these findings?**

   Dorsoventral (DV) and left lateral recumbent projections are supplied.

   There appears to be a very large (10 × 15 × 24 cm³), homogeneous, round, well marginated, soft tissue mass within the left cranial thorax, though on both the DV and the lateral projection (mid-thorax, intercostal spaces 4–6 on the lateral projection, intercostal spaces 4–7 to the left of midline on the DV view) a rounded soft tissue structure bordered by an inflated lung is seen superimposed on this larger structure; this may represent a second soft tissue mass or a lobulated area of the larger structure, partly surrounded by inflated lung. The inflated left caudal lung lobe is seen tracking between the mass and the lateral body wall (excluding an extrapleural mass). The mass is solid in appearance without intralesional air bronchograms. There is a marked mass effect resulting in marked right lateral and dorsal tracheal displacement and a marked mediastinal shift towards the right hemithorax (with the cardiac silhouette almost in apposition with the right lateral thoracic wall and severely elevated from the sternum). The remaining lung lobes are largely unremarkable. There is no evidence of a concurrent nodular pattern elsewhere in the lung field. There is a mild interstitial opacification in the unaffected lung lobes likely reflecting minor atelectasis due to the mass effect. The cardiac silhouette (though displaced) is subjectively unremarkable. The trachea is also otherwise unremarkable. The bronchial tree is unremarkable aside from the left cranial lobar bronchus, which cannot be detected. Very faint and slender pleural fissure lines are seen bilaterally in DV but the pleural space is otherwise unremarkable. The visible portion of the cranial abdominal field is unremarkable. There is moderate to marked osteophytic change around both elbows (much more marked in the right elbow). Otherwise skeletally it is unremarkable.

The principle differential diagnosis is of a pulmonary mass lesion of the left cranial lung lobe, but given the marked cardiac and tracheal displacement a mediastinal mass is not completely excluded. Differential diagnoses for pulmonary and mediastinal masses are listed in **Table 29.1**.

2. **Are haematological or biochemical findings likely to be helpful in distinguishing between these possibilities and if so in what way?**

By-and-large laboratory findings are not especially helpful in determining either the tissue of origin or the aetiology of thoracic masses. Expected haematological changes might include

- Presence of appropriate secondary polycythaemia if the mass lesion has resulted in prolonged hypoxaemia, or conversely anaemia if it is associated with local blood loss.
- Presence of neutrophilia +/− a band shift if the mass is associated with a significant inflammatory component or necrosis.
- Presence of circulating lymphocytosis, which is associated with up to 19% of dogs with thymoma and a similar proportion of dogs with lymphoma, with circulating atypical lymphocytes suggesting lymphomatous involvement of the bone marrow.
- Mild thrombocytopenia may be seen in a minority of patients with thoracic mass lesions and this may be consumptive, related to secondary immune-mediated destruction or reflect multi-systemic effects of lymphoma if bone marrow infiltration is present. Conversely a reactive thrombocytosis is frequently seen in the presence of inflammation or where prior bleeding has occurred.

Biochemical changes are equally non-specific and only variably present.

Table 29.1 Differential diagnosis for pulmonary or cranial mediastinal mass lesions

Principal differential diagnoses for pulmonary mass lesions:	• Primary lung tumour
	◦ Bronchoalveolar carcinoma
	◦ Adenocarcinoma
	◦ Adenosquamous carcinoma and squamous cell carcinoma
	• Histiocytic sarcoma
	• Lymphoma
	• Granuloma or abscess
	• Haematoma
Principal differential diagnoses for mediastinal mass lesions	• Cranial mediastinal lymphoma
	• Thymoma
	• Branchial cyst
	• Ectopic thyroid carcinoma
	• Heart base mass

Hypercalcaemia in cranial mediastinal mass lesions

In the presence of cranial mediastinal mass lesions, hypercalcaemia is frequently seen and whilst many veterinary surgeons commonly (and correctly) associate the presence of hypercalcaemia with cranial mediastinal lymphoma (it has been reported to be the form of lymphoma most commonly associated with hypercalcaemia of malignancy and up to 40% of dogs with the cranial mediastinal form will have hypercalcaemia) it should be borne in mind that 28% of dogs with thymoma are also reported to be hypercalcaemic, and in about half of these ionised calcium levels are also elevated. Where evaluated this has been most commonly associated with increased parathyroid-related peptide concentrations.

Curiously, mild to moderate rises in hepatocellular and cholestatic markers have been reported in a significant minority of patients with cranial mediastinal masses, but also in other patients with significant airway disease; the mechanism of this is obscure.

3. **How would you investigate this patient further?**

Further diagnostic imaging may help determine better both the site of origin, extent and anatomical relations of this mass than the initial radiographs. Diagnostic ultrasound has advantages that it is cost effective, widely available and may help determine the tissue of origin by observing for respiratory movement of the mass, lesions originating in lung parenchyma usually demonstrating respiratory 'lung slide' whilst extra-pleural and mediastinal lesions are generally static. Diagnostic ultrasound can also be performed without general anaesthesia and allows cytological material to be collected by fine needle aspiration under ultrasound guidance if mass lesions abut the thoracic wall (as here). Large solid lesions may be amenable to ultrasound-guided tissue core biopsy techniques for histopathology. Lastly, since mass lesions of the pulmonary parenchyma and the cranial mediastinum are commonly associated with the presence of mass lesions elsewhere, ultrasound evaluation of the mass may also be combined with abdominal ultrasound performance and evaluation of the cardiac base. A potential disadvantage of ultrasonography in the presence of very large mass lesions is that their anatomical origin may not be as apparent as with smaller lesions, since most of the thoracic contents may be displaced, and aforementioned respiratory movement may be decreased or absent in very large lesions, even if they are of respiratory origin.

Cross-sectional imaging techniques such as thoracic computed tomography (CT) allow greater detail of anatomic relationships to be determined and may offer higher sensitivity in detecting additional lung parenchymal lesions and lymph node pathology, which may represent metastasis. Reformatting of such images in a variety of planes is possible allowing even greater flexibility in determining these anatomical relationships. Increased expense, lack of availability and need for general anaesthesia are principle disadvantages.

Cytological diagnosis for intrathoracic mass lesions

Cytological evaluation is useful in dogs with **primary pulmonary mass** lesions though a confident diagnosis can be made in between 38% and 90% of cases based on cytology. The presence of extensive necrosis often hampers cytological interpretation and it should be borne in mind that, whilst uncommon, tumour 'seeding' of malignant primary pulmonary neoplasia has been reported along the needle tracts of dogs undergoing fine needle aspiration, and it may be argued that with solitary, peripheral and surgically amenable lesions, excisional biopsy at surgery without prior aspiration may be more appropriate.

In **cranial mediastinal mass** lesions, differentiation between the two most common types, lymphoma and thymoma, is frequently possible on the basis of cytological evaluation, thymoma being characterised by the presence of neoplastic epithelial cells and mature (small) lymphocytes, often with mast cells present as well. The presence of large numbers of lymphoblastic lymphocytes suggest mediastinal lymphoma. However, in many cases the cytological yield is either poor (often due to the presence of a cystic morphology of the mass) or samples are lacking in epithelial cells and contain a predominance of small lymphocytes, a cytological picture common to both thymomas and many 'lymphocytic' lymphomas. In such a setting, flow cytometry has been shown to be useful since thymic-origin lymphocytes, uniquely, co-express CD4 and CD8 and the presence of >10% CD4/CD8 co-expressing lymphocytes has been shown to reliably distinguish between lymphoma and thymoma in one study (Lana et al. 2006); very occasionally mediastinal lymphoma may co-express CD4 and CD8 in a small number of lymphocytes but is readily distinguished from thymoma on light-scatter properties.

Up to 17% of dogs with thymoma may have concurrent paraneoplastic myasthenia gravis, most commonly manifest as focal myasthenia causing megaoesophagus. Assessment of an edrophonium response test in those patients exhibiting generalised weakness and evaluation of an acetylcholine receptor antibody test is appropriate if myasthenia gravis is suspected but the proportion of false negative patients by antibody testing in dogs is poorly characterised.

Diagnosis

In this patient, haematological and biochemical findings are shown below:

Haematology

Parameter	Value	Units	Range
RBC	5.71	$\times 10^{12}/l$	(5.5–8.5)
Haemoglobin	14.4	g/dl	(12.0–18.0)
Haematocrit	0.42	l/l	(0.37–0.55)
Mean cell volume	74.2	fl	(60–77)
Mean cell haemoglobin concentration	25.2	g/dl	(29.0–38.0)
Mean cell haemoglobin	25.2	pg	(19.5–25.5)
Total white cell count	**16.94**	$\times 10^{9}/l$	(6.0–15.0)
Neutrophils	8.17	$\times 10^{9}/l$	(3.0–11.5)
Lymphocytes	**7.77**	$\times 10^{9}/l$	(1.0–4.8)

(Continued)

Parameter	Value	Units	Range
Monocytes	0.57	$\times 10^9/l$	(0.2–1.4)
Eosinophils	0.35	$\times 10^9/l$	(0.1–1.2)
Basophils	0.08	$\times 10^9/l$	(0.0–0.1)
Platelets	305	$\times 10^9/l$	(200–500)
Film comment:		Lymphocytes are normal in morphology	

Biochemistry

Parameter	Value	Units	Range
Total protein	60	g/l	(54–77)
Albumin	32	g/l	(25–40)
Globulin	28	g/l	(23–45)
Urea	6.7	mmol/l	(2.5–7.4)
Creatinine	82	µmol/l	(40–145)
Potassium	4.8	mmol/l	(3.4–5.6)
Sodium	146	mmol/l	(139–154)
Chloride	115	mmol/l	(105–122)
Calcium	**3.1**	mmol/l	(2.1–2.8)
Ionised calcium	**1.5**	mmol/l	(1.18–1.40)
Inorganic phosphate	1.2	mmol/l	(0.60–1.40)
Glucose	5.7	mmol/l	(3.3–5.8)
ALT	40	IU/l	(13–88)
AST	31	IU/l	(13–60)
ALKP	43	IU/l	(14–105)
GGT	4	IU/l	(0–10)
Bilirubin	2	µmol/l	(0–16)
Cholesterol	4.5	mmol/l	(3.8–7.0)
Triglyceride	0.9	mmol/l	(0.56–1.14)
Creatine kinase	87	IU/l	(0–190)

- Thoracic and abdominal ultrasound was performed (the abdominal ultrasound was normal). Thoracic ultrasound demonstrated a very large inhomogenous soft tissue mass lesion of the left cranial thorax containing multiple anechoic-fluid filled lesions (**Figure 29.3**). Very subtle respiratory movement could be detected within the mass but overall the anatomical origin could not be determined other than that it did not appear to originate from cardiac structures. Fine needle aspiration cytology samples were taken for both cytology and flow-cytometry.
- Cytology demonstrated
  - A moderate cell harvest with nucleated cells comprising 85% small lymphocytes.
  - Remainder of cells were intermediate to large lymphocytes, occasional mast cells and macrophages, some exhibiting erythrophagocytosis.

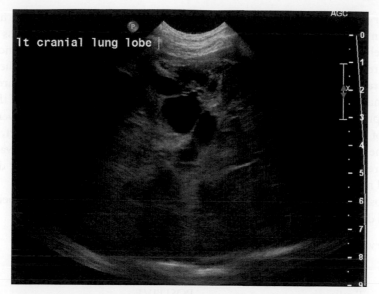

Figure 29.3 Intercostal ultrasound appearance of the mass lesion in this patient. Note that at the time of ultrasound it was wrongly considered that this mass might represent a lesion within the left cranial lung lobe – hence the incorrect label.

- ○ No epithelial cells were definitively identified though small aggregates of poorly preserved cells that might be epithelial cells or clusters of macrophages were observed.

  The cytological diagnosis was inconclusive but suggestive of thymoma or possibly lymphoma.

- • Pending flow-cytometry results a thoracic CT scan was performed.
- • Pre- and post-contrast transverse images of the thorax (**Figure 29.4**) were performed and re-constructed in a soft tissue, lung and bone algorithm. Within the cranial mediastinum was

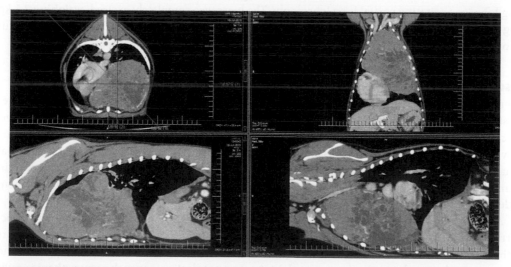

Figure 29.4 Multi-planar reconstructed (MPR) CT images of the thorax of the patient showing (clockwise from top left) transverse, dorsal, sagittal oblique and sagittal images through the mass lesion. The heart can be seen to be displaced to the right, caudally and dorsally, by the mass lesion occupying the left cranial thorax.

identified a very large, soft tissue attenuating (with pockets of fluid attenuating), homogeneously (except in the areas of fluid attenuation) contrast enhancing mass. This mass measured as approximately 11.7 cm in height, 14.5 cm in width and 17.7 cm in length and encompassed nearly the entire width of the cranial thorax and at least three-quarters of the left hemithorax. The caudoventral margin of the mass had a nodular appearance and extended towards the diaphragm. The mass caused nearly complete compression and dorsal displacement of the left cranial lung, compression and caudal displacement of the right cranial lung lobe and overall caudal displacement of the lung lobes, as well as caudal and rightward deviation of the heart, rightward deviation of the oesophagus and dorsal displacement of the trachea. The carina was caudally displaced. There was no evidence of vascular invasion or of pulmonary metastatic disease but there was mild multi-focal atelectasis.

- The CT diagnosis was of a cranial mediastinal mass with lymphoma or thymoma being principle differential diagnoses.

Flow cytometry report (see **Figure 29.5**)

CD3	T cells	10% positive
CD4	T helper cells	POSITIVE
CD5	T cells	POSITIVE
CD8	Cytotoxic T cells	POSITIVE
CD21	B cells	Negative
CD79a	All B cells	Negative
CD34	Early precursors	Negative
MHCII		Negative

The cells have low side scatter and forward scatter and co-express CD4 and CD8 and also express CD5, which is supportive of thymoma. Rarely, lymphoma can be CD4+/CD8+ but the scatter profile differs (high forward scatter, low side scatter).

After discussion with the dog's owners, attempted resection of the mass was performed and a median sternotomy performed. The mass was highly vascular and adherent to the left cranial lung lobe, necessitating partial lung lobectomy. The mass was completely excised, weighing 2.1 kg (**Figure 29.6**). Histopathology was consistent with a benign thymoma. The dog made an uneventful recovery from surgery.

Discussion

Thymomas are rare tumours though account for a significant proportion of dogs with cranial mediastinal mass lesions. Clinical signs associated with thymoma are usually related either to their space-occupying nature, and often large size, or due to paraneoplastic effects such as myasthenia gravis or hypercalcaemia. Thymomas may grow to a very large size and compression of the cranial vena cava (and subsequent reduction in venous return from the head and forelimbs) may result in 'cranial vena cava syndrome', manifested by head and neck or ventral neck oedema with or without oedema of one or both forelimbs.

Although thymoma is commonly reported to occur in older animals with a peak age of occurrence in dogs of 9 years, a recent case series demonstrated a range in age from 1.5 to 14 years with Labrador and Retriever breeds overrepresented. Clinical signs of lethargy, tachypnoea and weakness tend to predominate. As previously states paraneoplastic signs such as myasthenia gravis and hypercalcaemia occur in a significant number of dogs with thymoma. Although the presence of co-morbid conditions, especially myasthenia-induced megaoesophagus, has been previously

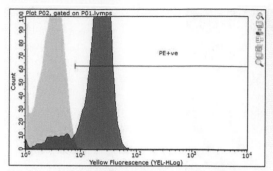
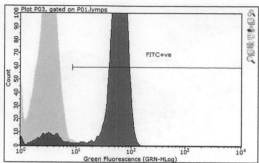
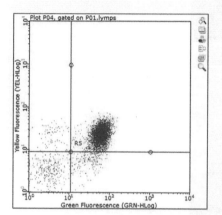
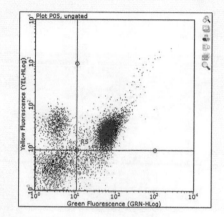

Figure 29.5 Flow cytometry performed on samples aspirated from the cranial mediastinal mass in this patient. The top-left trace shows negative control (yellow) and positive sample results for CD4-positive lymphocytes (yellow fluorescence, phycoerythrin) and the top-right trace shows negative control (yellow) and positive (dark pink) results for CD8-positive lymphocytes (green fluorescence, fluorescein). The bottom trace shows the scatter display plotting yellow fluorescence (CD4) on the y-axis against green fluorescence (CD8) on the x-axis. The upper left quadrant shows CD4 +ve/CD8 −ve, bottom left quadrant CD4 −ve/CD8 −ve, lower right quadrant CD4 −ve/CD8 +ve, upper right quadrant CD4 +ve/CD8 +ve. The highlighted (red) cells are those co-expressing CD4 and CD8.

reported to have a negative prognostic influence, a recent case series of 116 dogs with thymoma found no prognostic influence of the presence of either myasthenia gravis or hypercalcaemia on survival time. It has been reported that up to 27% of dogs with thymoma may have a concurrent tumour present at the time of diagnosis, emphasising that careful attention should be paid to diagnostic staging prior to making definitive treatment decisions.

Approximately 15% of dogs with thymoma are found to have local invasion into the cranial vena cava on diagnostic imaging and approximately 5% are found to have pulmonary metastases, though predominantly the biologic behaviour of thymomas is benign.

Where possible, surgical excision of thymoma is the treatment of choice and results in a median survival time of 635 days for those dogs in which surgery is performed versus 76 days for those dogs not treated surgically. Radiotherapy has been reported with variable success but overall a measurable response to thymoma is seen in 50–75% but with only a minority of patients showing a complete response and with a shorter median survival time than surgery of 248 days. The effects of chemotherapy are not well established with canine thymoma, though occasional satisfying responses have be seen.

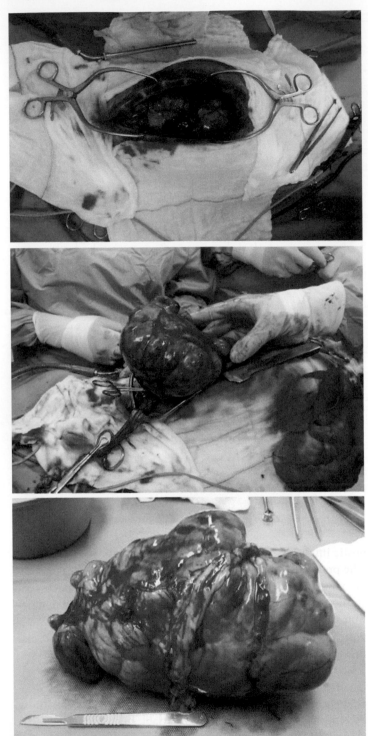

Figure 29.6 Intraoperative photographs of the thymoma being resected.

In one case series of those dogs undergoing attempted surgical excision of thymoma, approximately 10% of surgeries needed to be aborted due to the invasive/non-resectable nature of the tumour. One of the greatest difficulties in thymoma treatment planning is in attempting to predict, pre-operatively, the degree of local invasiveness and resectability, and in the same study 42% of dogs who had a pre-operative CT scan suggestive of a non-resectable tumour subsequently underwent successful surgery. Until pre-operative diagnostic imaging allows this determination to be made with greater accuracy it is advised that careful owner counselling, that the resectability of these tumours is best determined at the time of surgery, should be standard. Recurrence of thymoma may be seen in up to 14% of patients a mean of 518 days after surgery, with a good prognosis being described for those dogs in which a second surgery is undertaken.

Reference

Lana, S., Plaza, S., Hampe, K., Burnett, R. & Avery, A.C. (2006) Diagnosis of mediastinal masses in dogs by flow cytometry. *J Vet Intern Med* **20**, 1161–1165

Further reading

Aronsohn, M.G., Schunk, K.L., Carpenter, J.L. & King, N.W. (1984) Clinical and pathologic features of thymoma in 15 dogs. *J Am Vet Med Assoc* **184**, 1355–1362

Atwater, S.W., Powers, B.E., Park, R.D., Straw, R.C., Ogilvie, G.K. & Withrow, S.J. (1994) Thymoma in dogs: 23 cases (1980–1991). *J Am Vet Med Assoc* **205**, 1007–1013

Bellah, J.R., Stiff, M.E. & Russell, R.G. (1983) Thymoma in the dog: two case reports and review of 20 additional cases. *J Am Vet Med Assoc* **183**, 306–311

Day, M.J. (1997) Review of thymic pathology in 30 cats and 36 dogs. *J Small Anim Pract* **38**, 393–403

Meleo, K.A. (1997) The role of radiotherapy in the treatment of lymphoma and thymoma. *Vet Clin North Am Small Anim Pract* **27**, 115–129

Robat, C.S., Cesario, L., Gaeta, R., Miller, M., Schrempp, D. & Chun, R. (2013) Clinical features, treatment options, and outcome in dogs with thymoma: 116 cases (1999–2010). *J Am Vet Med Assoc* **243**, 1448–1454

Smith, A.N., Wright, J.C., Brawner, W.R., Jr, LaRue, S.M., Fineman, L., Hogge, G.S., Kitchell, B.E., Hohenhaus, A.E., Burk, R.L., Dhaliwal, R.S. & Duda, L.E. (2001) Radiation therapy in the treatment of canine and feline thymomas: a retrospective study (1985–1999). *J Am Anim Hosp Assoc* **37**, 489–496

Zitz, J.C., Birchard, S.J., Couto, G.C., Samii, V.F., Weisbrode, S.E. & Young, G.S. (2008) Results of excision of thymoma in cats and dogs: 20 cases (1984–2005). *J Am Vet Med Assoc* **232**, 1186–1192

Clinical presentation

An 8 year-old male-neutered German Shorthaired Pointer is presented because of reduced appetite and slightly subdued demeanour and because the owner has noticed 'lumps' to have appeared under the dog's neck. The dog has shown no other constitutional signs of illness, although is reported to be drinking progressively more, now bordering on the excessive. He has not lost weight and continues to interact and play with the owner's other dog who is clinically healthy. The dog is annually vaccinated and receives routine ecto- and endoparasitic treatments, is fed a normal complete commercial diet and has not travelled outside the United Kingdom. Previous medical history is unremarkable.

Physical examination demonstrates a reasonably bright dog in normal body condition. Palpable, non-painful enlargement of the mandibular (3 cm diameter), prescapular (4 cm diameter) and popliteal (3 cm diameter) lymph nodes is detected (**Figure 30.1**). Lymph nodes are freely movable. The remaining physical examination is normal and no abnormalities of auscultation or abdominal palpation are noted.

A diagnosis of multicentric lymphoma is suspected.

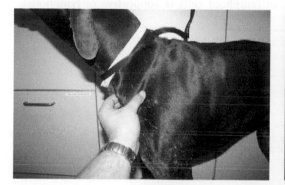
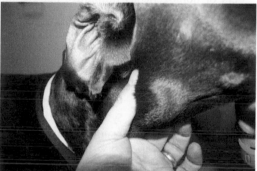
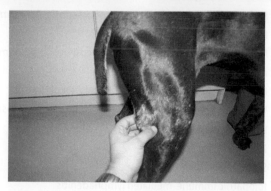

Figure 30.1 The patient at presentation, demonstrating lymphadenomegaly of the mandibular, prescapular and popliteal lymph nodes.

Canine Internal Medicine: What's Your Diagnosis? First Edition. Jon Wray.
© 2018 John Wiley & Sons Ltd. Published 2018 by John Wiley & Sons Ltd.

Questions

1. **Other than lymphoma, what other differential diagnoses for peripheral lymphadenomegaly should be considered? How can a diagnosis of lymphoma be confirmed?**
2. **What is meant by clinical 'staging' of lymphoma and by what criteria is canine lymphoma commonly 'staged'? What is the purpose of such 'staging'?**
3. **What is meant by the term 'paraneoplastic syndrome' and what such syndromes may be associated with canine lymphoma? Could the increase in thirst be attributable to any of these?**
4. **What broad treatment options exist for treatment of canine multi-centric lymphoma and what general guidance can be given to owners?**

Answers

1. **Other than lymphoma, what other differential diagnoses for peripheral lymphadenomegaly should be considered? How can a diagnosis of lymphoma be confirmed?**

The term lymphadenomegaly refers to enlargement of one or more lymph nodes. Though the term lymphadenopathy is often used interchangeably strictly this refers to lymph node pathology, which may include those disorders that actually decrease the size of lymph nodes.

Differential diagnoses for peripheral lymphadenomegaly are shown in **Table 30.1**.

A diagnosis of lymphoma can usually be confirmed cytologically by fine needle aspiration cytology of affected organs such as enlarged peripheral lymph nodes. The finding of large numbers of homogeneous immature populations of lymphoid cells is supportive of lymphoma,

Table 30.1 Differential diagnosis of peripheral lymphadenomegaly

Aetiology	Examples
N (Neoplastic)	Lymphoma
	Malignant histiocytosis
	Systemic mast cell neoplasia
	Multiple myeloma
	Leukaemias
	Metastatic neoplasia
I (Infectious)	Bacterial (e.g. streptococcosis, mycobacteriosis, *Actinomyces* infection)
	Rickettsial (e.g. anaplasmosis, ehrlichiosis)
	Fungal (e.g. Histoplasmosis, Blastomycosis, coccidioidomycosis)
	Algal (e.g. protothecosis)
	Protozoal (e.g. leishmaniosis, babesiosis, toxplasmosis)
	Viral (e.g. infectious canine hepatitis, canine herpesvirus)
I (Immune-mediated)	Immune-mediated polyarthritis
	Rheumatoid arthritis
	Systemic lupus erythematosus
	Idiopathic immune-mediated lymphadenitis
Miscellaneous	'Reactive' lymphadenopathy
	Post-vaccinal
	Mineral-associated lymphadenitis
	Generalised demodicosis

though there is some variability and histological examination of either excised tissue or tissue specimens collected with a biopsy device usually offer a definitive diagnosis where cytology is equivocal.

Immunohistochemical and immunocytochemical (flow cytometric) techniques may also be employed to both determine the homogeneity of the lymphoid population and to allow immunophenotyping (B-cell, T-cell or null cell). A PCR performed on fresh or preserved tissues for detection of antigen receptor rearrangements (PARR) may detect clonality in a population of lymphocytes, which is a hallmark of malignancy.

A number of potential serum biomarkers of lymphoma in the dog are currently under investigation and are even marketed as 'blood tests' for lymphoma, though the utility of such analytes is currently unclear. Some are based on alteration in acute phase proteins, which may have some utility, particularly in presaging relapse in previously diagnosed lymphoma that is in remission after therapy.

2. **What is meant by clinical 'staging' of lymphoma and by what criteria is canine lymphoma commonly 'staged'? What is the purpose of such 'staging'?**

Simply put, staging refers to the definition of severity, extent and effects of a tumour both locally and in locations remote to it. Many staging systems exist for different tumours in human and veterinary oncology, with most being based on the T/N/M, that is to say tumour (T, size), node (N, presence or absence of local lymph node involvement) and metastasis (M, presence or absence of distant metastasis) system. In the case of lymphoma, the site and extent of tumour involvement can be more variable than most other neoplasms and lymphoma is commonly referred to as 'nodal' or 'extranodal' and the latter frequently subdivided by anatomical site. An accepted WHO-based staging system for canine lymphoma is described in **Table 30.2**. Note that in addition to the principle stages, I through V, a substage designation of either substage (a) or substage (b) is given depending on the animal showing no quality of life-limiting constitutional signs of disease (a) or showing such constitutional signs (b). Practically speaking, staging is accomplished by a combination of a thorough clinical history and meticulous physical examination, routine laboratory tests such as haematology and biochemistry, and by performing diagnostic imaging to detect the extent of disease (which may be combined with tissue cytology or biopsy to confirm involvement). Some debate exists as to the necessity of performing bone marrow sample evaluation for the purposes of clinical staging since this diagnostic step is more intrusive and such increased risk of patient discomfort must be balanced against the utility of

Table 30.2 Veterinary staging system for canine lymphoma

Stage	Description
I	Single node or single organ involved, not including bone marrow
II	Involvement of many lymph nodes confined to a single anatomic area
III	Generalised lymph node involvement
IV	Liver and/or splenic lymphoma (with or without generalised lymph node involvement)
V	Evidence of circulating malignant lymphoid cells or bone marrow involvement (with or without features of stages I–IV)
Substage	*Subclassification of each stage*
a	Without systemic constitutional signs of illness
b	With systemic constitutional signs of illness

the information it provides in informing clinical and treatment decision making. Principle indications for bone marrow aspiration are the presence of circulating atypical lymphocytes, anaemia, lymphocytosis or peripheral 'cytopenias'. It should be noted, however, that in one study, whereas 28% of dogs evaluated and going on to have bone marrow aspiration had peripheral evidence of circulating malignant cells, 57% of dogs sampled had direct evidence of bone marrow involvement on aspiration cytology and clinical stage may be underestimated without bone marrow aspiration.

Why stage?

Like any single diagnostic test, a combination of diagnostic endeavours, such as clinical staging for lymphoma, must be utilised in the best interests of the patient, that is to answer a clinical question that is of importance, relevance and ultimately of benefit to the patient and its treatment to know the answer. Fundamentally, to do otherwise is to perform diagnostic testing for dogmatic rather than pragmatic purposes and generates unwarranted expense and medical intrusiveness. In order for staging not to be simply a knee-jerk and dogmatic approach to a diagnosis of lymphoma, it is important to continually bear in mind the purposes behind it. These may include

- To help guide in prognostication so that owners may make an informed decision as to whether or not to pursue therapy and to foster realistic expectations in those patients in whom therapy is pursued. For example, the owners of a patient who exhibits several negative prognostic indicators (such as substage b), stage V disease, T-cell immunophenotype and concurrent hypercalcaemia might reasonably use such information to reinforce a consideration not to pursue therapy.
- To identify additional morbidities, either directly related to tumour local effects, related to paraneoplastic syndromes (see later) or unrelated co-morbidities that may either substantially impact on prognosis, may alter expected longevity of the patient, may impact upon the safety of proposed treatments or may require additional management.
- To help guide appropriate treatment or alternatively to provide information to support that a variety of treatment strategies could potentially be undertaken without contraindications.

The influence of the clinical stage of lymphoma on prognosis is not necessarily an intuitive case of a continuum of worsening prognosis from stage I through to stage V. The current identified factors that are strongly associated with prognosis (which may refer to odds of induction of remission or survival time or both) are summarised in **Table 30.3**.

Table 30.3 Factors associated with prognosis in canine lymphoma

Clinical stage	• More favourable prognosis with stages I and II tumours
	• Unfavourable prognosis with stage V tumours
Clinical substage	• Unfavourable prognosis associated with clinical substage b, i.e. associated with constitutional signs of systemic illness

Immunophenotype	• More favourable prognosis with B-cell immunophenotype
	• Reduced survival associated with T-cell immunophenotype
Histological grade	• High response rate but reduced survival associated with high- and medium-grade histological findings. More prolonged (indolent) clinical course associated with low-grade tumours
Anatomical location	• Unfavourable prognosis associated with cranial mediastinal location, diffuse gastrointestinal, diffuse cutaneous, hepatosplenic and leukaemic forms
Clinicopathological features	• Unfavourable prognosis associated with hypercalcaemia, especially if accompanied by decreased renal function (though hypercalcaemia is more common in T-cell immunophenotype)
	• Unfavourable prognosis in presence of anaemia
Treatment factors	• Prolonged corticosteroid use prior to onset of cytotoxic chemotherapy is associated with shortened response duration, but critical length of this is unknown
	• Episodes of chemotherapy-induced neutropenia are associated with prolonged first remission duration

3. **What is meant by the term 'paraneoplastic syndrome' and what such syndromes may be associated with canine lymphoma? Could the increased thirst be attributable to any of these?**

Paraneoplastic syndromes

A paraneoplastic syndrome is any biologically significant effect, due to the presence of a tumour, either remotely or systemically, that is not due to anatomical infiltration of the tumour but due to remote tumour effects. Paraneoplastic syndromes do not invariably occur with all tumours but may be responsible for the initial or most clinically obvious presenting signs and their presence may often therefore raise clinical suspicion of neoplasia. Similarly, since their presence and magnitude usually parallels tumour burden, their resolution usually indicated successful therapy of the primary neoplasm and recurrence often heralds tumour relapse.

Common paraneoplastic syndromes associated with lymphoma are summarised in **Table 30.4**.

Hypercalcaemia in patients with lymphoma who exhibit it will often cause polyuria/polydipsia (see **Case 4, Table 4.1**) because of renal interference of ADH activity, and this may be the cause of the patient's increased thirst in this case. Although humoral hypercalcaemia of malignancy is an important cause of hypercalcaemia, when identified other differential diagnoses of hypercalcaemia should be considered (see below).

Table 30.4 Summary of paraneoplastic syndromes associated with canine lymphoma

Hypercalcaemia	Humoral hypercalcaemia of malignancy (HHM), associated with elevated plasma parathyroid hormone-related peptide (PTHrP) is identified in approximately 15% of cases of canine lymphoma, moreso (30–40% of cases) with the cranial mediastinal form and those with T-cell immunophenotype (of which 35% are hypercalcaemic)
Cancer cachexia	Profound malnutrition and rapid loss of body lean tissue mass may be seen in a minority of lymphoma patients due to cytokine-mediated excessive lipolysis and tissue proteolysis
Hyperglobulinaemia	Marked hyperglobulinaemia, which on protein electrophoresis may appear or be reported as a monoclonal gammopathy spike (but is sometimes due to a restricted migration polyclonal response due to inflammation), is identified in approximately 6% of canine lymphoma patients
Anaemia	Anaemia may develop as a paraneoplastic syndrome in lymphoma patients due to features of anaemia of chronic/inflammatory disease (ACD) or secondary immune-mediated haemolysis, though the relative contribution of these can be difficult to ascertain, particularly in the presence of stage V lymphoma where infiltrative neoplastic bone marrow disease is also present
Erythrocytosis	Lymphoma may occasionally be reported in association with paraneoplastic erythrocytosis but this is seen most commonly in renal lymphoma in which elevation of serum erythropoietin levels may be demonstrated (both due to direct tumour production of erythropoietin and production due to local tissue hypoxia)
Thrombocytopenia	Thrombocytopenia may be demonstrated in approximately 30–50% of dogs with lymphoma and may be a paraneoplastic effect (e.g. due to a secondary immune-mediated mechanism) or may be a manifestation of bone marrow myelophthesis
Myasthenia gravis	Generalised weakness due to myasthenia gravis has been rarely reported in dogs with lymphoma

Hypercalcaemia: approach and differential diagnoses

The homeostatic control of serum calcium and the calcium/PTH 'axis' was discussed in **Case 2** (see **Figures 2.2** and **2.4**). When hypercalcaemia is identified it is sensible to first verify that it is a genuine and repeatable finding and to ensure that the biologically active 'free' (ionised) calcium is also elevated. The differential diagnosis of hypercalcaemia is more extensive than that for hypocalcaemia whose differential diagnosis is restricted.

Differential diagnoses for hypercalcaemia are listed in **Table 30.5**.

When approaching the hypercalcaemic patient it should be borne in mind that the results of some diagnostic tests (such as measurement of PTH and PTHrP) may take some days to be available and there may be need to interim medical therapy provided to manage excessive hypercalcaemia, which may induce progressive renal injury and lead to soft tissue calcification, especially of the upper gastrointestinal tract and kidneys. Such therapy should not interfere with future diagnostic attempts or treatment and, though they may be calciuretic and ultimately part of treatment strategies in many of the above disorders, corticosteroids are best initially avoided lest they render diagnosis of lymphoproliferative disorders impossible. Judicious use of saline diuresis, loop diuretics such as furosemide and possibly salmon calcitonin may often alleviate hypercalcaemia whilst diagnostic evaluation is performed without prejudice to diagnostic efforts.

Initial assessment of hypercalcaemia should involve analysis of free (ionised) calcium and evaluation of the serum phosphate level. In conjunction with the PTH and PTHrP levels, when available these can help differentiate some of the major differential diagnoses of hypercalcaemia (**Figure 30.2**).

Table 30.5 Differential diagnosis of canine hypercalcaemia

Causes and association with clinical signs	Examples	Appropriate investigations
Non-pathogenic reasons	• Lipaemia • Growth • Spurious single result • Iatrogenic due to calcium-additive containing fluids	Repeat sample, ensure adequate fasting, consider patient age and concurrent drug therapy
Pathogenic but not normally associated with clinical signs due to hypercalcaemia	• Hypoadrenocorticism	ACTH stimulation test
	• Kidney disease	Urea, creatinine, urine SG
	• Granulomatous disease	Clinical investigation
	• Angiostrongylus vasorum	Antigen ELISA, faecal analysis, clinical investigation

Pathogenic and often associated with clinical signs due to hypercalcaemia	*Neoplastic*
	• Humoral hypercalcaemia of malignancy (HHM)
	  ○ Lymphoma
	  ○ Anal sac apocrine carcinoma
	  ○ Thymoma
	  ○ Leukaemias
	  ○ Carcinomas
	• Local tumour osteolysis
	  ○ Multiple myeloma
	  ○ Osteosarcoma
	  ○ Bone metastases
		Physical examination including palpation of external lymph nodes, liver, spleen, rectal examination and palpation of bones for pain. Palpation of ventral neck for nodular parathyroid lesions (though most are non-palpable and only occasionally are they large)
		
		Assessment of PTHrP
		
		Diagnostic imaging (thorax, abdomen, skeleton) for
		– Intracavitary lymph node enlargement or hepatosplenic infiltrative disease
		– Cranial mediastinal masses
		– Osteolytic/expansile bone lesions

	Endocrine • Primary hyperparathyroidism	Assessment of plasma PTH *at same time that calcium known to be elevated* Parathyroid ultrasound

Causes and association with clinical signs	Examples	Appropriate investigations
Toxicity	• Grapes, raisins • Vitamin D-containing medicated skin products and rodenticides	Clinical history of exposure

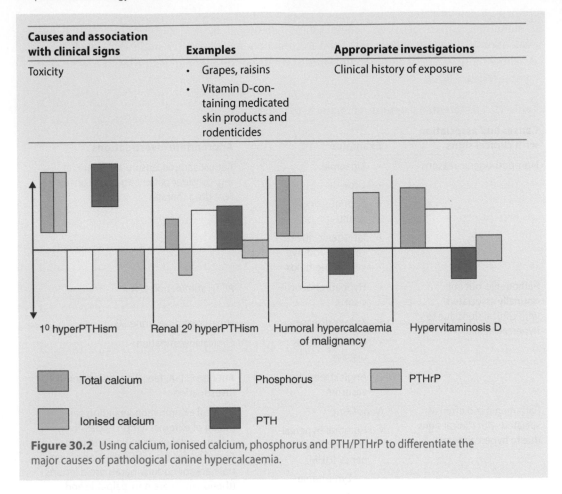

Figure 30.2 Using calcium, ionised calcium, phosphorus and PTH/PTHrP to differentiate the major causes of pathological canine hypercalcaemia.

4. **What broad treatment options exist for treatment of canine multi-centric lymphoma and what general guidance can be given to owners?**

A checklist for discussion points with owners of dogs with lymphoma, who are considering treatment, is shown in **Table 30.6**. Canine lymphoma is, generally speaking, a widespread disease process and surgical treatment options are not appropriate in this setting, with few exceptions (those dogs with localised disease only or where significant local mass effect, e.g. gastrointestinal obstruction due to an intestinal mass, is causing morbidity). Treatment options include

- No treatment with euthanasia upon diagnosis or when the quality of life declines.
- Provision of corticosteroid therapy for at-home palliation.
- Attempted induction of remission with systemic drug therapy (chemotherapy).

The option of no/palliative treatment

Untreated, most dogs with lymphoma will develop progressive clinical signs resulting in death or euthanasia on average 4–8 weeks after diagnosis. The provision of oral prednisolone therapy may improve the quality of life and induce a reduction in lymph node size, and even on occasion remission, that is generally short in duration (weeks) but may be appropriate in some circumstances.

Table 30.6 Checklist for discussion with owners considering treatment for lymphoma

Treatment option	• Setting out aims
	• Ensuring that owners are realistically appraised that clinical cure is not achieved in the majority of patients
	• Discussion of broad treatment options:
	◦ Euthanasia
	◦ No treatment
	◦ Palliative corticosteroids
	◦ Chemotherapy with view to inducing remission
Setting out treatment goals and prognosis	• Aim and meaning of remission
	• Odds of obtaining remission
	• Likely duration of remission
	• When and what to do upon relapse
	• The aim of rescue therapy, the diminished odds of durable rescue, the option of not pursuing rescue therapy
Risks of therapy	• General predictable risks common to chemotherapy agents and frequency with which they occur
	• Specific medication risks applicable to the individual protocol
	• Measures taken to avoid such risks; introducing rationale for haematological monitoring
	• Risks to personnel
	• Reassurance of the option to stop chemotherapy should adverse effects exist
Practicalities of therapy	• Costs
	• Time-course
	• Frequency and length of time-commitment
	• Possibility of dose adjustment/dose delay/treatment 'holidays'
	• Where, when and by whom will therapy be given
	• Assessment of response
	• Contingency planning
Expectations and understanding	• Discussion of what owners can expect to see
	• Provision of time and patience in soliciting questions from the owner (this should be repeated whenever possible)
	• Provision of a clear plan in writing and clear, concise written information to discuss at home
	• Provision of adequate time for family discussion and decision making that is not deleterious to patient health
	• Veterinary reassurance of validity of all the broad options discussed without prejudice or pressure.

Aims and practicalities of medical treatment for lymphoma

The decision to treat lymphoma with chemotherapy aimed at inducing remission is based on the clinical status of the patient (including tumour stage, prognostic factors and co-morbidities), owner-related practical factors such as financial and time constraints and owner considerations of likelihood of treatment success/failure, possibility of side effects and expectations of tumour relapse.

The decision to undertake treatment is a large one and can be a prodigious commitment and it is encouraged to take time counselling owners through this decision-making process and to provide written information to digest in the family setting. Nonetheless, canine lymphoma can be very rewarding to treat and benefits the vast majority of patients by tangible improvement in quality and length of life. Many forms of drug therapy (chemotherapy 'protocols') are available for treatment of canine lymphoma and a complete discussion is beyond the scope of this case description. See Further reading for comprehensive reviews on the subject. A greater odds of both achieving complete remission and of patients enjoying prolonged remission duration are generally seen with those protocols that employ multiple agents with antitumour activity, which act with differing mechanisms and multi-agent chemotherapy protocols, and are therefore considered superior to single-agent ones. Choice must also, however, be strongly influenced by pragmatic concerns such as clinician experience, the presence of facilities to handle cytotoxic chemotherapy agents safely and protect in-contact personnel (including protection of those personnel not directly involved in administration within the veterinary hospital and pet owners), costs and time constraints as there is little point in undertaking a chemotherapy protocol that is not practical for that individual patient or owner.

The odds of achieving remission and remission duration

One of the most commonly used multi-agent protocols is a 'CHOP' (Cyclophosphamide (C), Hyroxydaunorubicin (Doxorubicin)(H), 'Oncovin'(Vincristine)(O), Prednisolone (P)), which results in remission being achieved in approximately 80–95% of patients and an overall median survival time of 10–12 months. A less complex 'COP'-based protocol is commonly used and is popular and whilst it results in inferior remission responses and duration, it is not so inferior as to render it anything less than a very good treatment option for lymphoma provided at less cost than CHOP-based protocols. The majority of veterinary oncologists no longer recommend continuous treatment of patients in remission with chemotherapy, but employing discontinuous protocols, usually continuing for no longer than 6 months without apparent prejudice to remission duration or rate/timing of relapse.

Discussion of relapse and rescue

The majority of dogs who achieve complete remission with a multi-agent protocol will suffer tumour relapse, though a small but significant proportion (perhaps 20–25%) may enjoy prolonged disease-free survival in excess of 2 years. Relapse is usually thought to occur due to development of tumour cells that are inherently more resistant to chemotherapy agents. In patients exhibiting signs of relapse a decision is made to either not pursue further attempts at reinduction of remission ('rescue') or to employ further treatment strategies in an attempt to reachieve a state of remission. Such 'rescue' therapy is often governed by a 'law of diminishing returns' whereby successive remissions are both less commonly achieved and of generally shorter duration than the preceding one. This should be discussed with owners at the outset of deciding upon treatment for lymphoma.

Risks to the patient

Owners should be counselled that cytotoxic chemotherapy in veterinary patients is generally undertaken with a view to minimising patient-experienced side effects in species that cannot make this decision for themselves, but with some degree of trade-off in reduced rates of permanent remission in favour of quality-of-life considerations. Cytotoxic chemotherapy drugs may have individualised toxicity profiles but the major dose-limiting side effects common to many cytotoxic agents are of gastrointestinal toxicity and myelotoxicity. Toxicities are defined as those that are acute (at or within 48 hours of treatment), acute-delayed (2–14 days post-treatment) or cumulative/chronic (over weeks to months).

Gastrointestinal toxicity may manifest in a relatively benign and 'self-limiting' manner such as a brief period of inappetence or brief small intestinal diarrhoea unaccompanied by constitutional signs or may be more pronounced. Gastrointestinal toxicity manifests as overt nausea, vomiting or markedly increased frequency of diarrhoeic faeces requires both empirical therapy and some-times intravenous fluid therapy to limit the risk of dehydration. Antidiarrhoeal adsorbants (such as Kaolin-based products) and motility modifiers such as loperamide may be useful to manage diarrhoea and antiemetics, such as maropitant, metoclopramide and ondansetron, may be helpful in managing nausea and vomiting. Myelotoxicity is usually seen 5–12 days after administration of a cytotoxic chemotherapy agent (but may sometimes be delayed, especially with carboplatin) and is best prevented by ensuring an adequate neutrophil count prior to administration of a cytotoxic chemotherapy agent. As a rule, any illness developing during this time-frame after administration of chemotherapy, especially if accompanied by fever, should be presumed to be due to myelotox-icity and the patient potentially at risk of neutropenic sepsis, until proven otherwise. Assessment of a complete blood count should allow this possibility to be confirmed or refuted and appropriate action should be planned based on the absolute neutrophil count, presence/absence of constitu-tional signs of illness such as fever and the risk of sepsis. Supportive measures may range from watchful monitoring to hospital-based intravenous fluid and broad-spectrum antibiotic admin-istration as appropriate to that case. For an in-depth discussion of such management see Further reading. When significant toxicity is encountered it is common practice to decrease the dose of the next subsequent administration of that drug by 20–25%. Drug-specific toxicities, which are also relevant to CHOP-based protocols, are that of cyclophosphamide-induced cystitis (which is caused by accumulation and contact irritation of its metabolite acrolein in the urinary bladder) and car-diotoxicity due to doxorubicin. The former should be suspected if clinical signs of pollakiuria, dy-suria or haematuria develop in any animal that has received cyclophosphamide and should prompt replacement of cyclophosphamide with chlorambucil. Doxorubicin cardiotoxicity, which causes myocardial dysfunction and dilated cardiomyopathy phenotype, is cumulative and is seen most commonly with cumulative doses above 150 mg/m^2. Practically, this risk is greater in those breeds with a predisposition to myocardial systolic dysfunction, such as Dobermann Pinschers and Great Danes, and it is sensible to pursue echocardiographic assessment in at-risk dogs prior to instituting therapy and to carefully evaluate all dogs for alteration in cardiac parameters (especially onset of heart murmurs, poor pulse quality or arrhythmia) and to pursue further evaluation should these be detected prior to further dose administration.

Owners should be reassured that the decision to continue with a proposed chemotherapy pro-tocol is a collaborative decision that must be based on all parties being convinced of the worth of treatment to the patient. Embarking on chemotherapy to treat lymphoma is not a 'rollercoaster ride' where one can only get off at the end, no matter what occurs in between; should unacceptable side-effects be encountered stopping therapy is always a consideration.

Risks to personnel

It is incumbent on any veterinary surgeon prescribing cytotoxic chemotherapeutics not only to ensure that veterinary personnel involved either directly or indirectly with administration are properly trained and protected but also that the risks of exposure to agents are properly discussed with owners. Owners should also be counselled that minute amounts of cytotoxic and potentially carcinogenic agents will be secreted in body fluids and solid waste for 3–4 days on average after treatment and they should be specifically instructed in safe-handling of accidental eliminations in the house, hygiene precautions after contact with saliva highlighted and particular discussion should be given to the special risks of vulnerable individuals such as children and pregnant women. In these latter situations it may be more appropriate for cytotoxic chemotherapy not to be given. Any tablets to be administered at home should be dispensed in a secure and clearly labelled fashion with instructions not to split or crush tablets and with safety gloves and explicit instructions on administration.

Outcome

In the case reported here fine needle aspirate cytology from prescapular lymph nodes was taken and both cytology and, if appropriate based on the results of this, flow cytometry for immunphenotyping. Once lymphoma was confirmed, further staging by performance of haematology and biochemistry (see below) and thoracic radiography and abdominal ultrasound was performed. Bone marrow aspiration cytology was not performed.

Haematology

Parameter	Value	Units	Range
RBC	6.16	$\times 10^{12}$/l	(5.5–8.5)
Haemoglobin	14.7	g/dl	(12.0–18.0)
Haematocrit	0.44	l/l	(0.37–0.55)
Mean cell volume	71.7	fl	(60–77)
Mean cell haemoglobin concentration	33.2	g/dl	(30.0–38.0)
Mean cell haemoglobin	23.8	pg	(19.5–25.5)
Total white cell count	6.05	$\times 10^9$/l	(6.0–15.0)
Neutrophils	3.17	$\times 10^9$/l	(3.0–11.5)
Lymphocytes	1.16	$\times 10^9$/l	(1.0–4.8)
Monocytes	0.25	$\times 10^9$/l	(0.2–1.4)
Eosinophils	0.46	$\times 10^9$/l	(0.1–1.2)
Basophils	0.01	$\times 10^9$/l	(0.0–0.1)
Platelets	224	$\times 10^9$/l	(200–500)
Film comment:	Red cell morphology normal		
	White cell morphology normal		

Biochemistry

Parameter	Value	Units	Range
Total protein	59	g/l	(54–77)
Albumin	29	g/l	(25–40)
Globulin	30	g/l	(23–45)
Urea	4.9	mmol/l	(2.5–7.4)

Parameter	Value	Units	Range
Creatinine	141	µmol/l	(40–145)
Potassium	4.5	mmol/l	(3.4–5.6)
Sodium	153	mmol/l	(139–154)
Chloride	115	mmol/l	(105–122)
Calcium	**3.4**	mmol/l	(2.1–2.8)
Ionised calcium	**1.8**	mmol/l	(1.18–1.40)
Inorganic phosphate	1.22	mmol/l	(0.60–1.40)
Glucose	5.5	mmol/l	(3.3–5.8)
ALT	53	IU/l	(13–88)
AST	55	IU/l	(13–60)
ALKP	114	IU/l	(14–105)
GGT	1	IU/l	(0–10)
Bilirubin	2	µmol/l	(0–16)
Cholesterol	3.79	mmol/l	(3.8–7.0)
Triglyceride	0.8	mmol/l	(0.56–1.14)
Creatine kinase	88	IU/l	(0–190)

Thoracic radiographs (see **Figure 30.3**, left lateral not displayed) showed an ovoid soft tissue opacity dorsal to the second sternebrae felt to be consistent with sternal lymphadenomegaly and subsequently confirmed with transthoracic ultrasound.

Abdominal ultrasound examination (**Figure 30.4**) demonstrated a generalised hypoechoic mottling to the spleen with variably sized hypoechoic nodules, one of which was subsequently aspirated

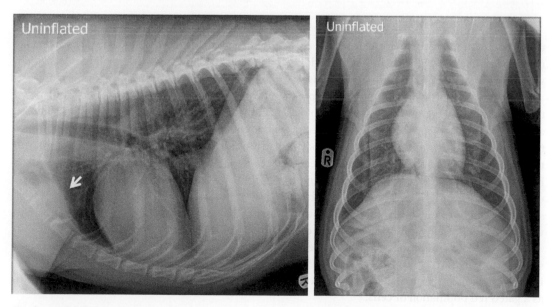

Figure 30.3 Right lateral and dorsoventral thoracic radiographs showing sternal lymphadenomegaly (arrow).

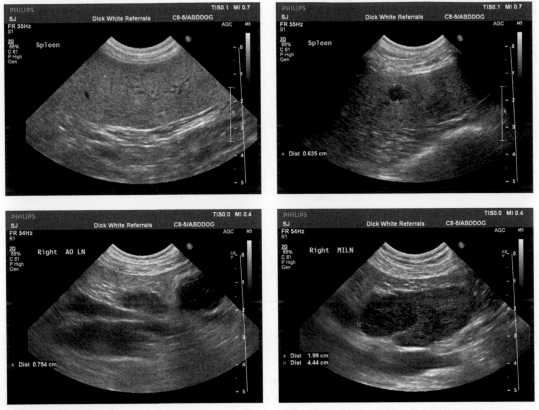

Figure 30.4 Abdominal ultrasound examination. Top row: spleen showing mottled appearance and hypoechoic nodule. Bottom row: enlarged right aortic lymph node (left), enlarged right medial iliac lymph node (right).

under ultrasound guidance for cytological evaluation. Generalised intra-abdominal lymphadeno-megaly was determined with all lymph nodes being hypoechoic and rounded, the largest of which was the right medial iliac lymph node, being 4 × 3 cm in diameter. The liver appeared normal.

Fine needle aspiration cytology of the prescapular lymph node and spleen yielded similar cytological findings (**Figure 30.5**, splenic cytology) demonstrating hypercellular samples with nucleated cells comprising primarily large lymphocytes that measured approximately up to 1.5–2 times the diameter of a neutrophil. These lymphocytes had a small amount of dark basophilic cytoplasm that commonly exhibited a pale staining perinuclear region. The nucleus was round and eccentric in position, with dispersed chromatin and multiple prominent marginal nucleoli. One mitotic figure was seen in 5 high-power fields (×50 objective). Low numbers of scattered small lymphocytes and a few tingible body macrophages were also present. These cytological findings were consistent with a centroblastic lymphoma, likely of B-cell origin.

Flow cytometry findings from fine needle aspirates of the prescapular lymph node demonstrated a population of larger (greater forward scatter, x-axis) lymphocytes with a more granular internal structure (greater side scatter, y-axis), which can be seen in the scatter plot in **Figure 30.6** as a gated red population of cells.

An immunopenotype was derived from the fluorescence-activated cell sorting (FACS) method and was as follows:

CD45	All leukocytes	POSITIVE
CD3	T-cells	Negative
CD4	T-helper cells	Negative
CD5	T-cells	Negative
CD8	Cytotoxic T-cells	Negative
CD21	B-cells	POSITIVE
CD79a	All B-cells	POSITIVE
CD34	Early precursors	Negative
MHCII		POSITIVE

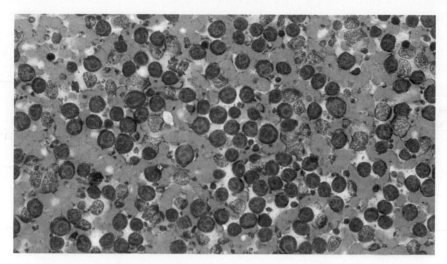

Figure 30.5 Fine needle aspiration cytology of the spleen of the patient (×50, Wright-Giemsa). Many large lymphocytes, which are about 1.5–2 × the diameter of a neutrophil, are seen with darkly basophilic cytoplasm, eccentric nuclei and multiple prominent nucleoli.

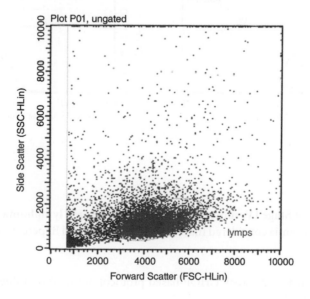

Figure 30.6 Scatter plot of cell size and granularity from flow cytometry of patient's lymph node.

Flow cytometry

Flow cytometry is a powerful diagnostic method in which cells are suspended in a stream of liquid and passed through a system of impedence detectors and laser light coupled to an analogue to digital detector/convertor interface. This allows cells to be 'sorted' by measurement of the scattering of light after it encounters cells and the structures they contain (forward scatter and side scatter) and by the use of fluorescent markers (fluorophores), which are attached to antibodies with specific affinity for a particular cell structure. Fluorescence-activated cell sorting (FACS) allows the binary detection of cells labelled with a fluorophore and the production of a histogram, which shows either a population of positive cells or a 'null' result. The plots below (**Figure 30.7**) show the histograms for CD45 (all leukocytes), CD3 (T-cell marker), CD21 (B-cell marker) and CD79a (B-cell marker) for the patient in this case. The 'control' peak is to the left of each plot and the region of positive cells is shown under the red band (PE = Phycoerythrin, FITC = Fluoroscein, both fluorophores).

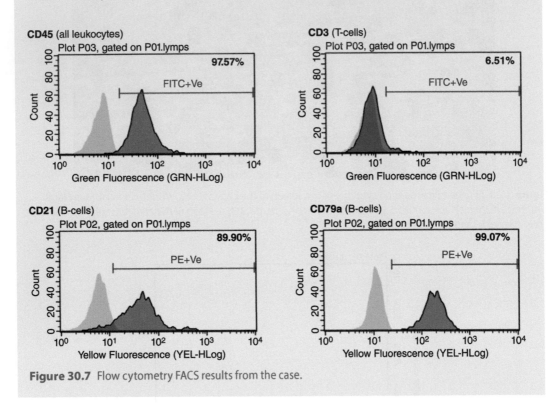

Figure 30.7 Flow cytometry FACS results from the case.

A final diagnosis of **Stage IV, substage (a) multicentric B-cell lymphoma** was made with total and ionised hypercalcaemia considered likely to be due to humoral hypercalcaemia of malignancy.

Treatment

The dog was treated with a 25-week CHOP-based protocol outlined in **Table 30.7** and remission was successfully induced.

Table 30.7 A 25-week chemotherapy protocol for canine multi-centric lymphoma used in the author's clinic

Week	Treatment given*
1	Vincristine[§] 0.5–0.7 mg/m² i.v. through preplaced intravenous cannula
	Prednisolone 2 mg/kg p/o SID for 7 days
2	Cyclophosphamide[#] 200–250 mg/m² p/o or i.v. through preplaced intravenous cannula
	Prednisolone 1.5mg/kg p/o SID for 7 days
3	Vincristine 0.5–0.7 mg/m² i.v. through preplaced intravenous cannula
	Prednisolone 1 mg/kg p/o SID for 7 days
4	Doxorubicin 30 mg/m² (1 mg/kg if <15 kg) i.v. through preplaced intravenous cannula
	Prednisolone 0.5 mg/kg p/o SID for 7 days then stop
5	*No treatment*
6	Vincristine 0.5–0.7 mg/m² i.v. through preplaced intravenous cannula
7	Cyclophosphamide 200–250 mg/m² p/o or i.v. through preplaced intravenous cannula
8	Vincristine 0.5–0.7 mg/m² i.v. through preplaced intravenous cannula
9	Doxorubicin 30 mg/m² (1 mg/kg if <15 kg) i.v. through preplaced intravenous cannula
10	*No treatment*
11	Vincristine 0.5–0.7 mg/m² i.v. through preplaced intravenous cannula
12	*No treatment*
13	Cyclophosphamide 200–250 mg/m² p/o or i.v. through preplaced intravenous cannula
14	*No treatment*
15	Vincristine 0.5–0.7 mg/m² i.v. through preplaced intravenous cannula
16	*No treatment*
17	Doxorubicin 30 mg/m² (1 mg/kg if <15 kg) i.v. through preplaced intravenous cannula
18	*No treatment*
19	Vincristine 0.5–0.7 mg/m² i.v. through preplaced intravenous cannula
20	*No treatment*
21	Cyclophosphamide 200–250 mg/m² p/o or i.v. through preplaced intravenous cannula
22	*No treatment*
23	Vincristine 0.5–0.7 mg/m² i.v. through preplaced intravenous cannula
24	*No treatment*
25	Doxorubicin 30 mg/m² (1 mg/kg if <15 kg) i.v. through preplaced intravenous cannula
	Treatment ends. Watchful monitoring for relapse

*A complete blood count is performed and assessed prior to each chemotherapy dose.

[§]Vincristine planned to be given at 0.7 mg/m² but downward dose adjustment may be necessary.

[#]If cyclophosphamide-induced cystitis develops, subsequent doses replaced with chlorambucil at a dose of 1.4 mg/kg p/o.

Discussion

Lymphoma is the most common haematopoietic tumour commonly seen in small animal practice in both dogs and cats and may present in a multitude of ways, reflecting the broad distribution of tissues containing lymphoid cells. In our clinic it is the most common reason for patients to attend for chemotherapy and whilst clinical cure compared with prolonged remission is relatively uncommon, most clients feel vindicated in their decision to pursue chemotherapy and it is gratifying to see patients benefit to an extent that their quality of life is usually normal after receiving treatment.

The key to successful management is good communication and contingency planning, coupled with watchful and proactive monitoring for development of adverse effects of chemotherapy and knowledge of safe handling of such agents.

Further reading

Mellanby, R.J., Herrtage, M.E. & Dobson, J.M. (2003) Owners' assessments of their dog's quality of life during palliative chemotherapy for lymphoma. *J Small Anim Pract* **44**, 100–103

Vail, D.M. (2009) Supporting the veterinary cancer patient on chemotherapy: neutropenia and gastrointestinal toxicity. *Topics in Companion Anim Med* **24**, 122–129

Vail, D.M. (2010) Chapter 324: Hematopoietic tumours. In *Textbook of Veterinary Internal Medicine*, 7th edn, eds S.J. Ettinger and E.C. Feldman, Elsevier Saunders, St Louis, pp. 2148–2152

Vail, D.M., Pinkerton, M.E. & Young, K.E. (2013) Chapter 32: Hematopoietic tumours. In *Small Animal Clinical Oncology*, 5th edn, eds S.J. Withrow, D.M. Vail and R.L. Page, Elsevier Saunders, St Louis, Pp. 608–638

Neurology

Canine Internal Medicine: What's Your Diagnosis? First Edition. Jon Wray.
© 2018 John Wiley & Sons Ltd. Published 2018 by John Wiley & Sons Ltd.

Neurology

Clinical presentation

A 9 year-old male-neutered Labrador Cross is presented with a history of breathing abnormalities, persistent gulping/retching after eating, episodes of regurgitation and altered appearance of the eyes.

Clinical signs have been noted to progress over the last 2 weeks and the dog's owner reports that he has become aware of the dog breathing with considerable effort with a rapid and forceful pattern that appears to involve some abdominal effort. This effort appears to be increased when the dog is in a recumbent position. After eating, the dog shows signs of repetitive gulping, more with dry food than with wet food, and there does not seem to be any problem with prehension or initial swallowing of food. Four episodes of regurgitation of food have occurred and these have been within 5–10 minutes of eating and have occurred during these past two weeks. Appetite has been normal to slightly decreased and no vomiting or diarrhoea has been noted. Water intake and urinating have been normal, no weakness, incoordination, weight loss or muscle wastage has been reported and no cough or dysphonia has been noticed.

In the last 2 days the owners have noticed that the dog's right eye appears slightly closed compared with the left and that the third eyelid is protruding on the right. The right pupil is considerably smaller than the left.

Physical examination demonstrates a slightly quiet dog with normal mentation and normal body condition. Anisocoria is present (**Figure 31.1**) with the right pupil smaller than the left. The right pupil is miotic and there is ptosis and enophthalmos of the right eye with concurrent protrusion of the third eyelid. The left eye appears normal and both menace and pupillary light responses

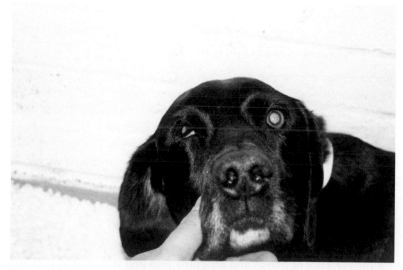

Figure 31.1 The patient at presentation.

Canine Internal Medicine: What's Your Diagnosis? First Edition. Jon Wray.
© 2018 John Wiley & Sons Ltd. Published 2018 by John Wiley & Sons Ltd.

(both direct and consensual) are present in both eyes, though the anisocoria remains and is more pronounced when the dog is examined in dim light. Both globes appear a similar size and examination of the anterior segment of both eyes is normal. The dog's respiratory effort is abnormal and the respiratory rate is 40/min with a shallow, restrictive pattern and with marked abdominal expansion during inspiration and contraction during expiration. Marked flaring of the nostrils occurs during inspiration. Heart rate is normal at 116/min and peripheral pulse rate and quality are normal. Thoracic auscultation demonstrates normal heart sounds and bronchovesicular respiratory sounds bilaterally. Percussion of the thorax is normal. Rectal temperature is 38.4 °C.

A brief neurological examination demonstrates the following:

- Examination of the cranial nerves other than the ocular abnormalities already described is normal and a gag reflex is present.
- Assessment of proprioception of all four limbs and of spinal myotatic reflexes is normal.
- The panniculus reflex is present bilaterally.
- No neck or spinal pain is identified on manipulation or palpation.

Questions

1. **What is the most likely cause of the anisocoria in this dog?**
2. **What is the relevant neuroanatomy of this lesion in the dog? What are the principle differential diagnoses and how can pharmacologic testing be used to distinguish these further?**
3. **What is the likely relevance of the respiratory abnormalities? How can these be investigated further?**

Answers

1. **What is the most likely cause of the anisocoria in this dog?**

Common causes of anisocoria in the dog

The presence of miosis, enophthalmos, third eyelid protrusion and ptosis of the upper eyelid is most likely due to **Horner's syndrome**, caused by interruption of the sympathetic innervation to the eye and adnexa. Post-ganglionic sympathetic neurones innervate the iris dilator muscle, the smooth muscle of the peri-orbital and Muller's muscle of the upper and lower eyelids. Conjunctival hyperaemia due to local vasodilation may also be seen.

When anisocoria is present differentiation should be made as to whether the larger or smaller pupil is abnormal. Pupillary enlargement (mydriasis) may be present with ipsilateral loss of vision, iris atrophy or with oculomotor nerve deficits.

Other considerations for the presence of miosis and enophthalmos and third eyelid protrusion include
- Anterior uveitis
- Space occupying lesions of the orbit
- Reduction in globe size
- Ocular surface pain

2. **What is the relevant neuroanatomy of this lesion in the dog? What are the principle differential diagnoses and how can pharmacologic testing be used to distinguish these further?**

The sympathetic innervation to the eye comprises three neurones (**Figure 31.2**):

- **First order** neurones originate in the brainstem, course dorsolaterally in the tectotegmental pathway of the spinal cord and preganglionic cell bodies synapse within the lateral horn of spinal cord grey matter in the thoracic spinal segments T1–T3. Lesions of these are often referred to as *central* Horner's syndrome.
- **Second order** neurones leave the spinal cord via ramus communicans and pass through the paired cervicothoracic ganglia and caudal cervical ganglia where they join the vagus nerve within the vagosympathetic trunk. This courses cranially within the cranial mediastinum synapsing on the post-ganglionic cell body within the cranial cervical ganglion adjacent to the tympanic bulla. Lesions of these are often referred to as *pre-ganglionic* Horner's syndrome.
- **Third order** neurones penetrate the petrous temporal bone (where they course in close association with the trigeminal nerve ganglion and the internal carotid artery) and then follow the ophthalmic nerve being distributed with ciliary branches of the ophthalmic nerve. Lesions of these are often referred to as *post-ganglionic* Horner's syndrome.

The anatomic route over which a lesion may produce Horner's syndrome is long and complex and anatomical neurolocalisation (and thence consideration of differential diagnoses) is aided by

- Recognition of concurrent neurological abnormalities, especially those affecting other cranial nerves, brainstem or spinal cord segments with overlapping anatomy to the course of the sympathetic nerves.

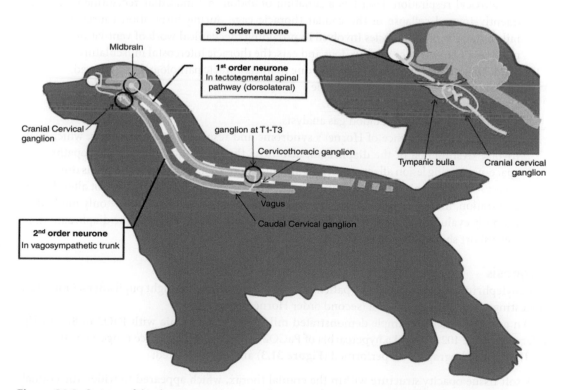

Figure 31.2 Cartoon of the three neurones involved in sympathetic innervation of the eye.

Pharmacologic testing in Horner's syndrome

- This relies on the phenomenon of 'denervation hypersensitivity', that is in the presence of autonomic dysfunction the receptor density is significantly increased at the post-synaptic receptor site. The effect of this is that pharmacological stimulation with an autonomic agonist results in an exageratedly rapid response, more so in post-ganglionic lesions than with pre-ganglionic (which in turn elicit a more rapid response than central lesions).
- The agent used most commonly is phenylephrine at 0.5–1%, a direct acting sympathomimetic, which under normal circumstances causes slow pupillary dilation over 1–2 hours.
- In post-ganglionic lesions, pupillary dilation occurs rapidly, usually in <20 minutes.
- In pre-ganglionic lesions, pupillary dilation takes longer, usually 40–60 minutes
- In both, third eyelid protrusion usually resolves before the miosis.
- Caution should be applied since there is considerable overlap between patients with different 'order' Horner's syndrome and the results are not always reliable.

3. **What is the likely relevance of the respiratory abnormalities? How can these be investigated further?**
   - The respiratory pattern is a restrictive/choppy one, but there is considerable abdominal effort, which implies that paradoxical respiration is occurring (see **Case 17, Table 17.1**).
   - Paradoxical respiration describes a situation of abdominal muscular recruitment and frequently inward collapse of the caudal thoracic cage during inspiration caused by either failure/fatigue of the muscles involved in providing mechanical work of ventilation (the diaphragm and to a lesser extent in dogs and cats, the thoracic intercostal musculature) or where caudal displacement of the diaphragm due to intrathoracic pathology has occurred.
   - Initial steps in diagnosis might include
     ◦ Performing thoracic radiographs.
     ◦ Performing an arterial blood gas analysis.
   - In this case, the presence of Horner's syndrome and respiratory abnormalities, which may involve dysfunction of the diaphragm, also raise the possibility of a polyneuropathy or a space-occupying lesion affecting control of ventilation. Diaphragmatic function is difficult to assess – radiographic doming of one or both hemi-diaphragms, which does not alter during inspiration, may be suggestive but dynamic imaging with fluoroscopy is the only method to properly evaluate this (in humans this is accomplished by evaluation of the diaphragm during a short sharp intake of breath, the 'sniff test').

Diagnosis

A phenylephrine response test in this patient resulted in dilation of the right pupil after 45 minutes, suggesting a pre-ganglionic lesion (second order Horner's syndrome).

An arterial blood gas sample demonstrated mild atrial hypoxaemia with PaO_2 of 88 mmHg (reference range 102 ± 7) and a hypercarbia of $PaCO_2$ of 44 mmHg (reference range 37 ± 3).

Thoracic radiography was performed (**Figure 31.3**) and demonstrated:

- A soft tissue opacity structure within the cranial thorax, which appeared to widen the cranial mediastinum.

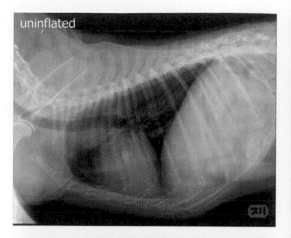

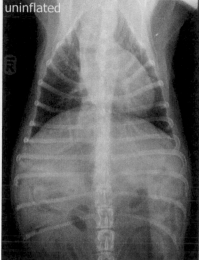

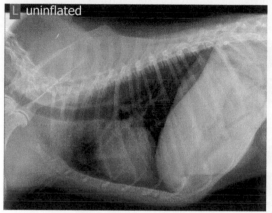

Figure 31.3 Right and left lateral and dorsoventral thoracic radiographs.

- A 1.5 cm diameter nodular interstitial soft tissue opacity structure visible on the right lateral radiograph overlying the fifth intercostal space and the central portion of the cardiac silhouette.
- Less distinct soft tissue interstitial nodular structures in the perihilar location on the left lateral radiograph.

A fluoroscopic assessment of diaphragmatic function (**Figure 31.4**) demonstrated bilateral diaphragmatic paralysis.

An intercostal ultrasound examination of the cranial thorax was not diagnostically rewarding.

Computed tomography (CT, **Figure 31.5**) was undertaken. This demonstrated two cranial mediastinal mass lesions, one extending from the level of the heart base along the dorsal and lateral aspect of the cranial vena cava at the level of the vagus nerve and a second arising in the region of the left subclavian artery and extending towards the sternum. The mass associated with the cranial vena cava was seen to partially invade it. Within the caudal subsegment of the left cranial lung lobe a well-defined soft tissue attenuating nodule 1 cm in diameter was noted. The cranial mediastinal lymph nodes were seen to be enlarged and contrast-enhancing. An anomalous right subclavian artery arising directly from the aortic arch was noted as an incidental finding.

Given the appearance of two mass lesions, one of which appeared vasculoinvasive, a pulmonary nodule suspected to be a metastasis, cranial mediastinal lymphadenomegaly and the co-morbidity caused by diaphragmatic paralysis, metastatic and locally invasive neoplasia of

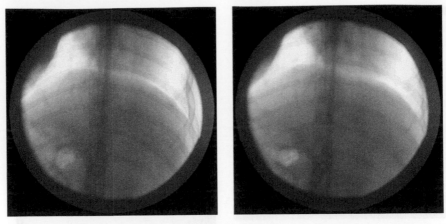

Figure 31.4 Fluoroscopic dorsoventral view of the diaphragmatic crura at end expiration (left image) and at peak inspiration (right image). Note the lack of change in the diaphragmatic positon.

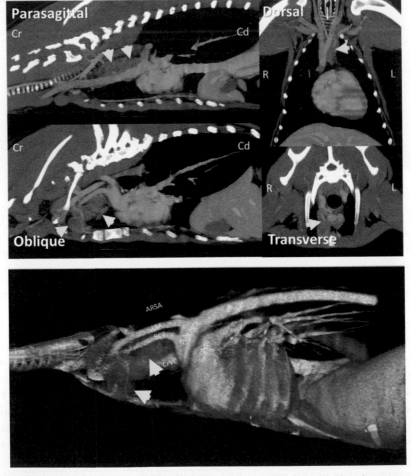

Figure 31.5 Multiplanar reconstruction (MPR) CT images (top) and 3D volume-rendered reconstruction (below) orientating the vascular anatomy. Two mass lesions (arrowheads) are noted, one associated with the cranial vena cava (CrVC), which it invades, and one associated with the left subclavian artery (LSA) and extending ventrally towards the sternum on the right of the midline. (BCT = brachiocephalic trunk, ARSA = anomalous right subclavian artery, AA = aortic arch, PA = pulmonary artery, CdVC = caudal vena cava).

the cranial mediastinum was suspected. Ectopic thyroid carcinoma, malignant thymoma and haemangiosarcoma were the most likely differential diagnoses considered. Given the associated poor prognosis, the dog's owners elected for humane euthanasia. Post-mortem examination was not permitted.

Discussion

Horner's syndrome is caused by lesions affecting the sympathetic nerve supply to the eye, part of the lower motor neurone: the general visceral efferent (LMN:GVE) system. Idiopathic Horner's syndrome is common in dogs, especially in Golden Retrievers and localises to the third order neurone. Third order Horner's syndrome in animals is frequently associated with disease affecting the tympanic bulla and is often associated with concurrent signs of ipsilateral peripheral vestibular syndrome and ipsilateral facial nerve paralysis. First order lesions are frequently accompanied by concurrent severe motor deficits such as tetraparesis or tetraplegia or hemiplegia; injuries and diseases of the T1–T3 ventral nerve roots (such as may be seen in brachial plexus avulsion and brachial plexus tumours) are accompanied by lower motor neurone paresis or paralysis ipsilaterally.

The long second order neurone is vulnerable to damage along its length from extension of intrathoracic or cervical pathology, traumatic injury and neoplasia (both external to the sympathetic nerve but which may invade it and intrinsic nerve tumours). The innervation of the diaphragm is via somatic efferent phrenic nerves bilaterally arising from the 5th to 7th cervical nerves. These course caudally through the cranial mediastinum adjacent to the left subclavian artery and the sympathetic trunk before attaining more lateral positions within narrow plica of pleura, coursing over the basilar structures of the heart before dividing and spreading over the diaphragmatic musculature. Presumably in this patient, given the distribution and apparently invasive nature of the cranial mediastinal mass lesions, bilateral phrenic nerve involvement was due to the local effects of the mass lesions at the site of the left subclavian artery/sympathetic trunk, though whilst a bilateral phrenic nerve dysfunction was present only unilateral second order sympathetic nerve dysfunction was found.

Further reading

deLahunta, A. & Glass, E. (2009) Chapter 7: Lower motor neuron: general visceral efferent system. In *Veterinary Neuroanatomy and Clinical Neurology*, 3rd edn, eds A. deLahunta and E. Glass, WB Saunders, St Louis, pp. 168–191

Featherstone, H. & Holt, E. (2011) Chapter 10: The abnormal pupil. Case 1. In *Small Animal Ophthalmology. What's Your Diagnosis?* Wiley-Blackwell, Oxford, pp. 181–188

Penderis, J. (2002) Chapter 15: Neuro-ophthalmology. In *Canine Ophthalmology: An Atlas and Text*, eds K.C.Barnett, J.Sansom & C. Heinrich, WB Saunders, St Louis, pp. 181–195

Clinical presentation

A 1 year-old male-neutered Labrador retriever (**Figure 32.1**) is presented for development of stiffness, reluctance to walk and dysphagia. The dog had experience an unwitnessed trauma to the top of its tail 2 weeks previously and despite conservative management (topical antiseptic bathing, bandaging) repeated self-trauma had led to a partial tail amputation being undertaken 1 week previously.

Five days after amputation, the dog started to develop a stiff and stilted gait in all four limbs, coarse generalised tremors that appeared to be exacerbated by noise or other stimulation, hypersalivation, an altered facial expression and progressive dysphagia on trying to prehend and swallow food.

Physical examination demonstrates a very anxious dog with extensor rigidity in all four limbs. Bilateral enophthalmos, protrusion of the third eyelids and miosis is present. The ears are held semi-erect bilaterally and the forehead has a wrinkled appearance. The mouth is held partly open and lips retracted ('risus sardonicus'). Marked hypersalivation is present. Rectal temperature is 39.4 °C, heart rate is 116/min and respiratory rate 20/min. Evaluation of proprioception and spinal myotatic reflexed demonstrates normal positioning and reflexes in all limbs but rigidity of all limbs resulting in poor flexion.

Questions

1. What condition does the history and clinical examination findings in this dog suggest?
2. What is the pathogenesis of this condition and how is diagnosis confirmed?
3. How is this condition managed and what is the prognosis?

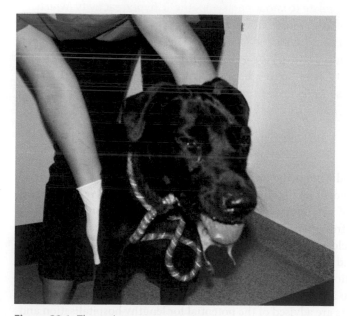

Figure 32.1 The patient at presentation.

Canine Internal Medicine: What's Your Diagnosis? First Edition. Jon Wray.
© 2018 John Wiley & Sons Ltd. Published 2018 by John Wiley & Sons Ltd.

Answers

1. What condition does the history and clinical examination findings in this dog suggest?

The history of recent injury and surgery followed by progressive generalised stiffness, anxious facial expression, ear rigidity, characteristic facial tetany and dysphagia are all highly suggestive of generalised tetanus.

2. What is the pathogenesis of this condition and how is diagnosis confirmed?

Tetanus develops from introduction into wounds of spores of *Clostridium tetani*. Dogs are relatively resistant to tetanus compared with other species such as horses and man, which are much more susceptible. Tetanospasmin, a toxin produced by *C. tetani*, comprises two components, a light chain that blocks release of neurotransmitters and a heavy chain that binds to neuronal cells and transport proteins. Retrograde axonal transport of tetanospasmin in motor nerves results in progressive peripheral nerve, spinal cord and brain effects but haematogenous spread of toxin also occurs. Tetanospasmin causes inhibition of neurotransmitters of inhibitory interneurons within the brain and spinal cord, mainly glycine and gamma-aminobutyric acid (GABA). The net result of this is CNS hyperexcitability and muscle rigidity/spasm.

Diagnosis of tetanus

A diagnosis of tetanus is usually made on characteristic clinical signs developing on average 5–10 days after a wound. Localised tetanus may simply result in extensor rigidity of one limb adjacent to the wound site, or more generalised signs may develop. It appears that younger dogs are more severely affected than older dogs. Occasionally autonomic nervous system signs can also be seen and these may relate to vagal-parasympathetic hyperreactivity (which may result in bradycardia) but conversely exaggerated catecholamine release may occur in response to sympathetic stimulation, resulting in tachycardia and hypertension.

Isolation of *C. tetani* from wounds is possible provided that samples are cultured strictly anaerobically for prolonged periods of time, but this has very low sensitivity and is rarely undertaken successfully. Similarly, measurement of serum antibodies to *C. tetani* is feasible but of limited specificity. Diagnosis is therefore routinely made on clinical grounds only.

---

3. How is this condition managed and what is the prognosis?

Management of tetanus is dependent on the timing, severity and focal or generalised nature of the clinical signs. The degree of veterinary care needed is hugely variable and severity of presenting signs may run a gamut from those mildly affected animals who may have focal limb rigidity only, to those patients developing generalised tetanus and associated recumbency, dysphagia, respiratory compromise and inability to urinate, who require intensive supportive management for several weeks. Prediction of this at the time of presentation may be difficult as it is not uncommon for clinical signs to initially progress despite rapid institution of therapy. These factors make it essential that owners are advised of the potential for lengthy hospitalisation and expense associated with the frequent development of complications associated with tetanus. Therapy may be specific and supportive.

A classification scheme of severity of tetanus has been reported by Burkitt et al. (2007) and is shown in **Table 32.1**.

Table 32.1 Classification of tetanus severity reported by Burkitt et al. (2007)

Class I	Any or all of the following:
	• Miosis, enophthalmos, risus sardonicus, erect ears or trismus
	• Hypersensitivity to noise, light or touch
	• Ambulatory
	Absence of any class II, III or IV signs
Class II	May include any or all class I signs
	Any or all of the following:
	• Dysphagia
	• Stiff gait, sawhorse stance or erect tail
	• Ambulatory
	Absence of any class III or IV signs
Class III	Must have class I or class II signs (requirement)
	Any or all of the following:
	• Recumbency
	• Muscle fasciculations or spasms
	• Seizures
	Absence of any class IV signs
Class IV	Must have class I, II or III signs (requirement)
	Any or all of the following:
	• Bradycardia (heart rate <60 beats/min) or bradyarrhythmia
	• Sinus tachycardia (heart rate >140 beats/min) or tachyarrhythmia
	• Labile hypertension (mean arterial blood pressure >130 mmHg or systolic arterial blood pressure >150 mmHg)
	• Labile hypotension (mean arterial blood pressure <60 mmHg or systolic arterial blood pressure <80 mmHg)
	• Periods of apnoea or respiratory arrest

Specific therapy may comprise:

- Administration of tetanus antitoxin (TAT)
  - Either equine serum-derived antitoxin or human tetanus immunoglobulin has been used with the latter not advised for intravenous use.
  - Intravenous use is associated with a more rapid and marked increase in circulating antitoxin but is associated with risk of anaphylaxis and an initial test dose of 0.1 ml intradermally or subcutaneously and observation for a subsequent wheal/flare reaction has been recommended prior to slow intravenous administration. However, in one study (Burkitt et al. 2007) there was little association between development of reaction to intravenous infusion of antitoxin (largely vomiting, retching, tachypnoea) and prior skin reaction.
  - Doses of 100–1000 units/kg to a maximum of 20 000 units have been recommended as a single treatment.
  - The efficacy and effect of timing on progression and severity of tetanus signs has not been demonstrated with tetanus antitoxin; nonetheless, it continues to be recommended as specific treatment.

- Systemic antimicrobial therapy
  - Penicillin G and metronidazole administration, parenterally initially, are the two antimicrobials most commonly recommended. There is little rationale in giving both although this is commonly done. Dosage recommendations are
    - Penicillin G (benzylpenicillin) 20 000–40 000 units /kg i.v., i.m. q6–8 hours for 10 days*
    - Procaine penicillin 20 000–40,000 units/kg i.m. q6–10 hours for 10 days
    - Metronidazole 10–15 mg/kg i.v. q12 hours**

- Local therapy
  - Surgical debridement of local wounds and topical therapy with hydrogen peroxide may be of benefit but should not be undertaken prior to institution of antimicrobial therapy and tetanus antitoxin.
  - There is some rationale in local intramuscular administration of benzylpenicillin to achieve local tissue levels.

Supportive care may include
- Provision of a quiet comfortable environment as free as possible from noise and light stimulation.
- Use of muscle relaxants and sedatives to control tetanic muscle spasm, reduce sensory hypersensitivity and reduce muscle spasm-induced hyperthermia. Many empirical recommendations exist including:
  - Acepromazine 0.01–0.03 mg/kg i.v. q2–6 hours prn
  - Chlorpromazine 0.5 mg/kg i.m., s.c. q6–8 hours prn
  - Diazepam 0.2–0.5 mg/kg i.v. or 5–10 mg total p/o q4–6 hours prn
  - Midazolam 0.1–0.2 mg/kg i.v., i.m. q2–4 hours prn
  - Phenobarbital 1–6 mg/kg i.m. q6–12 hours
  - Methocarbamol 22–44 mg/kg p/o, i.v. q8 hours
  - Dantrolene 1–5 mg/kg p/o q8 hours

In most patients a combination of a phenothiazine and a barbiturate or benzodiazepine appears reasonably effective but it is recommended that blood pressure assessments and serial monitoring for development of bradycardia is frequently performed.
- Nutritional support and oral hygiene
  - Tetanic dogs can frequently feed themselves by sucking at soupy consistency foodstuffs or being handfed small meatballs.
  - Lack of prehension and oral/pharyngeal dysphasia as well as copious salivation frequently leads to food debris accumulation and cheilitis and regular nursing care of the mouth and lips is usually needed.
  - Development of oesophageal dysphagia, megaoesophagus, hiatal herniation are all seen in some tetanic animals and feeding tube placement (percutaneous endoscopic gastrostomy tube, PEG) is useful in these patients.
  - Gastro-oesophageal reflux may be seen and may be exacerbated by prolonged recumbency and gastric prokinetic agents such as metoclopramide and ranitidine may be helpful in this setting.

---

*Note that this agent is not licenced for use in dogs in the United Kingdom.
**At higher doses metronidazole may be associated with development of reversible CNS toxicity. This usually manifests as central vestibular signs but there is considerable overlap (extensor rigidity, ataxia, tremor) between this and signs of tetanus.

- ◦ Parenteral nutrition may also be given but is not recommended as a sole means of nutrition since the absorptive parts of the gastrointestinal tract are working normally in these patients. Parenteral nutrition is expensive and assiduous attention to sterility is required if nosocomial infection of delivery lines is not to occur.
- Respiratory management
  - ◦ In recumbent patients, frequent turning and monitoring for respiratory compromise, both due to the primary effects of tetanus on musculature associated with ventilation but also due to aspiration pneumonitis (from which such patients are at risk) are important.
  - ◦ Provision of oxygen supplementation is often of benefit.
  - ◦ Tetanic patients should be monitored closely for the development of obstructive respiratory disease both due to laryngeal spasm and due to occlusion of the pharynx/larynx by copious oral secretions. Suction equipment and materials for emergency intubation should always be adjacent to these patients.
  - ◦ In some patients ventilation assistance is required and this may also result in markedly increased expense and hospitalisation time.
- Regular dermal hygiene assessment, provision of padded bedding and regular turning to avoid development of decubitus ulcers and intertrigo dermatopathies in recumbent patients.
- Urinary bladder management is often required and a degree of dyssynergia complicates spontaneous bladder voiding in many patients. Gente manual bladder expression may be possible though in many patients intermittent sterile urinary catheterisation is needed or use of indwelling urinary catheters (though this latter is associated with increased risk of ascending urinary tract infections).
- Hyperthermia may frequently occur secondary to tetanic muscle spasm though it should be borne in mind that developing hyperthermia may also be caused by development of nosocomial infections of the respiratory or urinary tract or intravenous cannula sites.

Prognosis

Prognosis is variable with mortality rates in studies in dogs varying between 8% and 50%. Time of hospitalisation can vary considerably (and thus the associated expense of treatment) with a mean of approximately 20 days reported. For some severely affected patients the costs associated with treatment may be prohibitive and euthanasia may be considered by owners of these patients. Most animals surviving initial treatment have a good long-term prognosis and persistence of neurological signs beyond 2–3 months is very uncommon.

Outcome

Due to the severity of clinical signs and the likely costs associated with predicted management, the owners of this dog elected for humane euthanasia.

Discussion

Tetanus is an uncommon condition that may, anecdotally, be seen in some regional areas more commonly than others. Whilst definitive diagnosis is difficult, the classical presenting signs and physical examination findings when combined with a history of a recent wound combine to allow a confident clinical diagnosis in most cases.

Treatment of tetanus cases can be rewarding but often lengthy and labour-intensive (and thus costly) and it is not uncommon for clinical cases to worsen over the first few days after diagnosis before improvement is seen.

Reference

Burkitt, J.M., Sturges, B.K., Jandrey, K.E. & Kass, P.H. (2007) Risk factors associated with outcome in dogs with tetanus: 38 cases (1987–2005). *J Am Vet Med Assoc* **230**, 76–83

Further reading

Adamantos, S. & Boag, A. (2007) Thirteen cases of tetanus in dogs. *Vet Rec* **161**, 298–302

Bandt, C., Rozanski, E.A., Steinberg, T. & Shaw, S.P. (2007) Retrospective study of tetanus in 20 dogs: 1988–2004. *J Am Anim Hosp Assoc* **43**, 143–148

Dieringer, T.M. & Wolf, A.M. (1991) Esophageal hiatal hernia and megaesophagus complicating tetanus in two dogs. *J Am Vet Med Assoc* **199**, 87–89

Greene, C.E. (2012) Chapter 41: Tetanus. In *Infectious Diseases of the Dog and Cat*, 4th edn, ed. C.E. Greene, Elsevier Saunders, St Louis, pp. 423–431

Infectious Diseases

Clinical presentation

An adult male-neutered German Shepherd Cross (**Figure 33.1**) of unknown age is presented for investigation of anaemia, azotaemia and proteinuria. The dog was imported from Spain 8 weeks previously by a British rescue charity but very scant information is available regarding the dog's previous history and disease status. The dog had initially presented to another veterinary surgeon with a peracute history of vomiting and colitic diarrhoea four weeks previously that had improved spontaneously within three days of onset with empirical therapy comprising oral metronidazole and a kaolin-based adsorbent paste. However, the new owner reported that the dog remained rather lethargic and appeared polyuric.

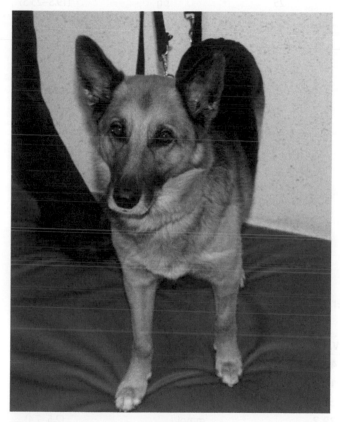

Figure 33.1 The patient at presentation.

Canine Internal Medicine: What's Your Diagnosis? First Edition. Jon Wray.
© 2018 John Wiley & Sons Ltd. Published 2018 by John Wiley & Sons Ltd.

A haematology and biochemistry sample obtained recently at the previous veterinary practice demonstrated the following:

Haematology at previous veterinary surgeon (sample analysed at reference laboratory)

Parameter	Value	Units	Range
RBC	**3.8**	× 10¹²/l	(5.5–8.5)
Haemoglobin	**9.5**	g/dl	(12.0–18.0)
Haematocrit	**0.29**	l/l	(0.37–0.55)
Mean cell volume	77.0	fl	(60–77)
Mean cell haemoglobin concentration	32.5	g/dl	(30.0–38.0)
Mean cell haemoglobin	25	pg	(19.5–25.5)
Total white cell count	11.53	× 10⁹/l	(6.0–15.0)
Neutrophils	9.10	× 10⁹/l	(3.0–11.5)
Lymphocytes	1.67	× 10⁹/l	(1.0–4.8)
Monocytes	0.63	× 10⁹/l	(0.2–1.4)
Eosinophils	**0.09**	× 10⁹/l	(0.1–1.2)
Basophils	0.02	× 10⁹/l	(0.0–0.1)
Platelets	353	× 10⁹/l	(200–500)
Film comment:	**White cell morphology.** Unremarkable. No infectious agents are seen		
	Red cell morphology. Unremarkable. No infectious agents are seen		
	Platelets. Marked platelet clumping present; actual count may be higher than measured number		

Biochemistry at previous veterinary surgeon (sample analysed at reference laboratory)

Parameter	Value	Units	Range
Total protein	**40**	g/l	(54–77)
Albumin	**10**	g/l	(25–40)
Globulin	30	g/l	(23–45)
Urea	**29.2**	mmol/l	(2.5–7.4)
Creatinine	**263**	µmol/l	(40–145)
Potassium	4.5	mmol/l	(3.4–5.6)
Sodium	151	mmol/l	(139–154)
Chloride	122	mmol/l	(105–122)
Calcium	**2.0**	mmol/l	(2.1–2.8)
Magnesium	**0.61**	mmol/l	(0.62–0.90)
Inorganic phosphate	**2.4**	mmol/l	(0.60–1.40)

Parameter	Value	Units	Range
Glucose	5.8	mmol/l	(3.3–5.8)
ALT	14	IU/l	(13–88)
AST	26	IU/l	(13–60)
ALKP	17	IU/l	(14–105)
GGT	3	IU/l	(0–10)
Bilirubin	1	µmol/l	(0–16)
Cholesterol	**10.6**	mmol/l	(3.8–7.0)
Triglyceride	1.1	mmol/l	(0.56–1.14)
Creatine kinase	131	IU/l	(0–190)

On the advice of the laboratory and in light of the azotaemia and prior gastrointestinal upset, a urinalysis (from a free-catch sample) and an ACTH stimulation test to exclude hypoadrenocorticism were performed. The ACTH stimulation test showed normal stimulation of cortisol production in response to an exogenous secretagogue, excluding hypoadrenocorticism. Urinalysis demonstrated the following:

Urinalysis at previous veterinary surgeon (sample analysed at reference laboratory)

Parameter	Value	Units	Range
Appearance	Clear, mid-yellow		
Chemistry			
Specific gravity	1.015		
pH	7.0		
Protein	Trace		
Nitrite	Negative		
Blood/Hb	Negative		
Glucose	Negative		
Ketones	Negative		
Bilirubin	Negative		
Urobilinogen	Negative		
Cytology			
Red cells	**4–5**	/hpf	(0–2)
White cells	1–2	/hpf	(0–2)
Epithelial cells	Occasional	/hpf	(0–5)
Casts	Negative		
Crystals	Negative		
Bacteria	Negative		
Urine culture	Negative		
Quantitative protein			
Urine protein:creatinine	**6.67**	Ratio	<0.5

On physical examination the dog is bright and in normal body condition. Oral mucous membranes are very slightly pale with a normal capillary refill of <2 seconds and are moist to the touch. Heart rate is normal at 116/minute, respiratory rate 12/minute and auscultation is normal. Abdominal palpation is unremarkable and both kidneys can be palpated as being of normal size and contour and palpation does not elicit discomfort. Rectal temperature is 38.7 °C. No lymphadenomegaly or hepatosplenomegaly is palpated. Small crusting lesions (**Figure 33.2**) are noted on the tips of the pinnae, which have not been previously mentioned. The lesions are hairless and comprise focal crust, scale and mild excoriation, which the owner feels has not been associated with pruritus at any stage.

Questions

1. Interpret the clinical pathology data presented from this patient.
2. From the history, physical examination findings and the laboratory results, construct a problem list and determine what the principle or 'pivotal' problems are. What are the main differential diagnoses for these pivotal problems?
3. How would you propose to investigate this case?

Answers

1. Interpret the clinical pathology data presented from this patient.

Haematology

An anaemia is present that is moderate in severity (we classify canine anaemias as mild when HCt is 0.30–0.37, moderate when 0.20–0.29, severe when 0.13–0.19 and very severe when <0.13). It is normocytic, normochromic, which does not support the presence of a regenerative response, in which anisocytosis due to the presence of macrocytes and polychromasia due to the presence of hyperchromatic cells would be expected. However, this analysis alone can neither refute nor confirm the presence of a regenerative response and one must also take into account factors such as timing

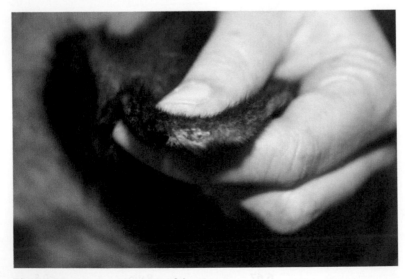

Figure 33.2 Lesion on margin of the pinna.

of onset of anaemia as to whether development of a reticulocyte response has had adequate time to be seen (see Case 6). It is also helpful to evaluate anaemias in the context of the clinical time course (always asking the questions):

- 'Has this animal's clinical signs been present long enough that I would expect to find evidence of a regenerative response, were one to be likely to develop?' and also
- 'Does the severity of the anaemia match the severity of the clinical signs (or is the anaemia much worse than one might suspect, suggesting time for clinical adaptation has occurred)?'

In this case the animal's clinical signs are of moderate lethargy and this would indeed be in keeping with the moderate nature of the anaemia. The remaining haemogram findings are normal except for a borderline eosinopenia, which at this marginal level may be of questionable significance but may simply reflect a typical eosinopenia of the illness/stress leukogram. There is absence of both neutropenia and thrombocytopenia, the presence of which in addition to the anaemia might strongly implicate a bone marrow pathology.

Biochemistry

The most striking biochemical findings are the azotaemia and severe hypoalbuminaemia.

Interpretation of azotaemia

It is always helpful to evaluate the presence of azotaemia in light of the clinical hydration status of the patient (whilst bearing in mind that physical examination may fail to detect early evidence of dehydration) and the concurrent urine specific gravity before any fluid therapy has been given. Following the accepted strategy of classifying azotaemia as being pre-renal, post-renal or renal (see **Case 24**) is sensible and a good starting point in evaluation of any azotaemic animal provided that one is wary of common pitfalls and of overinterpretation. Most commonly post-renal azotaemia develops in patients with lower urinary obstruction and clinical signs of dysuria are evident. However, in patients in whom prior obstruction has been recently relieved or in whom the site of obstruction is at the ureteral level, this may confound clinical assessment.

In this patient there was no clinical evidence of dehydration and the urine SG was 1.015, i.e. is *just* hypersthenuric but well below the threshold (approximately 1.030 in dogs) where adequate tubular concentrating ability is demonstrable. This would suggest that the azotaemia is renal in origin. Whilst evaluation of strict ratios between urea and creatinine may be easy to overinterpret, a broader assessment of the difference in relative magnitude of increases in urea and creatinine may be helpful and in this case the relative magnitude of the increase in urea (approximately 4 times the upper limit of the reference range) is proportionally higher than the magnitude of the creatinine raise (just under twice the upper limit of the corresponding reference range). Creatinine is the preferred analyte for assessment of renal function because it is less commonly affected by non-renal factors such as dehydration, recent feeding or gastrointestinal bleeding (whereas urea levels can be affected by all of these factors).

The hypoalbuminaemia is striking in a number of respects. Not only is it severe (we generally class hypoalbuminaemia as being mild when below the reference interval but >20g/l, moderate when 15–20 g/l and severe when <15 g/l) but it is unaccompanied by changes in the serum globulin level.

Hypoalbuminaemia

Mild hypoalbuminaemia may be seen with acute whole blood loss (in which situation mild hypoglobulinaemia – i.e. panhypoproteinaemia – is commonly also seen) as an accompanying biochemical feature of chronic disease and as a 'negative acute phase' response when an inflammatory response is seen, this latter usually accompanied by other evidence of inflammation such as an inflammatory leukogram and/or hyperglobulinaemia.

Hypoalbuminaemia is also commonly encountered in situations of protein-losing nephropathy (where it is usually decreased without any reduction in globulin), in fulminant hepatic failure or severe hepatocellular dysfunction, and in protein-losing enteropathy (where it commonly is associated with concurrent hypoglobulinaemia, though this is not an invariable finding and sometimes hypoalbuminaemia precedes globulin loss or a markedly inflammatory gastrointestinal pathology offsets any intestinal loss of protein see Case 13).

Due to the major contribution of albumin to colloid oncotic pressure, albumin levels <15 g/l (or thereabouts) are commonly accompanied by development of transudative ascites. The absence of this, at least as definable on physical examination, with an albumin of 10 g/l might suggest that either forces opposing fluid extravasation due to low colloid oncotic pressure may be present or that time to adapt to this very low protein level may have elapsed, or a combination of the two.

There is marginal reduction in the total calcium and magnesium, both of which would be expected in the presence of such marked hypoalbuminaemia. Reduction in these analytes may also be seen in gastrointestinal disease but the reduction in this case is both extremely marginal and unassociated with current gastrointestinal signs in the patient (although gastrointestinal signs have been noted previously and further monitoring of these parameters would be sensible). The phosphate elevation is likely to relate to failure of excretion in the presence of azotaemia, though may also occur with increased phosphate absorption from the intestine and shift of phosphate from the intracellular space (e.g. in acidosis or cellular lysis). The hypercholesterolaemia may, provided that recent feeding has been excluded as a potential cause, reflect an undetermined endocrinopathy (of which diabetes mellitus, hypothyroidism and hyperadrenocorticism are the most frequently causative), pancreatitis, protein-losing nephropathy or dyslipidaemia.

Urinalysis

Mild microscopic haematuria is present. The source of the haematuria cannot be inferred. Haematuria may increase the urine protein:creatinine ratio to a degree commensurate with the degree of haemorrhage, but at this marginal degree of haematuria and in the absence of more severe inflammatory debris, such an influence is likely to be small. There is substantial proteinuria indicating *in the absence of a more active urinary sediment* a loss of glomerular 'permselectivity', meaning that the ability of the glomerular apparatus to resist filtration of protein into Bowman's capsule has been lost. It is important not to equate this with the term glomerulonephritis. Glomerulonephritis is one cause of protein-losing nephropathy and is not a diagnosis implicit in the finding of proteinuria.

2. From the history, physical examination findings and the laboratory results, construct a problem list and determine what the principle or 'pivotal' problems are. What are the main differential diagnoses for these pivotal problems?

From the information presented a problem list for this patient might read:

- Vomiting
- Large intestinal diarrhoea
- Lethargy
- Copious urination
- Anaemia
- Azotaemia
- Hypoalbuminaemia
- Proteinuria
- Haematuria
- Hypercholesterolaemia
- Crusting/scaling ear-tip lesions

This is a long problem list and attempting to problem-solve based on such an extensive list is fraught with difficulty. It is sensible to try and marshal this differential diagnosis list and focus on those problems that are both consistent/reproducible (rather than being historical and now resolved) and that may be 'pivotal' (pivotal problems are those that are both clinically important and that have a limited differential diagnosis list, or at least an approach that is well-defined See Case 3.). Problems that are either logically explicable by others (provided that one keeps an open mind as to other confounding causes) or that are so vague as to have very lengthy differential diagnoses, may assume secondary importance. In this case it might be appropriate to reconfigure the list as:

Pivotal problems (see **Table 33.1**)
- Anaemia, moderate, normocytic/normochromic and unaccompanied by other 'cytopenias'
- Azotaemia, moderate, renal
- Hypoalbuminaemia
- Proteinuria

Problems
- Hypercholesterolaemia
- Haematuria
- Crusting/scaling ear-tip lesions, non-pruritic
- Copious urination

Historical or non-specific problems
- Vomiting and large intestinal diarrhoea, which occurred as a single self-limiting event 4 weeks previously and which have not recurred
- Lethargy

Table 33.1 Differential diagnoses for 'pivotal' problems

Moderate, normocytic/ normochromic anaemia	Regenerative anaemias (though accompanying evidence of anisocytosis due to the presence of macrocytes and polychromasia due to the presence of hyperchromatic cells would be expected)	• Blood loss • Haemolysis

	Non-regenerative anaemias	○ Ineffective erythropoiesis due to effects of non-bone marrow disease on erythropoiesis
		   - Chronic kidney disease
		   - Chronic inflammatory disease
		   - Endocrine deficiencies (especially hypothyroidism)
		○ Primary bone marrow disease
		   - Failure of production/release of red cells, e.g. aplastic anaemia, myelofibrosis with myeloid metaplasia, myelodysplastic syndrome, pure red cell aplasia, non-regenerative immune-mediated anaemia
		   - Myelophthisis due to
		     -- Leukaemias (note that these need not be accompanied by evidence of circulating abnormal cells since evidence of an 'aleukaemic leukaemia' may be confined to the marrow compartment)
		     -- Multiple myeloma
		     -- Lymphoma
		• Infectious disease processes affecting the bone marrow, especially
		○ Ehrlichiosis
		○ Leishmaniosis

Renal azotaemia	Acute intrinsic renal azotaemia	Renal Ischaemia Nephrotoxins Infectious renal disease (pyelonephritis, leptospirosis, borreliosis, babesiosis*, leishmaniosis*) Immune-mediated renal disease Vasculitis Neoplasia Renal effect of systemic disease states • Systemic inflammatory response syndrome • Sepsis • DIC • Pancreatitis • Hypertension

		• Polycythaemia
		• Hypercalcaemia
Chronic intrinsic renal azotaemia		Familial/inherited/congenital disease, e.g.
		• Amyloidosis in the Shar Pei
		• Glomerulopathy of Cocker Spaniels, Bull Terriers, Dobermann Pinscher, Samoyed
		• Polycystic kidney disease of Cairn Terriers
		• Fanconi syndrome in Basenjis
		• Renal dysplasia in any breed but especially Boxer and Labrador Retriever
		Infectious renal disease (pyelonephritis, leptospirosis, borreliosis, babesiosis, leishmaniosis*)
		Immune-mediated renal disease
		Vasculitis
		Neoplasia
		Hydronephrosis due to long-standing post-renal obstruction (e.g. ureterolithiasis, spay granulomas, lower urinary tract neoplasia)
		Polycystic kidneys
		Renal effect of systemic disease states
		• Systemic inflammatory response syndrome
		• Sepsis
		• DIC
		• Pancreatitis
		• Hypertension
		• Polycythaemia
		• Hypercalcaemia
		Idiopathic/cause undetermined before development of chronic kidney disease
Acute-on-chronic intrinsic renal azotaemia		

*Not endemic to the United Kingdom.

Hypoalbuminaemia	Mild hypoalbuminaemia	Chronic inflammatory disease
		Negative acute-phase response *and*
	Severe hypoalbuminaemia	Protein-losing nephropathy
		Protein-losing enteropathy
		Hepatic dysfunction

Significant proteinuria has been established suggesting that protein-losing nephropathy is the likely cause of this. Since hypercholesterolaemia is also commonly seen in patients with protein-losing nephropathy, we can reasonably consider that this is also likely to be due to a protein-losing nephropathy.

The crusting ear lesions are non-pruritic and alopecic. Differential diagnoses include dermatophytosis, keratinisation defects, leishmaniasis and actinic keratitis. Sometimes crusting pinnal lesions may result from vasculitis or from crusting of previously ruptured vesicular diseases, such as pemphigus foleaceus. Parasitic dermatitis is less likely due to the absence of pruritus. Lastly, neoplastic conditions such as actinic squamous cell carcinoma and epitheliotrophic lymphoma should not be discounted.

3. How would you propose to investigate this case?

Initial diagnostic priorities should include:

- Establishment of whether the anaemia is regenerative or non-regenerative.
- Exclusion of causes of the profound hypoalbuminaemia other than protein-losing nephropathy of which a bile-acid stimulation test to evaluate hepatic function would be the most immediately practical.
- Performing diagnostic imaging of the upper urinary tract to evaluate for structural diseases affecting the renal architecture (such as renal neoplasia).
- Performing skin scrapes and potentially dermatophyte culture of the crusting pinnal lesions.
- Given the dog's travel history, considering diagnostic evaluation for infectious diseases non-endemic to the UK that might be associated with protein-losing nephropathy, especially leishmaniosis, ehrlichiosis and babesiosis and the heartworm *Dirofilaria immitis*.

In this patient a reticulocyte count of $73 \times 10^9/l$ (0–80) and a reticulocyte percentage of 1.6% were established, suggesting that the anaemia was non-regenerative. Since the clinical time-course was such that, were a regenerative response to have developed it would have had time by referral presentation to have done so, it would be unlikely that this represented a 'pre-regenerative' response. A bile acid stimulation test was normal, suggesting that hypoalbuminaemia was not contributed to by hepatocellular dysfunction.

Diagnostic imaging of the urinary tract was performed by ultrasound examination (**Figure 33.3**), which demonstrated bilaterally normal renal size and architecture. The bladder also appeared normal and a urine sample collected by cystocentesis was cultured and produced no bacterial growth. The remaining abdominal organs including the liver and spleen appeared normal.

Skin scrapes of the pinnae demonstrated moderate numbers of superficial anucleated squamous epithelial cells and keratin bars, these often being in clusters. There were low numbers of

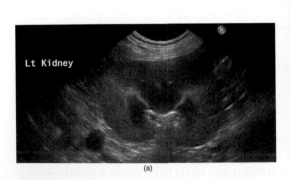

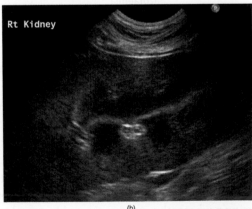

Figure 33.3 (a) Left renal ultrasound and (b) right renal ultrasound.

neutrophils and histiocytes/macrophages. A few cells containing green pigment (melanin: melanophages or melanocytes) were seen but no intracellular organisms were detected.

Due to a high index of suspicion for leishmaniosis given the dog's travel history, crusting/scaling non-pruritic pinnal lesions and the severe protein-losing nephropathy, peripheral blood was submitted for assessment by polymerase chain reaction (PCR) for *Leishmania*, *Ehrlichia* and *Babesia* and for *Dirofilaria immitis* antigen testing and Knott's test for microfilariae of *D. immitis*. Though leishmaniosis was the principle consideration, co-infection with other arthropod-borne diseases is frequently encountered in infected dogs and hence the panel of tests performed. Bone marrow aspiration cytology and PCR for *Leishmania* was also performed under a brief general anaesthetic in light of the non-regenerative anaemia, and at the same time fine needle aspiration cytology of the spleen and peripheral lymph nodes was undertaken (even though these were normal in appearance / size) to try and increase the likelihood of identification of *Leishmania* amastigotes.

The results are shown below and in **Figure 33.4**.

***Babesia* PCR** (peripheral blood)	Negative
***Ehrlichia* PCR** (peripheral blood)	Negative
Leishmania* qPCR (peripheral blood)	**DETECTED @ CT 33.91****
***Dirofilaria immitis* antigen** (peripheral blood)	Negative
Knott's test for *D. immitis* microfilariae (peripheral blood)	Negative
Leishmania* qPCR (bone marrow)	**DETECTED @ CT 25.12****

*qPCR denotes quantitative PCR analysis.

**CT denotes 'cycle threshold' – this is the number of thermal cycles required to cross the threshold value. CT values are inversely proportional to the amount of target nucleic acid in the sample.

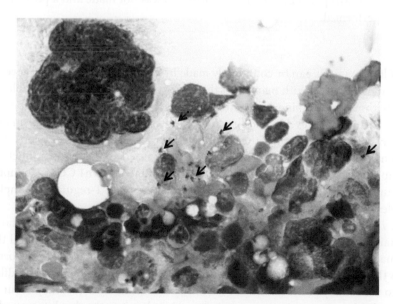

Figure 33.4 Bone marrow aspirate cytology (stained with Wright stain) demonstrating *Leishmania* amastigotes (arrows) with intensely-staining kinetoplasts within the macrophages.

Spleen FNA cytology	Normal cytology; no organisms seen
Lymph node FNA cytology	Normal cytology; no organisms seen
Bone marrow aspiration cytology	Both myeloid and erythroid cell lines are present and mature to segmented neutrophils and metarubricytes respectively. There are also frequent macrophages and these often contain multiple *Leishmania* amastigotes. The amastigotes are also seen free in the background in low numbers. Low numbers of small lymphocytes and plasma cells are seen.

Diagnosis and treatment

A diagnosis of leishmaniosis was confirmed. The patient was treated with a combination of allopurinol at a dose of 15 mg/kg p/o BID initially and creatinine was monitored weekly. After 14 days serum creatinine had decreased to 176 μmol/l (from 263 μmol/l, reference interval 40–145) and at this time meglumine antimonate was introduced at a dose of 100 mg/kg s.c. Although this latter is, often in combination with allopurinol, the most successful treatment for visceral leishmaniosis in dogs, a potential for nephrotoxicity exists, which is an important consideration since (as in this patient) concurrent nephropathy is often present. In this patient the risk of nephrotoxicity was weighed up against the benefit of killing the organisms likely to be causing the protein-losing nephropathy in the first place and the reduction in creatinine seen initially with allopurinol alone. Mild clinical improvement was seen initially but progressively worsening proteinuria was seen without evidence of worsening azotaemia and over the first 6 weeks of therapy the urine protein:creatinine ratio was seen to progress to 12.67 and then 15.55. Additional therapy in the form of benazepril 0.5 mg/kg p/o SID and clopidogrel at a dose just exceeding 1 mg/kg p/o SID was introduced. However, 7 weeks after diagnosis the patient developed sudden onset abdominal pain, haemorrhagic diarrhoea, weakness and shock. An acute vascular abdominal thromboembolic event was suspected based on clinical description and the dog was euthanased. It was suspected that worsening protein-losing nephropathy leading to a hypercoagulable state had initiated a vascular thrombotic catastrophe, but a definitive diagnosis was not made and a post-mortem examination was not performed.

Discussion

A diagnosis of leishmaniosis can be confidently made in this patient. The clinical spectrum of disease in leishmaniosis is broad with many dogs that are exposed to infection being able to eliminate the organism without succumbing to the disease. The level of host immunity appears to dictate whether clinical illness will develop and the complex interaction between organism and host immune system in itself can dictate whether elimination or clinical disease develops. Whether the immune response to infection is of a Th1 or Th2 type (this refers to the distinct functional subsets of CD4+ T lymphocytes, cell-mediated immunity being mediated by Th1 CD4+ T-lymphocytes and humoral immunity by Th2 CD4+ T-lymphocytes), the expression of T-regulatory lymphocytes and genetic variables all play a part in the pathogenicity of the infection.

In Europe *L.infantum* is transmitted by the sandfly *Phlebotomus*. The sandfly takes up macrophages containing amastigotes from an infected animal during a blood meal and these are released from macrophages during digestion in the sandfly gut. Amastigotes transform to motile promastigotes that multiply by binary fission and these continue to divide in the sandfly gut, being regurgitated to the sandfly proboscis from where infection of the new host may occur during further feeding. In the dog, promastigotes are transferred in saliva into the skin bite wound where they are phagocytosed by macrophages. Within the macrophage the organism multiplies as amastigotes

Table 33.2 Common clinical signs of systemic leishmaniosis in dogs

Clinical signs of leishmaniosis
• Crust, scale, alopecia and non-pruritic exfoliative dermatitis
• Mucocutaneous ulceration
• Lethargy, decreased activity
• Anorexia and weight loss
• Vomiting and diarrhoea
• Epistaxis
• Lymphadenomegaly
• Splenomegaly
• Uveitis and keratitis
• Pyrexia
• Icterus

(non-motile form) within phagolysosomes where they are relatively protected from host immunity. Dissemination around the body in the haemolymphatic system then ensues.

The pathological consequences depend on the organism load, the integrity of the host immune response and the tissues to which organism dissemination principally occurs. Common clinical signs are shown in Table 33.2.

However, as in this case, clinical signs may be subtle and variable combinations of these may be seen. Hyperglobulinaemia is commonly detected on serum biochemistry but is not invariably present and a concomitant hypoalbuminaemia (both due to a negative acute-phase response and if proteinuria is present) is often seen. Sometimes hyperglobulinaemia may be very marked and in such cases serum protein electrophoresis (SPE) may help distinguish between monoclonal and polyclonal rises in serum globulins.

Hyperglobulinaemia in arthropod-borne infections

Although not present in this case, often very marked hyperglobulinaemia may accompany arthropod-borne infectious diseases and is seen most commonly in leishmaniosis and ehrlichiosis caused by *E. canis* infection. Hyperglobulinaemia has also been reported in some cases of *Dirofilaria immitis*. In these diseases a polyclonal rise in globulins is seen but their migration on serum protein electrophoresis (SPE) is restricted, leading to a relatively narrowed 'spike' in the gamma-globulin region of the SPE trace, distinct from the more 'broad-based' gamma globulin rise seen in many inflammatory responses (particularly to infection). This restricted migration gammopathy is often referred to as an 'oligoclonal' gammopathy and is distinct from the 'monoclonal' gammopathy that occurs when increased κ- or λ-light chains accumulate due to B-lymphocyte neoplasia (multiple myeloma, plasmacytoma, lymphoma, lymphocytic leukaemia). Caution should be applied to interpretation of SPE as many laboratories interpret narrow-based protein spikes as 'monoclonal', which may simply reflect restricted migration of multiple globulin fractions, and without assessment of light chains by immunocytochemical or histochemical analysis this conclusion may be erroneous. The differential diagnosis for marked hyperglobulinaemia is shown in **Table 33.3.**

Table 33.3 Differential diagnosis of marked hyperglobulinaemia

Broad-based hyperglobulinaemia

- Inflammation due to infection: bacterial, viral, fungal, protozoal
- Inflammation due to non-infectious process: necrosis, neoplasia, immune-mediated disease

Narrow-based hyperglobulinaemia

- Infection (usually oligoclonal spike in γ-globulin region): leishmaniasis, ehrlichiosis, dirofilariasis
- B-cell neoplasia (usually true monoclonal): multiple myeloma, plasmacytoma, lymphoma, lymphocytic leukaemia

An example is shown in **Figure 33.5** of a serum protein electrophoresis trace from a dog with leishmaniosis that had a serum globulin of 69 g/l and a serum albumin of 18g/l.

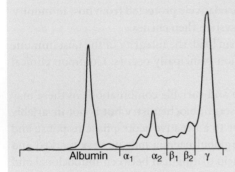

Figure 33.5 Serum protein electrophoresis trace from a dog with leishmaniosis.

The trace shows an apparent narrow-based hyper-gammaglobulinaemia.

Azotaemia and rises in hepatic transaminases are also common, as are anaemia (which is usually non-regenerative and moderate as in this case) and proteinuria. Some animals may display variable leukopenia and thrombocytopenia.

Diagnosis of leishmaniosis may rely on

- Detection of antibodies to *Leishmania infantum*
  - This is highly specific for exposure to the organism but does not necessarily imply that clinical disease is due to leishmaniasis since after seroconversion dogs may remain positive for many months even after successful elimination of the organism.
  - There may be a lag of several months after infection before seroconversion occurs but nearly all infected dogs will seroconvert.

- Detection of organism DNA
  - PCR tests to detect *Leishmania* DNA (commonly kinetoplast DNA) are useful in documenting the presence of *Leishmania* organisms, though it should be borne in mind that PCR tests are more commonly positive from infected tissues of the haemolymphatic system, such as bone marrow, spleen and lymph nodes, than from peripheral blood samples, which may sometimes yield false negative results.
- Identification of the organism
  - *Leishmania* amastigotes are relatively easy to identify in tissue macrophages but the presence of low numbers of organisms may hamper detection. Assessment of deep skin scrapings from any dermatological lesions as well as fine needle aspiration cytology from infected bone marrow, splenic and lymph node tissue is invaluable.

Treatment of leishmaniasis is not straightforward and a clinical cure is frequently not achieved. Owners should be counselled as to the commitment involved in treatment and monitoring of a dog with leishmaniasis and be forewarned that eradication may not be possible. Nonetheless, clinical control of disease and improvement in clinical signs can be achieved in the majority of cases. The prognosis is noticeably poorer in patients such as the one described where azotaemia and protein-losing nephropathy have developed. Anecdotally, cases treated in non-endemic regions such as the UK, provided that progressive protein-losing nephropathy has not developed, appear to have a fair chance of parasitological cure if treated early and appropriately.

The two most commonly employed treatment options are

1. Meglumine antimoniate 100 mg/kg s.c. q24 hours for 3–4 weeks
   Allopurinol 10–20 mg/kg p/o q12–24 hours indefinitely
2. Miltefosine 2 mg/kg p/o q24 hours for 3–4 weeks
   Allopurinol 10–20 mg/kg p/o q12–24 hours indefinitely

Pentavalent antimonials such as meglumine antomoniate selectively inhibit those protozoal enzymes required for fatty acid oxidation and glycolysis. Miltefosine is an alkylphosphocholine derivative and protein kinase B inhibitor. Both drugs appear effective in reducing parasite load and reducing clinical signs but neither routinely results in successful elimination of parasitaemia. Combining therapy with indefinite administration of allopurinol appears to increase efficacy. The author has encountered instances where rescue charities have advised therapy with allopurinol alone and does not support this treatment strategy, which is inferior to the treatments described and appears to be a recommendation based on cost rather than with sound medical foundation. Other therapeutic options include the use of amphotericin B, though the potential for nephrotoxicity in this agent would make this an unsuitable choice in the patient described.

Other agents with clinical efficacy but which do not result in parasitological cure include fluoroquinolones and combinations of spiramycin and metronidazole.

Further reading

Baneth, G., Koutinas, A.F., Solano-Gallego, L., Bourdeau, P. & Ferrer, L. (2008) Canine leishmaniosis – new concepts and insights on an expanding zoonosis: Part one. *Trends Parasitol* **24**, 324–330

Barbieri, C.L. (2006) Immunology of canine leishmaniasis. *Parasite Immunol* **28**, 329–337

Miro, G., Cardoso, L., Pennisi, M.G., Oliva, G. & Baneth, G. (2008) Canine leishmaniosis – new concepts and insights on an expanding zoonosis: Part two. *Trends Parasitol* **24**, 371–377

Saridomichelakis, M.N. (2009) Advances in the pathogenesis of canine leishmaniosis: epidemiologic and diagnostic implications. *Vet Dermatol* **20**, 471–489

Solano-Gallego, L., Koutinas, A., Miro, G., Cardoso, L., Pennisi, M.G., Ferrer, L., Bourdeau, P., Oliva, G. & Baneth, G. (2009) Directions for the diagnosis, clinical staging, treatment and prevention of canine leishmaniosis. *Vet Parasitol* **165**, 1–18

Torres, M., Bardagi, M., Roura, X., Zanna, G., Ravera, I. & Ferrer, L. (2011) Long term follow-up of dogs diagnosed with leishmaniosis (clinical stage II) and treated with meglumine antimoniate and allopurinol. *Vet J* **188**, 346–351

Clinical presentation

A 7 year-old female-neutered Weimaraner is presented to a colleague with an acute history of lethargy, inappetence, vomiting and jaundice for the previous 48 hours. Physical examination shows a depressed dog in normal body condition. Mucous membranes, sclerae and inner ear pinnae are icteric. The dog is estimated to be 5% dehydrated and rectal temperature is elevated at 39.8 °C. Laboratory findings found at initial investigation are shown below. The dog lives in a rural environment and has not been recently vaccinated. Your colleague suspects the dog may have leptospirosis.

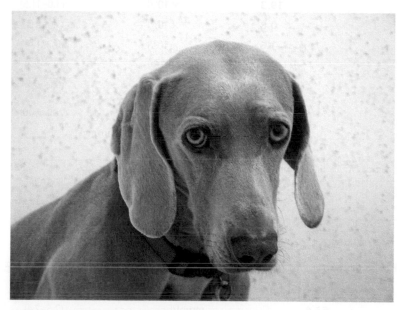

Figure 34.1 The patient at presentation.

Canine Internal Medicine: What's Your Diagnosis? First Edition. Jon Wray.
© 2018 John Wiley & Sons Ltd. Published 2018 by John Wiley & Sons Ltd.

Haematology

Parameter	Value	Units	Range
RBC	5.16	$\times 10^{12}/l$	(5.5–8.5)
Haemoglobin	11.2	g/dl	(12.0–18.0)
Haematocrit	0.36	l/l	(0.37–0.55)
Mean cell volume	69.1	fl	(60–77)
Mean cell haemoglobin concentration	31.4	g/dl	(30.0–38.0)
Mean cell haemoglobin	21.7	pg	(19.5–25.5)
Total white cell count	22.7	$\times 10^9/l$	(6.0–15.0)
Neutrophils	19.3	$\times 10^9/l$	(3.0–11.5)
Lymphocytes	0.8	$\times 10^9/l$	(1.0–4.8)
Monocytes	1.6	$\times 10^9/l$	(0.2–1.4)
Eosinophils	1.0	$\times 10^9/l$	(0.1–1.2)
Basophils	0	$\times 10^9/l$	(0.0–0.1)
Platelets	134	$\times 10^9/l$	(200–500)
Film comment:	Red cells are normocytic and normochromic		
	White blood cell morphology normal		
	Platelet count appears accurate		

Biochemistry

Parameter	Value	Units	Range
Total protein	69	g/l	(54–77)
Albumin	23	g/l	(25–40)
Globulin	46	g/l	(23–45)
Urea	63.4	mmol/l	(2.5–7.4)
Creatinine	856	µmol/l	(40–145)
Potassium	5.6	mmol/l	(3.4–5.6)
Sodium	153	mmol/l	(139–154)
Chloride	111	mmol/l	(105–122)
Calcium	3.2	mmol/l	(2.1–2.8)
Magnesium	–	mmol/l	(0.62–0.90)
Inorganic phosphate	2.6	mmol/l	(0.60–1.40)
Glucose	5.5	mmol/l	(3.3–5.8)
ALT	589	IU/l	(13–88)
AST	165	IU/l	(13–60)
ALKP	1243	IU/l	(14–105)
GGT	52	IU/l	(0–10)
Bilirubin	856	µmol/l	(0–16)

Parameter	Value	Units	Range
Cholesterol	4.5	mmol/l	(3.8–7.0)
Triglyceride	1.1	mmol/l	(0.56–1.14)
Creatine kinase	**549**	IU/l	(0–190)

Urinalysis (free catch sample)

Parameter	Value	Units	Range
Appearance	Clear, pale straw coloured		
Chemistry			
Specific gravity	1.012		
pH	6.5		
Protein	++		
Nitrite	–		
Blood/Hb	++		
Glucose	–		
Ketones	-		
Bilirubin	++		
Urobilinogen	–		
Cytology			
Red cells	**10**	/hpf	(0–2)
White cells	1	/hpf	(0–2)
Epithelial cells	0	/hpf	(0–5)
Casts	–		
Crystals	–		
Bacteria	–		
Other	–		
Quantitative protein			
Urine protein:creatinine	**2.5**	ratio	<0.5

Questions

1. Interpret the clinical and pathological findings in this patient.
2. What clinical presentations are commonly reported with leptospirosis and what animals are at risk?
3. How could a diagnosis of leptospirosis be confirmed?
4. What treatment recommendations exist for the management of suspected leptospirosis cases?

Answers

1. Interpret the clinical and pathological findings in this patient.

A problem list for this patient is:

Based on history/physical examination

- Jaundice
- Elevated rectal temperature
- Vomiting
- Inappetence
- Dehydration

Jaundice reflects hyperbilirubinaemia and may be further defined as pre-hepatic, hepatic or post-hepatic (see **Case 12** and **Table 12.1**). In the presence of only very mild anaemia (below) and the moderate rise in liver enzymes a hepatic or post-hepatic cause is implicated. The elevated rectal temperature may represent hyperthermia or true fever/pyrexia; in the absence of excessive muscular or seizure activity or evidence of respiratory obstruction true fever is most likely. For a complete discussion see **Case 23** and **Table 23.1**. Vomiting should be distinguished from regurgitation based on the clinical history, and broadly primary gastrointestinal, systemic and abdominal diseases local to the gastrointestinal tract should be considered as causes.

Based on laboratory findings

- Very mild anaemia that is normocytic, normochromic. This might suggest a non- or pre-regenerative anaemia but assessment of a reticulocyte count and, if appropriate and a pre-regenerative response is suspected, repeating this after 3–4 days.
- Mild mature neutrophilia accompanied by mild monocytosis and lymphopenia suggest components of an established inflammatory response and stress leukogram.
- Thrombocytopenia. The platelet count is modestly reduced and clinical bleeding tendency is not expected at this level. The thrombocytopenia may be due to consumption of platelets (including as part of disseminated intravascular coagulation), destruction, sequestration or reduced production.
- Hypoalbuminaemia that is mild. This may reflect reduced production as a 'negative acute phase' response in the presence of inflammation (which may contribute to mild hyperglobulinaemia, below), reflect reduced production due to hepatic dysfunction, or excessive loss through the kidneys or GI tract or sequestration ('third space loss' in any cavitary effusions).
- Hyperglobulinaemia that is mild and may reflect an inflammatory response but should also be considered may presage a developing more marked hyperglobulinaemia (see **Table 33.3**).
- Azotaemia that is marked and in which elevation of urea and creatinine are of a broadly similar magnitude (6–9 × upper reference limit). Interpreted in conjunction with the isosthenuric urine SG of 1.012 suggests a true renal azotaemia.
- Hypercalcaemia that is mild but that should be interpreted in the light of a free (ionised) calcium assessment. Differential diagnoses of hypercalcaemia were discussed in **Case 30**. In this case there is significant azotaemia and renal secondary hypercalcaemia is considered the most likely possibility.
- Hyperphosphataemia most commonly results from a decreased glomerular filtration rate. Whilst levels may also increase due to increased intestinal absorption, transcellular shift or release from cellular damage, in the setting of marked azotaemia, reduced GFR is the most likely cause.
- Moderate rise in liver enzymes. A description of interpretation of liver enzymes was given in **Case 12**. In this case the magnitude of elevation is significantly greater than might be expected in a 'secondary' or 'reactive' hepatopathy and both markers of hepatocellular damage and cholestasis are raised.

- A very marked rise in bilirubin, which is the cause of the jaundice. An approach to hyperbilirubinaemia was discussed in **Case 12**.
- Rise in creatine kinase. Creatine kinase is generally held to be an indicator of muscular injury though the level in this case is only very modestly raised.
- Microscopic haematuria and proteinuria. Haematuria on a free catch urine sample may originate from the upper urinary (kidneys, ureters), lower urinary (bladder, urethra) or genital tracts and may result from disease processes causing local denudation of urininary/genital epithelium, be due to vascular pathology or may arise due to a bleeding tendency. Proteinuria may be defined as prerenal (e.g. in systemic paraproteinaemias), renal (reflecting loss of glomerular 'permselectivity') or post-renal in the presence of haemorrhage or inflammation in the lower urinary tract. In this case the degree of proteinuria is significant but may be contributed to by the presence of haemorrhage.

2. What clinical presentations are commonly reported with leptospirosis and what animals are at risk?

Anorexia, vomiting, lethargy and dehydration with variable occurrence of fever are the most common presenting clinical signs in dogs with acute leptospirosis, with approximately one-third of patients also exhibiting icterus. Abdominal and musculoskeletal pain are also commonly reported. Some patients may present with evidence of primary or secondary coagulation deficits and may display petechiation, haematemesis, haematochezia, epistaxis and overt cardiovascular collapse. Increased respiratory rate and effort and uveitis are also intermittently reported.

Common laboratory findings include mild anaemia, leucocytosis (usually comprising neutrophilia and monocytosis), thrombocytopenia, azotaemia (seen in most affected dogs), increases in hepatic transaminases and bilirubin (seen in about one-third to two-thirds of affected dogs) and mild hypoalbuminaemia.

Urinalysis usually demonstrates isosthenuria or hyposthenuria and proteinuria is common. Presence of haematuria, leukuria and granular casts in urine are all variable findings.

Middle-sized to larger breeds of dogs of working types that are young and live in rural environments with frequent access to water courses have been reported to be predisposed, though epidemiological studies have yielded conflicting information. Leptospirosis may appear as a seasonal disease with many outbreaks being temporally and location-associated. Vaccine status of the patient may have some bearing though many recent cases are reported in dogs vaccinated against some serovars, infected with a different one.

3. How can a diagnosis of leptospirosis be confirmed?

Leptospirosis is caused by pathogenic spirochaete bacteria of the genus *Leptospira*, which are gram negative, coiled, motile bacteria. The nomenclature describing Leptospires is complex, most pathogenic organisms described as being of the species *Leptospira interrogans*. Subclassification has traditionally been based on a serovar, the reaction of a member of the genus with a specific monoclonal antiserum that is specific for a carbohydrate antigen of leptospiral lipopolysaccharide. Groups of closely related serovars may all agglutinate in the presence of the same antiserum and are grouped as a 'serogroup'. Specific species (9 pathogenic to date) have been identified by genotypic classification but these do not correlate with seroreactivity.

Confirmation of leptospirosis is difficult. Organism culture is difficult and may take up to six months. Darkfield microscopy (to identify intact motile leptospires in urine) is limited by poor sensitivity. Confirmatory tests are therefore largely based on either the detection of anti-leptospiral serum antibodies (microscopic agglutination testing, MAT) or use of the polymerase chain reaction (PCR) for detection of leptospiral DNA in blood, urine or both. A patient-side

Leptospira antibody ELISA test is also available. The limiting features of all tests for leptospirosis are that many dogs may be exposed to leptospiral organisms and seroconvert without becoming overtly affected, many unaffected dogs will shed viable leptospiral organisms in urine and both vaccinal and non-vaccinal serovars are often positive in recently vaccinated dogs. Whilst the majority of these have been shown to become antibody negative by 15 weeks post-innoculation, in some individuals vaccinal titres may persist for 12 months. Conversely, many dogs in early stages of infection are yet to seroconvert and it is recommended (a) to perform diagnostic testing in those animals in whom a likelihood of leptospirosis exists, (b) to consider utilising both antibody and PCR-based testing to establish a diagnosis and (c) to perform 'convalescent' titres by assessing paired serum antibody tests at time of presentation and 2–4 weeks later. Obviously this latter approach has the disadvantage that clinical patients may be acutely ill and may have been deceased or better by the time a second sample is planned.

Interpretation of MAT tests may be difficult and no consensus is established. However, many sources recommend a single titre of >1:800 in unvaccinated dogs, a titre >1:1600 in vaccinated dogs or an increase in titre between initial and convalescent of 4 times (2 dilutions) should be interpreted as highly suspicious for leptospirosis.

PCR tests target the *lipL32/hap1* gene, which is specific for pathogenic *Leptospira*. Leptospiral DNA is usually found in blood during the first 10 days post-infection and thereafter in urine. Testing of both substances (separately) before antibiotic administration is therefore recommended to increase sensitivity. The specificity of PCR testing would be predicted to be high since the target gene is specific for pathogenic leptospires, but bear in mind the phenomenon of asymptomatic carriers.

4. **What treatment recommendations exist for the management of suspected Leptospirosis cases?**

Antibiotic therapy is recommended in all dogs suspected to have leptospirosis. Doxycycline (5 mg/kg q12 h or 10 mg/kg q24 h) for 14 days has been shown to be effective in both eliminating infection and eliminating intrarenal persistence and long-term carriage. In the acute phase or in vomiting animals poorly tolerant of doxycycline, intravenous penicillin derivatives are the treatments of choice.

Acute kidney injury should be managed by correction of fluid and electrolyte imbalances with assiduous monitoring for development of oliguria/anuria and for iatrogenic fluid overload. Provision of extracorporeal dialysis may be required in some patients. Haemostatic disorders may require blood product component therapy and other supportive measures.

Outcome

In this case a serum ionised calcium was measured and was 0.8 mmol/l (1.18–1.4), suggesting that the hypercalcaemia was due to renal insufficiency. The patient was managed with intravenous crystalloid (Hartmann's solution) fluid therapy and, due to a high index of suspicion for leptospirosis, therapy with doxycycline at a dose of 10 mg/kg/24 hours orally for 4 weeks in total and clavulanate-amoxycillin at a dose of 20 mg/kg intravenously every 8 hours for the first seven days were given. Supportive management with antiemetic therapy (metoclopramide) was also administered and an indwelling urinary catheter was placed in order to monitor for development of oliguria.

After institution of therapy the dog rapidly brightened and azotaemia steadily improved. Reduction in hepatocellular and cholestatic markers occurred ahead of reduction in hyperbilirubinaemia and at a rate commensurate with the biological half-life of the analyte concerned.

Serial evaluation of serum biochemistry over the 7 days of hospitalisation demonstrated the following alteration in parameters:

Parameter	Value d1	Value d2	Value d3	Value d5	Value d7	Units	Range
Urea	63.4	46.8	42.3	30	12.7	mmol/l	(2.5–7.4)
Creatinine	856	566	397	162	57	µmol/l	(40–145)
Calcium	3.2	2.89	2.9	3	2.7	mmol/l	(2.1–2.8)
Phosphate	2.6	2.8	2.7	2.2	1.8	mmol/l	(0.60–1.40)
ALT	589	192	202	157	135	IU/l	(13–88)
AST	165	130	165	150	122	IU/l	(13–60)
ALKP	1243	610	587	385	299	IU/l	(14–105)
GGT	52	35	24	22	14	IU/l	(0–10)
Bilirubin	856	913	179	128	99	µmol/l	(0–16)

The patient eventually made a full recovery and was discharged home after 8 days. Follow-up examination at days 10 and 21 showed resolution of the dog's jaundice and normalisation of remaining biochemical parameters. A urine protein:creatinine ratio on day 21 was normal. A complete recovery was reported (**Figure 34.2**).

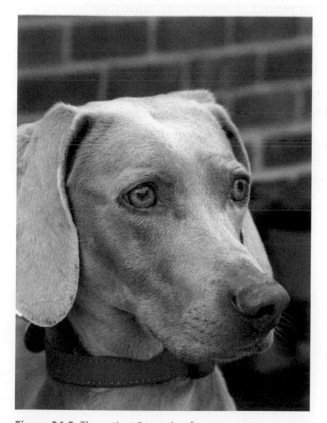

Figure 34.2 The patient 2 months after treatment.

A patient-side ELISA test was not available at the time of this case presentation and samples were submitted for leptospirosis MAT testing initially and as convalescent titres, with the following results being obtained:

Serovar	Day 1	Day 10	Day 21
L. canicola	Negative	1/200	1/200
L. icterohaemorrhagica	Negative	1/400	1/400
L. copenhageni	Negative	1/400	**1/1600**
L. ballum	Negative	Negative	Negative
L. zanoni	Negative	Negative	Negative
L. javanica	Negative	Negative	Negative

A retrospective diagnosis of clinical **leptospirosis caused by** *Leptospira copenhageni* was made.

Discussion

A diagnosis of leptospirosis remains one of the most difficult to make with certainty in small animal practice and environmental history and vaccination status may offer important clinical clues. However, cases are frequently seen in vaccinated dogs due to non-vaccinal serovars and 'clusters' of cases may be seen confined to one geographical location. The presence of asymptomatic carriers, antibody persistence to vaccination and the lack of highly specific, sensitive and rapid diagnostic tests may add to the challenge of diagnosis.

Further reading

Schuller, S., Francey, T., Hartmann, K., Hugonnard, M., Kohn, B., Nally, J.E. & Sykes J. (2015) European consensus statement on leptospirosis in dogs and cats. *J Small Anim Pract* **56**, 159–179

Sykes, J.E., Hartmann, K., Lunn, K.F., Moore, G.E, Stoddard, R.A. & Goldstein, R.E. (2011) 2010 ACVIM small animal consensus statement on leptospirosis: diagnosis, epidemiology, treatment and prevention. *J Vet Intern Med* **25**, 1–13

Index of Tables and Figures, Pearls and Clinical Skills Generated

Section	Case	Figure or table	Contents	Blue box 'Pearls'	Clinical skills / knowledge developed
A	1	Figure 1.1	Picture of patient at presentation	• Overlap in biochemistry results between Diabetes Mellitus and Hyperadrenocorticism	• Assessment of hydration status
		Figure 1.2	Development of ketone bodies in DKA		• Development of a fluid therapy plan
		Table 1.1	Co-morbidities associated with DKA	• diagnostic pitfalls in hyperadrenocorticism when nonadrenal illness present	• Differential diagnosis of hyperglycaemia
		Table 1.2	Physical examination findings of hydration and perfusion	• fluid therapy as an 'iterative' process	
		Table 1.3	Estimating degree of dehydration		
		Table 1.4	Intravenous insulin regimen for treatment of diabetic ketoacidosis		
		Table 1.5	Potassium replacement rates		
	2	Figure 1.1	Picture of patient at presentation	• Components of a neurological examination	• Classification and initial assessment of seizures
		Figure 2.2	Calcium /PTH axis	• Spurious calcium measurements	• Differential diagnosis of hypocalcaemia
		Figure 2.3	Lenticular cataracts in primary hypoparathyroidism	• The differential diagnosis for hypocalcaemia is limited	• The calcium/PTH axis
		Figure 2.4	Calcium absorption and mobilisation	• Handling of PTH and the PTH axis	• Calcium absorption
		Table 2.1	Causes of seizures	• Use of activated vitamin D when PTH is lacking	
		Table 2.2	Differential diagnosis of hypocalcaemia		
	3	Figure 3.1	Picture of the patient at presentation	• Defining shock	• Differentiating causes of azotaemia
		Table 3.1	Stages of shock	• Significance of lymphocytosis and eosinophilia in ill dogs	• Differential diagnosis of hyperkalaemia and hyponatraemia
		Table 3.2	Classifying azotaemia	• Sorting out long differential diagnosis lists and the principle of Occam's razor	
		Table 3.3	Differential diagnosis of hyperkalaemia, hyponatraemia or both	• Exception to the rule in assessing urine specific gravity in dehydrated patients	

(Continued)

(Continued)

(Continued)

(Continued)

Section	Case	Figure or table	Contents	Blue box 'Pearls'	Clinical skills / knowledge developed
		Figure 22.7	Electrical alternans		
		Figure 22.8	Drainage of pericardial effusion		
		Figure 22.9	Pathogenesis of cardiac tamponade		
		Figure 22.10	Thoracoscopic pericardiectomy		
	23	Figure 23.1	The patient at presentation	• Continuous heart murmurs	• Differential diagnosis of PUO
		Figure 23.2	Echocardiographic views of aortic valve	• Hyperdynamic pulses	• Continuous heart murmurs
		Figure 23.3	Colour-flow Doppler echocardiography of aortic insufficiency	• Blood cultures	
		Figure 23.4	CW Doppler of aortic insufficiency		
		Table 23.1	Common causes of PUO in dogs		
H	24	Figure 24.1	The patient at presentation	• Azotaemia	• Approach to the azotaemic patient
		Figure 24.2	IRIS staging of chronic kidney disease (CKD) in the dog	• Introducing renal diets	• Staging of chronic kidney disease
		Figure 24.3	Radiography and ultrasound of gastric calcification		• Management of chronic kidney disease
		Figure 24.4	Ultrasound of the left and right kidneys		
	25	Figure 25.1	Radiographs of urolithiasis in the patient	• Radiographic appearance aiding assessment of urolith composition	• Distinguishing urolith types by radiographic appearance, signalment, urine pH and co-morbidities
		Figure 25.2	Ultrasound examination of the urinary bladder in the patient	• Crystalluria is not the same as urolithiasis	
		Figure 25.3	Surgical removal of uroliths by cystotomy	• Canine struvite uroliths are, for the most-part, infection-associated/induced	
		Table 25.1	Radiographic features of different uroliths		
		Table 25.2	Use of signalment, urine pH and comorbid conditions to 'guesstimate' urolith composition		

(Continued)

Section	Case	Figure or table	Contents	Blue box 'Pearls'	Clinical skills / knowledge developed
L	33	Figure 33.1	The patient at presentation	• Interpretation of azotaemia	• Approach to hypoalbuminaemia
		Figure 33.2	Lesion on the margin of the pinna	• Hypoalbuminaemia	• Approach to hyperglobulinaemia
		Figure 33.3	Renal ultrasound in the patient	• Hypergobulinaemias in arthro-pod-borne infections	• Differential diagnosis of hyperglobulinaemia
		Figure 33.4		• Diagnosis of leishmaniosis	
		Table 33.1	Differential diagnoses for 'pivotal' problems		
		Table 33.2	Common clinical signs of leishmaniosis in dogs		
		Table 33.3	Differential diagnosis of marked hyperglobulinaemia		
	34	Figure 34.1	The patient at presentation		• Approach to and management of Leptospirosis
		Figure 34.2	The patient 2 months after treatment		• Interpretation of diagnostic tests for Leptospirosis

Diagnosis by Case

	Subject	Cases
A	**Endocrinology**	1. Diabetic ketoacidosis
		2. Primary hypoparathyroidism
		3. Hypoadrenocorticism
		4. Hyperadrenocorticism
		5. Hypothyroidism
B	**Haematology and immunology**	6. Immune-mediated haemolytic anaemia (IMHA)
		7. Heinz body/iron deficiency anaemia
		8. Acquired coagulopathy
		9. Immune-mediated polyarthritis
C	**Hepatobiliary disease**	10. Gall bladder mucocoele
		11. Portosystemic shunt
		12. Chronic hepatitis
D	**Gastroenterology**	13. Protein-losing enteropathy
		14. Acute pancreatitis
		15. Exocrine pancreatic insufficiency
		16. Megaoesophagus
E	**Respiratory**	17. Eosinophilic bronchopneumonopathy
		18. Tracheal collapse
		19. Pyothorax
F	**Ear, nose and throat**	20. Laryngeal paralysis
		21. Sino-nasal aspergillosis
G	**Cardiovascular**	22. Pericardial effusion
		23. Bacterial endocarditis
H	**Urology and nephrology**	24. Renal dysplasia
		25. Urolithiasis
		26. Bladder urothelial carcinoma

Canine Internal Medicine: What's Your Diagnosis? First Edition. Jon Wray.
© 2018 John Wiley & Sons Ltd. Published 2018 by John Wiley & Sons Ltd.

	Subject	Cases
I	**Reproductive/ genital tract**	27. Benign prostatic hyperplasia
J	**Oncology**	28. Mast cell tumour
		29. Thymoma
		30. Multicentric lymphoma
K	**Neurology**	31. Horner's syndrome
		32. Tetanus
L	**Infectious diseases**	33. Leishmaniosis
		34. Leptospirosis

Conversion Table of SI to Common Units

Serum biochemistry (order as appears in tables in the cases)

Analyte	SI unit	Conversion factor	Common unit
Total protein	g/l	0.1	g/dl
Albumin	g/l	0.1	g/dl
Globulin	g/l	0.1	g/dl
Urea	mmol/l	2.8	mg/dl
Creatinine	μmol/l	0.011	mg/dl
Potassium	mmol/l	1	mEq/l
Sodium	mmol/l	1	mEq/l
Chloride	mmol/l	1	mEq/l
Calcium	mmol/l	4	mEq/l
Magnesium	mmol/l	2	mEq/l
Phosphate	mmol/l	3.1	mg/dl
Glucose	mmol/l	18	mg/dl
ALT	IU/l	1	IU/l
AST	IU/l	1	IU/l
ALKP	IU/l	1	IU/l
GGT	IU/l	1	IU/l
Bilirubin	μmol/l	0.058	mg/dl
Cholesterol	mmol/l	38.6	mg/dl
Triglyceride	mmol/l	88.5	mg/dl
Creatine kinase	IU/l	1	IU/l
Bile acids	μmol/l	0.39	mg/l

Canine Internal Medicine: What's Your Diagnosis? First Edition. Jon Wray.
© 2018 John Wiley & Sons Ltd. Published 2018 by John Wiley & Sons Ltd.

Endocrine tests

Analyte	SI unit	Conversion factor	Common unit
Cortisol	nmol/l	0.0362	ng/dl
ACTH	pmol/l	4.51	pg/ml
Thyroxine (T4)	nmol/l	0.078	µg/dl
Free-T4	pmol/l	0.078	ng/dl
Insulin	pmol/l	0.139	µU/ml
PTH	pmol/l	9.1	pg/ml

Index

Page numbers in "**bold**" indicate tables and those in "*italics*" indicate figures.

Canine Internal Medicine: What's Your Diagnosis? First Edition. Jon Wray.
© 2018 John Wiley & Sons Ltd. Published 2018 by John Wiley & Sons Ltd.

Printed and bound by CPI Group (UK) Ltd, Croydon, CR0 4YY

27/10/2024

14580356-0002

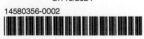